Diagnostic and Treatment in Voice Therapy

Springer Nature More Media App

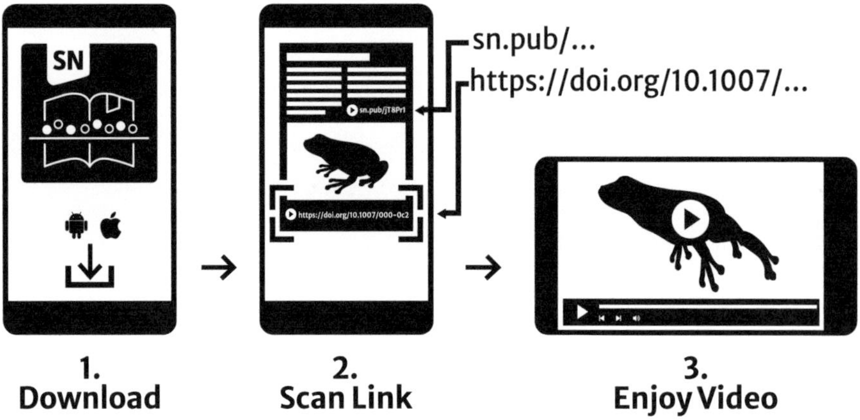

Ben Barsties v. Latoszek ·
Andreas H. Mueller · Ahmed Nasr

Diagnostic and Treatment in Voice Therapy

Quantifiable – Interdisciplinary – EBM based Criteria

Springer

Ben Barsties v. Latoszek
School of Health, Education and Social Science SRH University of Applied Sciences Heidelberg
Düsseldorf, Germany

Andreas H. Mueller
Dept. Otorhinolaryngology
SRH Wald-Klinikum Gera GmbH
Gera, Thüringen, Germany

Ahmed Nasr
The Voice Clinic Germany
Böblingen, Germany

Department of Otorhinolaryngology
Head and Neck Surgery Schwarzwald-Baar Klinikum
Villingen-Schwenningen, Germany

The online version of the book contains digital supplementary material, which is marked by a play symbol. The files can be viewed by readers of the printed book using the free Springer Nature "More Media" app. The app is available in the relevant app stores and allows the supplementary material marked accordingly to be opened with a mobile device.

ISBN 978-3-662-70161-4 ISBN 978-3-662-70162-1 (eBook)
https://doi.org/10.1007/978-3-662-70162-1

This book is a translation of the original German edition "Diagnostik und Behandlung in der Stimmtherapie" by Ben Barsties v. Latoszek et al., published by Springer-Verlag GmbH, DE in 2024. The translation was done with the help of an artificial intelligence machine translation tool. A subsequent human revision was done primarily in terms of content, so that the book will read stylistically differently from a conventional translation. Springer Nature works continuously to further the development of tools for the production of books and on the related technologies to support the authors.

This Springer imprint is published by the registered company Springer-Verlag GmbH, DE, part of Springer Nature.
The registered company address is: Heidelberger Platz 3, 14197 Berlin, Germany

Foreword 1

It is a great pleasure for me to introduce to you the innovative textbook by Prof. Dr. Ben Barsties v. Latoszek, Prof. Dr. Andreas Müller, and Dr. Ahmed Nasr. This innovative and unique work in its form opens the doors to a new era in evidence-based therapy for patients with voice disorders and offers a deep insight into the fascinating world of vocal health.

In a time when medical research and practice are constantly evolving, it is of crucial importance to have tools and resources that support us in ensuring the best possible care for our patients. The book by Prof. Dr. Ben Barsties v. Latoszek, Prof. Dr. Andreas Müller, and Dr. Ahmed Nasr undoubtedly has the potential to be one of these indispensable tools.

The special feature of this book is its interactive and digital nature. It not only enables readers to understand the theoretical foundations of vocal health but also to actively participate in diagnosis and therapy planning. The possibility of entering the results of speech therapy, ENT medical, and phoniatric examinations into the book and deriving individual action and therapy recommendations based on this is undoubtedly revolutionary.

The authors have succeeded in impressively integrating the five diagnostic pillars of the voice protocol of the "European Laryngological Society" from 2001. In doing so, established measurement methods are examined as well as newer methods that represent the current state of science. This book not only offers a comprehensive understanding of the background and interpretation of various subjective and objective measurements but also enables the practical application of this knowledge.

The significance of this work extends far beyond the field of voice therapy. It is a pioneering example of how digital technologies and interactive teaching aids can change our approach to medical diagnosis and therapy.

Overall, the textbook by Prof. Dr. Ben Barsties v. Latoszek, Prof. Dr. Andreas Müller, and Dr. Ahmed Nasr is an absolutely unique and valuable work that will serve as a guiding thread for evidence-based medical practice for trainees, students, beginners, but also experts in the field of voice care.

I would like to sincerely thank the authors for their great work and their important contribution to medical education and practice.

Regensburg,
November 2023

Prof. Christopher Bohr, MD
Head of the Clinic and Polyclinic for Ear, Nose and Throat Medicine, University Hospital Regensburg, Germany On behalf of the German Society of Oto-Rhino-Laryngology, Head and Neck Surgery

Foreword 1

Voice rehabilitation is a fascinating field of activity for therapists as well as for physicians . It is based, like so many areas of medicine, on the one hand on established knowledge, but on the other hand also on personal experience and empathy. As in many areas of medicine, the volume of research is rapidly increasing. It is not to be feared that the scientifically secured gain in knowledge will ever be able to replace individual experience, acquired intuition, and gut feeling. However, the latter suffer from the fact that we can only pass them on to our students to a very limited extent, that they have arisen to a considerable extent in random situations on our personal life paths, and that their development can be influenced by various types of cognitive biases.

Therefore, clear insights, as science can discover them, are a necessary complement. For beginners, because they provide support and direction during the familiarization phase, for the experienced, as constant control and to expand one's own thinking and actions. The book presented here, written by experienced practitioners from various professions involved in voice treatment, turns to the knowledge acquired through scientific methods and filters out the practice-relevant from the seemingly unmanageable mountain of publications.

It offers a compact yet never superficial summary of the published material, following a common thread: practical relevance. This includes readable chapters on modern diagnostic procedures, therapeutic approaches, and an introduction to clinical reasoning.

Special about this book is the approach of combining quantitative findings and therapy research into a practical guide and also practically demonstrating this using clinical examples. Additionally downloadable multimedia content usefully complements the practical part.

I can highly recommend the book for practitioners of voice treatment, and in this sense, I wish the book much success and wide dissemination.

Greifswald
im December 2023

Bernhard Lehnert, MD
PhoniatricianHead of Dept. of Phoniatrics and Pedaudiology in the Ears-, Nose-, Throat-Diseases, Head and Neck Surgery Clinic, University Medicine Greifswald, Germany
Member of the Deutschen Gesellschaft für Phoniatrie und Pädaudiologie (DGPP, German Society of Phoniatrics and Pediatric Audiology), German Society of Oto-Rhino-Laryngology, Head and Neck Surgery and German Society for Manual Medicine

Preface

"Meten is weten" (translated into English: "Measuring means knowing") is a maxim in the Dutch and Belgian educational culture in health professions. This guiding principle lays the foundation for a goal-oriented and successful therapy. Voice examination allows for many different procedures to test the various facets of voice production. This is done, among other things, through various visual analyses for laryngoscopy, perception, aerodynamics, acoustics, and patient self-evaluation. In clinical practice, there is a lack of comprehensive standardization for a minimal standard of measurement parameters for a voice examination. In particular, quantitative measurement parameters still need to find their place in practical clinical routine. With this book, we have made it our task to present those quantitative measurement methods whose quality has already been reliably proven based on research and to propose them as a necessary evidence-based minimal standard in voice diagnostics. Another advantage of quantitative measurement methods over qualitative measurement parameters is the precise documentation of treatment success control, calculation of the individual dysphonia severity degree, assessment of clinically significant improvements up to normophonia, and a clear tabular presentation of the examined facets of voice production as well as statistical evaluation of a before-and-after comparison of intra- or interindividual differences. Therefore, this book focuses exclusively on evidence-based, quantitative methods of voice diagnostics, which can be complemented in clinical practice by qualitative diagnostic means. Such a multidimensional approach to voice diagnostics first makes it possible to uncover the true extent of a voice disorder. We are convinced that the outlined minimal standard in voice diagnostics creates a basis for the therapeutic actions of physicians and therapists. The underlying measurement parameters demonstrate a proven high validity and reliability according to EBM (evidence-based medicine) standards. Providing an examination and acceptance protocol enables a structured approach in voice diagnostics as well as an easy interpretation of the results to identify the degree of a voice disorder and to detect deficits in phonation more precisely. Current scientific findings of recent years open up new possibilities in the care of voice patients at the highest EBM level.

Voice diagnostics and different voice treatments of heterogeneous voice disorders can thus be better integrated. Therefore, one of the book chapters summarizes new research findings on voice treatment from literature review. The clinical preferences of physicians and/or therapists (EBM level 5) are secondary in this work. Only results from the literature with a high level of evidence are considered. A reliable guarantee of success in voice treatment, which is significantly based on practical experience and knowledge, e.g., of recurring voice characteristics in the disorder patterns—which has also been developed over the years into various medical or therapeutic methods—is not assured when it comes to the extent of the voice disorder and the prognosis for the individual new patient.

In addition to the standardization of a minimal standard in voice examination and the latest research findings on the care of voice patients, close cooperation between otolaryngology, phoniatrics, and voice therapists is another success factor in voice treatment. This triple interdisciplinarity ensures optimal patient care with a more efficient and effective treatment outcome towards normophonia, which this work also aims to demonstrate.

The book is therefore intended to be a guide to optimizing medical-therapeutic actions based on evidence. In particular, for novices/beginners, the book provides a framework to initiate the beginning of voice treatment from the perspective of (Scientific) Clinical Reasoning. The contents are illustrated on various learning and application levels, and numerous videos and materials are available for download and/or streaming.

We would like to express our sincere thanks to all those involved from the SRH Schools for Speech and Language Therapy and the SRH University, who actively supported us in this project with feedback and input, such as students (including Ms. L. Schönfeld, Ms. M.C. Hintzen, Ms. E. Hecken, and Mr. D. Bergedieck), colleagues (including Ms. M. Humbert and Ms. I. Ritter), and faculty colleagues (including Prof. Dr. I. Ablinger-Borowski and Prof. Dr. J. Klann).

Our thanks also go to everyone who has read this book attentively and helped us with its further development.

Düsseldorf
Gera
Böblingen
in November 2023

Ben Barsties v. Latoszek, PhD
Andreas Müller, MD
Ahmed Nasr, MD

Address to the Readers

In consultation with the publisher and from the perspective of good readability of a technical book, the following gender rule is used for the designation of persons: Whenever possible, gender-neutral terms in the plural are used, which include the generic masculine and feminine and always refer to persons of both genders.

Contents

1 Voice Disorders—A Brief Overview 1
References. 2

2 Quantitative Measurement Methods in Voice Diagnostics 5
2.1 Voice Assessment Using Imaging Techniques. 6
2.1.1 Laryngoscopy. 6
2.1.2 Advanced Imaging Techniques 9
2.2 Voice Assessment through Perception 10
2.2.1 Auditory-Perceptual Voice Diagnostics 11
2.2.2 Tactile-Perceptual Voice Diagnostics. 12
2.3 Voice Assessment through Acoustics. 13
2.3.1 Guideline Requirements for Hardware 14
2.3.2 Other Factors for the Basis of Valid Results in Acoustics 15
2.3.3 Software Capabilities. 18
2.3.4 Acoustic Assessment Using Multiparametric Indices 18
2.3.5 Acoustic Assessment of Voice Function 27
2.4 Voice Assessment through Aerodynamics 44
2.5 Voice Assessment through Self-Perception 45
References. 48

3 Documentation and Objective Setting. 61
3.1 Procedure for Voice Diagnostics 68
3.2 ICF Model in Voice Disorders 76
3.3 Derivation of the Severity of a Voice Disorder 79
3.4 Therapeutic Goal Setting Based on Evidence-Based Voice Diagnostics. 80
References. 81

4 Clinical Reasoning: The Path to Effective and Efficient Primary Treatment 83
4.1 Clinical Reasoning in Voice Therapy. 83
4.2 The Systematic Path to the Appropriate Intervention in Three Steps. 86
References. 95

5 Treatment of Voice Disorders According to EBM Criteria 99
5.1 Primary Medical Interventions Depending on the Disorder 101
5.1.1 Acute Laryngitis 101
5.1.2 Vocal Fold Polyps 102
5.1.3 Laryngopharyngeal Reflux and Irritative Cough 102
5.1.4 Reinke's Edema 103
5.1.5 Spasmodic Dysphonia 105
5.1.6 Sulcus Vocalis 106
5.1.7 Vocal Fold Scars 107
5.1.8 Recurrent Respiratory Papillomatosis 107
5.1.9 Malignant Laryngeal Tumors 108
5.2 Surgical and Medicinal Therapy of Voice Disorders 110
5.2.1 Details on Surgical Techniques 110
5.2.2 Outpatient Intervention vs. Microlaryngoscopy 115
5.2.3 Voice Rest After Phonosurgery 115
5.2.4 Voice Disorders as a Side Effect of Medications 116
5.3 Conservative Voice Therapy 116
5.3.1 Concepts in Conservative Voice Therapy 116
5.3.2 Voice Therapy Programs Based on Systematic Literature Studies: EBP 122
References 153

6 Case Studies 167
6.1 Case 1: Chronic Laryngitis with Bilateral Leukoplakia 176
6.2 Case 2: Unilateral Vocal Fold Paresis (Right) 184
6.3 Case 3: Functional Dysphonia with Bronchial Asthma 187
6.4 Case 4: Functional Dysphonia with Suspected Allergy-Induced Laryngitis 189
6.5 Case 5: Vocalis Atrophy 192
6.6 Case 6: Reinke's Edema 194
6.7 Case 7: Mix of Various Organic Voice Pathologies: a) Chronic Laryngitis, b) Reinke's Edema, c) Vocal Fold Polyp with Crusting 197
References 200

Glossary 201

1 Voice Disorders—A Brief Overview

Voice disorders affect voice production (phonation) in terms of volume, quality, pitch, resonance, flexibility, and endurance. These vocal changes are expressions of disorders of the larynx, resonator, and vocal tract function, as well as breathing and respiratory mechanics, which can be attributed to heterogeneous local causes (Verdolini et al. 2006). Additionally, there are miscoordination of various parts of the vocal tract and systemic diseases such as hypothyroidism or hyperthyroidism, imbalance of sex hormones, or growth hormone disorders (Verdolini et al. 2006).

Classification of Voice Disorders into Organic, Functional, and Psychogenic Dysphonias (De Bodt et al. 2015a)

1) Organic voice disorders are based on morphological-pathological changes of the vocal folds and their movement, but also other parts of the vocal apparatus. They are usually acquired and are based, for example, on structural pathologies of the larynx, inflammatory diseases of the larynx, tumors, injuries of the larynx, systemic diseases (that affect the voice), immunological, non-laryngeal aerodigestive, and peripheral neurological diseases (that affect the voice), as well as central nervous system disorders (Verdolini et al. 2006).
2) Functional voice disorders are based on unfavorable voice techniques or habits, miscoordination in the interaction of the components of the phonation system, or an unphysiological compensation of vocal strain. They are named differently over time in the literature, e.g., Myasthenia Laryngis (1946), Hyperkinetic Dysphonia (1965), Laryngeal Tension-Fatigue Syndrome (1982), Muscle Tension Dysphonia (1983), Bogart-Bacall Syndrome (1988), Muscle Misuse Dysphonia (1993), Malregulative Dysphonia (2022), as well as general terms like

B. Barsties v. Latoszek et al., *Diagnostic and Treatment in Voice Therapy*,
https://doi.org/10.1007/978-3-662-70162-1_1

(functional) hyper-/hypotensive or hyper/hypofunctional dysphonia, musculoskeletal tension dysphonia, and laryngeal isometric dysphonia (De Bodt et al. 2015a; Hacki et al. 2022).

3) Psychogenic voice disorders are either acutely triggered by short-term conflict situations or are expressions of long-term feelings of stress or other psychopathological changes.

For example, according to data from a national health survey in the USA, one in 13 adults is affected annually by voice disorders (dysphonia) lasting longer than a week (Bhattacharyya 2014). Limited or effortful voice production represents a significant impairment of quality of life (Bhattacharyya 2014; Benninger et al. 2017). However, insurance claims for dysphonia diagnoses in the USA were only made by 1.7% of the population (Benninger et al. 2017). The overall prevalence rate is likely higher, as studies only capture those patients who seek medical care, while there are many affected individuals who do not seek help. The number of patients with voice problems who seek treatment is estimated to be up to 15% of the population (Bhattacharyya 2014). However, the values increase significantly when stratified, for example, by women (about twice as high) (Bhattacharyya 2014; De Bodt et al. 2015b; Cohen et al. 2012; Mozzanica et al. 2016), by people living in urban areas (85%) (Cohen et al. 2012), and by professional voice users (71.9%) (Mozzanica et al. 2016). The most commonly treated voice pathologies in ENT and/or phoniatrics clinics are functional voice disorders (non-structural voice disorders) and four of the following organic voice disorders: laryngitis, vocal fold nodules, vocal fold edema, and vocal fold paralysis. Vocal fold nodules and occasionally vocal fold edema are considered secondary-organic changes and expressions of (hyper)functional dysphonia (De Bodt et al. 2015b; Mozzanica et al. 2016). Many voice disorders are associated with or cause abnormal vibration patterns of the vocal folds. The resulting voice sound is variably sensitive to vibration changes in different areas of the vocal folds, but especially at the free edge of the vocal folds. The more a critical area of one or both vocal folds is affected by an organic laryngeal pathology, the more variations in voice sound are to be expected (Fleischer & Hess 2006).

References

Benninger MS, Holy CE, Bryson PC, Milstein CF (2017) Prevalence and occupation of patients presenting with dysphonia in the United States. J Voice 31(5):594–600. https://doi.org/10.1016/j.jvoice.2017.01.011

Bhattacharyya N (2014) The prevalence of voice problems among adults in the United States. Laryngoscope 124(10):2359–2362. https://doi.org/10.1002/lary.24740

Cohen SM, Kim J, Roy N, Asche C, Courey M (2012) Prevalence and causes of dysphonia in a large treatment-seeking population. Laryngoscope 122(2):343–348. https://doi.org/10.1002/lary.22426

De Bodt M, Heylen L, Mertens F, Vanderwegen J, Van de Heyning P (2015a) Stemstoornissen. Handboek voor de klinische praktijk, 6. Aufl. Garant-Uitgevers nv, Antwerpen

De Bodt M, Van den Steen L, Mertens F, Raes J, Van Bel L, Heylen L, Pattyn J, Gordts F, van de Heyning P (2015b) Characteristics of a dysphonic population referred for voice assessment and/or voice therapy. Folia Phoniatr Logop 67(4):178–186. https://doi.org/10.1159/000369339

Fleischer S, Hess M (2006) [The significance of videostroboscopy in laryngological practice]. HNO 54(8):628–634. https://doi.org/10.1007/s00106-006-1437-0

Hacki T, Moerman M, Rubin JS (2022) ‚Malregulative' Rather Than ‚Functional' Dysphonia: A new etiological terminology framework for phonation disorders-a position paper by the Union of European Phoniatricians (UEP). J Voice 36(1):50–53. https://doi.org/10.1016/j.jvoice.2020.04.032

Mozzanica F, Ginocchio D, Barillari R, Barozzi S, Maruzzi P, Ottaviani F, Schindler A (2016) Prevalence and voice characteristics of laryngeal pathology in an Italian voice therapy-seeking population. J Voice 30(6):774.e13-774.e21. https://doi.org/10.1016/j.jvoice.2015.11.018

Verdolini K, Rosen CA, Branski RC (2006). Classification manual for voice disorders-I. Special interest division 3, voice and voice disorders, American Speech-Language-Hearing Association. Mahwah: Lawrence Erlbaum Associates, Inc.

Quantitative Measurement Methods in Voice Diagnostics

2

The movement of the vocal folds is the result of complex muscular and aerodynamic processes with tissue displacements (Titze 1980). The associated result of the vibration of the vocal folds is a fundamental source of voice production according to the source-filter model of phonation (Rothenberg 1980). It thus makes a significant contribution to the resulting overall sound. However, only through a strong air column in the vocal tract and the resonators such as the chest and head-neck area, which are set into vibration, can the transmissions of these vibrations be registered as sound waves.

The complex phonation process encompasses various components, e.g., acoustics, aerodynamics, morphology, physiology, and external (self) perception, which can ultimately only be assessed with a multidimensional voice protocol. In the past, several attempts have been made in selecting methods for evaluating voice production. A conclusion of this research was that the voice examination protocol should be based on 5 independent but complementary pillars and should include them. One of the most established pillar systems thus includes the following 5 pillars/facets as a minimal standard for voice evaluation: a visual analysis of the vocal folds and larynx, an auditory-perceptual judgment, an aerodynamic analysis, an acoustic analysis, and a self-assessment (Dejonckere et al. 2001; Boominathan et al. 2014; Lechien et al. 2023). Such a multidimensional voice protocol should be quantifiable for all individual measurement parameters, enabling a more effective assessment, e.g., before and after treatment (using statistical evaluation, which is the basis of evidence-based medicine). All the evaluation facets described above in the voice protocol are independent of each other and are suitable for assessing voice disorders and their treatment outcomes (Dejonckere et al. 2003; Friedrich

Supplementary Information The electronic version of this chapter contains supplementary material, which can be accessed via the following link https://doi.org/10.1007/978-3-662-70162-1_2. The videos can be played by clicking on the DOI link in the legend of a corresponding figure, or by scanning this link with the SN More Media app.

B. Barsties v. Latoszek et al., *Diagnostic and Treatment in Voice Therapy*,
https://doi.org/10.1007/978-3-662-70162-1_2

and Dejonckere 2005). In Sects. 2.1 to 2.5, various measurement parameters under this successfully evaluated five-pillar system and considering the current state of research, evidence, and technology are listed and described. They are handled as a minimal standard to evaluate voice problems and voice disorders for the individual patient and to determine the extent to which dysphonia (dysphonia severity) is present through the deviating measurement parameters. Here too, the final criterion for a measurement parameter is that it is quantifiable, to make an assessment with a clear cutoff between physiological and pathological, and to have a general possibility to determine a grading of the severity of dysphonia from mild to severe, provided this grading has been evaluated in the measurement parameters (see further details in Sects. 3.3 and 4.2).

Additionally, all proposed measurement parameters from Sects. 2.1 to 2.5 are divided into three categories (see overview also in Sect. 3.1): voice quality (VQ), voice function (VF), or a combination of VQ and VF (VQ & VF). VQ parameters describe the voice sound at the glottis level, but further detailed information on objectivity is still undefined. In the literature on voice quality, there is only a consensus on voice characteristics or measurement methods that cannot measure VQ; thus, no pitch, no volume, or no phonetic categories (Barsties and De Bodt 2015). Furthermore, a voice quality parameter does not include a monodimensional equivalent, e.g., monodimensionality is given in pitch, volume, and phonetic characteristics, which are measured in Hz, dB, and a spectral formant analysis (Maryn 2010). Unlike voice quality, voice function parameters examine the performance of a voice, i.e., pitch, volume, and endurance. The combination of VQ & VF refers to parameters from voice diagnostics that do not have a clear assignment as primary VQ or VF, or can exhibit both characteristics in the individual result (i.e., sometimes concerning VF or sometimes VQ). Examples of this category of measurement parameters include self-assessment methods (see Sect. 2.5), or measurement parameters for the visual analysis of vocal fold vibration, which additionally constitute an essential component for diagnosing voice pathologies (see Sect. 2.1) or individual measurement parameters of perception such as palpation (see Sect. 2.2.2) or acoustics such as the Dysphonia Severity Index (see Sect. 2.3.4).

This feature classification of measurement parameters into VQ and VF is important for clinical reasoning to estimate and justify the choice, the claim of a specific (primary/initial) form of treatment, and its possibilities for the voice patient. The focus is thus on efficient and effective voice treatment with the greatest possible success for the patient, but also on the effective use of resources in the healthcare system.

2.1 Voice Assessment Using Imaging Techniques

2.1.1 Laryngoscopy

The classical indirect laryngoscopy with a laryngeal mirror, introduced by Türck and Czermak in 1858/1859 (Lübbers and Lübbers 2016), enabled the first view of the human vocal organ and shaped the public perception of the ENT doctor or phoniatrist. Today, this examination technique is largely uncommon thanks to easy-to-handle modern endoscopes with high image quality and video storage capability.

The best image of the larynx in voice diagnostics is obtained by the examiner using magnifying laryngoscopy with rigid optics (Boles et al. 2023). This involves a rod lens endoscope (Hopkins 1959) with a 70° or 90° view of the vocal folds with magnifying function and variable focusing. Using attachable cameras or integrated camera systems, laryngoscopies can be recorded in High Definition (HD) or 4K resolution, and even in 3D with specially calibrated laryngoscopes. This allows for the possibility of reviewing the recordings in slow motion and discussing the findings with patients, therapists, and physicians. Clinically, the respiratory and phonatory mobility (opening and closing of the vocal fold movement), as well as the texture, color, vascular pattern of the vocal folds, and the use of the ventricular folds can be assessed. Asymmetries of glottic motor function, functional voice disorders with their compensation mechanisms (such as surrounding muscular contractions that are additionally activated but not necessary), but especially epithelial neoplasms and pathological changes in the vocal folds can be detected early. The acquisition of rigid optics is economical, as they can be used directly with the eyepiece without expensive camera systems, and the hygiene requirements are easier to meet than for flexible endoscopes (DGHNO-KHC 2023).

The not always sufficient tolerance of patients (increased gag reflex) during transoral laryngoscopy and the significantly improved image quality with the introduction of the "Chip on the Tip" technology have led to an increased use of transnasal endoscopies with flexible rhinolaryngoscopes in laryngoscopy in recent years. These also provide images almost comparable to those of the magnifying laryngoscope when they have HD resolution, but they are then more expensive and more complex in hygienic processing. The use of frequency-controlled strobe light illumination of the vocal folds (adjusted to the speed of the vocal fold movement) in stroboscopy allows the vibratory processes of phonation to be viewed in slow motion. By carefully approaching the vocal folds during prolonged inhalation *(dipping maneuver)*, a detailed representation of the vocal fold surface and, with good illumination, also of the upper trachea is achieved. By rotating the endoscope 180° in the nasopharynx *(rotation maneuver)*, a better view of the Sinus Morgagni, the anterior commissure, and the undersides of the vocal folds is obtained (Fleischer 2020).

According to the basic protocol of the European Laryngological Society (Friedrich and Dejonckere 2005), the mucosal wave propagation relative to the lamina propria *(mucosal wave)*, the *amplitude* of the vocal fold vibration, the *regularity* and *symmetry* of the vibration, and the completeness of the *glottal closure* as well as the *supraglottic compensation* during phonation should be assessed and graded from 0 to 3 (see Table 2.1). For better understanding, these measurement parameters can be viewed in the following video (see Fig. 2.1), to better recognize and assess the features from Table 2.1 through the extremes 0 and 3.

These six measurement parameters have an impact on voice quality and/or voice function. The stroboscopic examination findings are influenced by pitch and

Table 2.1 Measurement parameters for videolaryngostroboscopy (Friedrich and Dejonckere 2005)

Measurement parameters for videolaryngostro-boscopy	Normal	Pathological		
Amplitude	**0:** normally wide 1/3 of the visible vocal fold width	**1**: slightly extended/ shortened	**2**: moderately extended/ shortened	**3**: resounding/ canceled (phona-tory stop)
MucosalWave	**0:** normal 1/2 of the visible vocal fold width	**1**: slightly reduced	**2**: moderately reduced	**3**: canceled (phonatory stopp)
Symmetry	**0**: normal (sym-metrical oscilla-tions according to location and phase)	**1**: slightly asym-metrical vibration pattern	**2**: moderately asymmetrical vibration pattern	**3**: severely asymmetrical vibration pattern
Regularity	**0**: regular vibra-tion pattern	**1**: slightly irregu-lar vibration pattern	**2**: moderately irregular vibra-tion pattern	**3**: severely irregular vibra-tion pattern
Glottal closure (forms: longitudi-nal gap, bowing, posteriorgap, hourglass shape, anterior gap)	**0**: complete	**1**: slightly incomplete	**2**: moderately incomplete	**3**: severely incomplete
Supraglottic compensation (during phonation)	**0**: no supraglottic contractions	**1**:slightly supraglottic contractions	**2**: moderately supraglottic contractions	**3**: supraglottic closure

volume, therefore these should be considered and documented. During laryngo-stroboscopy, patients should be asked to sustain the vowel /i/ or /e/ for a longer period (see Sect. 3.1). Additionally, speaking short sentences under stroboscopic observation can be considered to evaluate the position of the glottis and supraglottis during phonation for the evaluation of functional glottic closure insufficiencies, and to uncover hyperkinesias and pathological compensation mechanisms. When examining singers or professional speakers, a glissando maneuver should also be observed.

In addition to this consensus, there are numerous other national and international standard protocols for documenting videolaryngostroboscopy. For less experienced colleagues, the Italian SIFEL protocol (Ricci-Maccarini et al. 2018), which provides a guide for systematic documentation and illustration of pathological findings through graphically illustrated examination forms, is recommended.

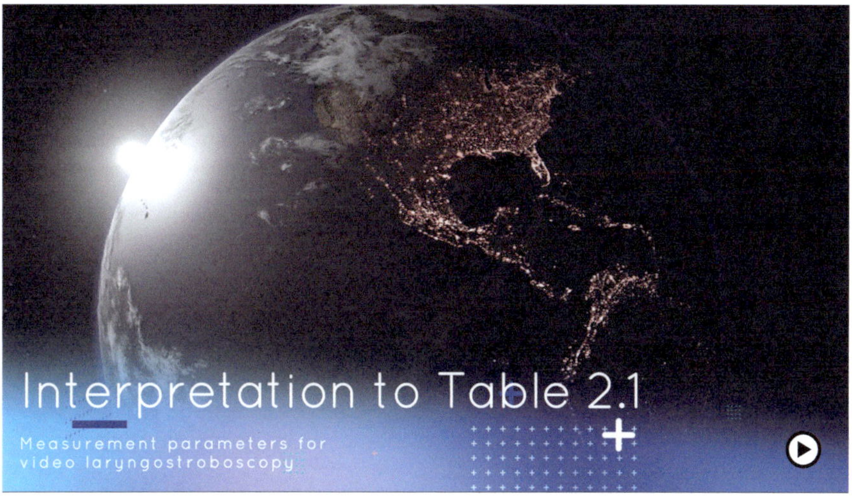

Fig. 2.1 Interpretation aid of stroboscopic recordings for the 6 measurement parameters from Table 2.1 (▸ https://doi.org/10.1007/000-dwj)

2.1.2 Advanced Imaging Techniques

In certain cases, it may be necessary to analyze the vertical vibration pattern at the point of maximum vibration of the vocal folds using the so-called *videokymography* (Saindani et al. 2023). Using cameras with a resolution of 4000 frames per second *(high-speed video laryngoscopy)*, the vibration behavior can also be examined during irregular cycles (Tsuji et al. 2014).

Less complex and without affecting the tension of the vocal folds through endoscopy, the regularity of the vocal fold vibrations can also be recorded and evaluated externally using *electroglottography* (Herbst 2020). Additionally, fundamental frequency and register boundaries can be determined.

By using narrow-band optical filters in the image processor of the endoscope (most commonly known as *narrow band imaging*), the microvascular architecture of the vocal folds can be better visualized (Davaris et al. 2017). The image resembles a histological staining.

Cross-sectional imaging of the neck and larynx, such as magnetic resonance imaging *(MRI)* and computed tomography *(CT)*, is particularly significant in oncology, less so in voice diagnostics. This involves detecting tumor infiltrations in the depth of the vocal folds using MRI or the laryngeal skeleton with CT. In cases of unclear vocal fold motility disorders, an MRI of the skull base and neck, as well as possibly a CT thorax, is performed to rule out tumors along the course of the vocal fold nerves.

The *laryngeal ultrasound* was long a little-noticed method, which, for example, allows the non-invasive detection of vocal fold motility disorders or voice disorders due to benign lesions on the anterior vocal folds in young children without the burdens of laryngoscopy (Ongkasuwan et al. 2017a, b). Similarly, tumor infiltrations of the laryngeal framework can be well recognized in adults (Klinge and Müller 2013). The method reaches its limits in the area of the posterior laryngeal sections and with severe calcification of the thyroid cartilage.

An example of a 62-year-old male patient with a T4 laryngeal carcinoma with paraglottic spread and infiltration of the laryngeal framework on the right serves to illustrate the various imaging techniques (see Fig. 2.2).

2.2 Voice Assessment through Perception

The assessment of the voice through perception can be divided into two areas in this chapter: on the one hand, the auditory-perceptual aspect, in the evaluation of voice quality from the sound of the voice, and on the other hand, the tactile-perceptual area through palpation of the larynx.

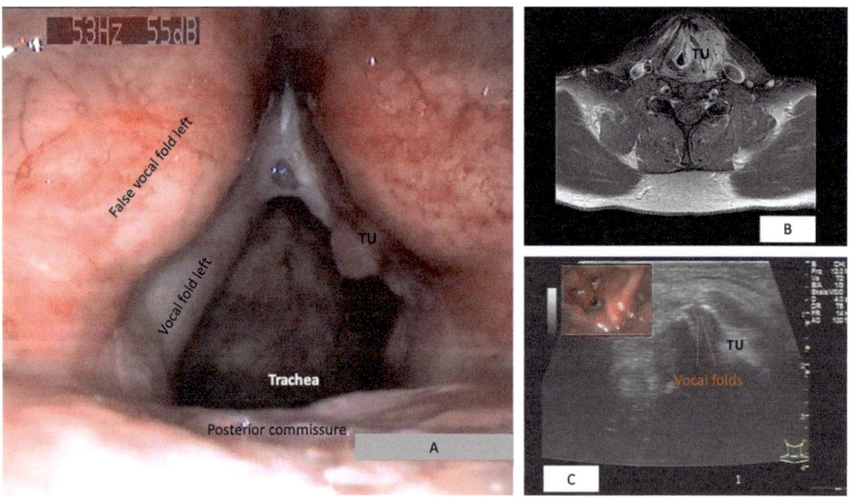

Fig. 2.2 Three different imaging techniques of a 62-year-old male patient with a T4 laryngeal carcinoma (TU) with paraglottic spread and infiltration of the laryngeal framework on the right. **Image A:** Magnified laryngostroboscopic image with defect and neoplasm in the area of the right vocal fold, limited mobility of the right vocal fold with incomplete glottic closure during phonation; **Image B:** MRI with marking of the tumor extent (white area; TU); **Image C:** Image fusion laryngoscopy/ultrasound, vocal fold edge in the anterior part (orange line) and paraglottic tumor (white) almost as clearly visible as in the MRI *Source* SRH Waldklinik Gera

2.2.1 Auditory-Perceptual Voice Diagnostics

The auditory-perceptual voice assessment is an important component of routine clinical voice diagnostics, which is used in phoniatrics, otorhinolaryngology, and by speech-language pathologists. The auditory assessment of voice quality is simple and efficient to measure. There are various measurement methods for standardizing the auditory-perceptual assessment of voice quality, i.e., the perception of deviations in voice sound, which are usually associated with the term hoarseness (Barsties and Maryn 2015). Internationally, several schemes or scales have been evaluated, such as the GRBAS scale or the GRB scale, the Consensus Auditory-Perceptual Evaluation of Voice (CAPE-V), Laver's voice profile analysis, the Stockholm consensus model of voice evaluation, the voice profile analysis scheme, the Buffalo voice profile, and the Hammarberg schema (De Bodt et al. 1996; Kreiman and Gerratt 2011). Three evaluation schemes that are frequently reported and have high acceptance are the GRBAS scale, the GRB scale, and CAPE-V (Carding et al. 2000; Dejonckere et al. 2001; Zraick et al. 2011). The GRBAS scale, developed by the Japan Society of Logopedics and Phoniatrics (Hirano 1981), consists of a five-dimensional scale that uses four unidimensional parameters to selectively direct the assessor to specific quality characteristics of the voice. These are referred to as Roughness (R), Breathiness (B), Asthenia (A), and Strain (S). The G (Grade), the fifth parameter, considers the overall severity of the impression of an abnormality in the voice.

► In the German-speaking and European regions, the GRB scale is used (Dejonckere et al. 2001; Friedrich and Dejonckere 2005) and is the subject of this quantitative voice diagnostics. Compared to the GRBAS scale, only three of the five dimensions are evaluated, but on the same 4-point ordinal scale; namely Roughness, Breathiness, and Hoarseness/Overall Severity/Grade. All parameters are evaluated on a four-level equal appearing interval scale, ranging from 0 (normal) to 3 (severe).

Thirdly, the CAPE-V (Consensus Auditory-Perceptual Evaluation of Voice) can be used, which was proposed by the American Speech-Language- and Hearing Association (Kempster et al. 2009). Here, comparable parameters to the GRBAS scale are considered in the standard analysis, as well as additional parameters such as pitch, loudness, and an individual selection of further parameters (e.g., diplophonia, glottal fry, falsetto, asthenia, aphonia, pitch instability, tremor, and wet/gurgling sound). Furthermore, CAPE-V uses a visual analog scale (a line whose endpoints represent extreme states and allows for multi-level assessment) and suggests specific speech tasks and criteria for the analysis (Shrivastav 2011). In the auditory-perceptual assessment of voice quality, speech tasks play an important role. Typically, one or more sustained vowels and/or continuous speech are evaluated. The type and severity of the perceived voice impairment differ significantly within these two types of speech tasks (Zraick et al. 2005; Maryn and Roy 2012).

Continuous speech represents daily language use, but the assessment of the voice through sustained vowels better reflects non-vocal phenomena (e.g., prosodic fluctuation, phonetic context, and compensatory relationships in the perceived degree of voice sound change) than the analysis of continuous speech. In general, the analysis of continuous speech is preferred over the use of sustained vowels in the assessment of perceptual voice quality.

In principle, it should be considered in the auditory-perceptual assessment that there are large differences in intra- and inter-rater reliability (Kreiman et al. 1993; Bele 2005). There are several reasons for this, which can be divided into three categories—(a) rater-based (e.g., number of expert group, concentration, experience, professional background), (b) stimulus-based (e.g., use of anchor voices), (c) scale-based (visual analog vs. ordinal assessment) (Barsties and De Bodt 2015). If the numerous influencing factors summarized by Barsties and De Bodt (2015) are not sufficiently considered, the results of the auditory-perceptual voice assessment should be interpreted with caution.

2.2.2 Tactile-Perceptual Voice Diagnostics

The assessment of muscle tension in and around the larynx is a key component in many voice disorders and can be evaluated using various instrumental or non-instrumental methods. One of the most clinically popular non-instrumental assessment methods is palpation (Khoddami et al. 2015). During palpation, the function of the larynx and the degree of muscle tone are documented, with the variability of muscle tone existing both at rest (i.e., static assessment) and during phonation (i.e., dynamic assessment). Examiners should have sufficient palpatory skills to assess the range of motion of the joint, the structural conditions of the surrounding tissue, and especially the muscles working at a particular joint (Lieberman 1998).

Palpation is a simple and useful clinical method to assess muscle tone with the hands. Additionally, it is a safe technique without known specific side effects for patients. However, the validity and reliability of the results depend on many different factors that can influence the assessment outcomes. Factors influencing the application of palpation include, for example, the experience and skills of the examiners as well as the clarity and definition of the descriptions and/or quantification for the palpated areas (Khoddami et al. 2015).

A proposal for a recent quantitative palpation procedure based on the palpation findings regarding the reliability and validity of the literature study by Khoddami et al. (2015) was developed by Barsties and Thede (2016) (see palpation assessment forms in Sect. 3.1).

During palpation, patients sit upright with a neutral head position (i.e., no lifting, lowering, retracting, or protruding of the chin). Examiners use their thumbs and index/middle fingers for all areas to be palpated. The examination begins with the static assessment. The palpated areas are the lateral laryngeal mobility, the thyroid space, and the cricothyroid space. Additionally, examiners ask the subjects in each of the three palpation areas whether there is any pain (excluding discomfort, unpleasant, or unfamiliar feelings). This is followed by the dynamic assessment. During the dynamic assessment, subjects sustain the vowel /a:/ at habitual pitch and loudness for a few seconds. The areas to be palpated for the dynamic assessment are the position of the larynx/hyoid bone as well as the two areas as in the static assessment, i.e., the thyroid space and the cricothyroid space. Additionally, examiners ask the patients again in each of the three palpation areas whether any pain is felt during palpation. The quantification refers to the palpation findings of the individual anatomical sections with the respective 3 aspects that are examined for the static and dynamic areas. Each of these areas has intermediate values, where the examined section is assigned a specific value (see Sect. 3.1). An exception is the pain cluster, where all pain findings are added to calculate the intermediate value. All intermediate values of an assessment are added to determine a total value for the static and dynamic assessment, respectively. In general, the higher the values, the greater the measured laryngeal muscle tone.

▶ The normal value for the static assessment of palpation is <1.25 points (sensitivity: 84%; specificity: 100%) and for the dynamic area <1.75 points (sensitivity: 68%; specificity: 93%) (Bargar 2024; Ippers 2024). The measurement instrument for palpation also shows high inter-rater reliability (ICC = 0.800 to 0.866) and intra-rater reliability (ICC = 0.840 to 0.966) (Bargar 2024; Ippers 2024).

2.3 Voice Assessment through Acoustics

Acoustic analyses of the voice signal are one of the most frequently used diagnostic tools for quantifying and describing voice disorders (Roy et al. 2013). They are primarily used to objectively measure the quality and function of the voice. Voice signal analyses for voice quality assessment can be acoustically analyzed in the domains of time, frequency, amplitude, and "quefrency." A large number of acoustic parameters exist to objectively describe types of dysphonia and their severity. This is illustrated and summarized, for example, by Buder's taxonomy (2000) with 15 signal processing-based categories, of which only a few parameters are suitable for voice quality assessment (Maryn et al. 2009a; Barsties v. Latoszek et al. 2018). Therefore, in this book, only the measurement parameters or indices that have evidence-based sufficient validity for assessing voice quality are detailed (see Sect. 2.3.4). Voice function includes vocal frequency/pitch (in Hz) and intensity/loudness (in dB) as well as the interaction between these two parameters, e.g., in a voice range profile (see Sect. 2.3.5; Heylen et al. 2002).

In addition to guideline requirements for hardware, room acoustics, patient voice behavior, and the influence of mouth-nose masks under appropriate hygiene standards (see Sects. 2.3.1 and 2.3.2), software capabilities (see Sect. 2.3.3) are also part of the acoustic assessment of voice quality and function. Since all these aspects influence reliability and measurement accuracy, these aspects are elaborated in more detail in the following Sects. 2.3.1 to 2.3.3 (Barsties and De Bodt 2015; Patel et al. 2018).

2.3.1 Guideline Requirements for Hardware

The validity of objective-acoustic analysis in research or clinical practice depends on various conditions that enable highly accurate and reliable measurements of a voice analysis (Barsties and De Bodt 2015; Patel et al. 2018).

Valid voice recordings for voice and speech analysis are mainly influenced by microphones and digitization processes. Microphones must meet seven different conditions to enable acceptable voice recordings for analyses: (1) condenser type, (2) cardioid characteristic, (3) frequency range of 20–20,000 Hz, (4) frequency response curve flat with a maximum deviation of 2 dB, (5) equivalent noise level 25 dB(A), (6) maximum sound pressure level (i.e., maximum volume) at 3% total harmonic distortion (THD) of 126 dB, and finally (7) high sensitivity. These details of the microphone properties described here are published in the manual of the respective microphone manufacturers and are thus explained in this book only from a voice diagnostic perspective.

Condenser microphones with a cardioid characteristic are recommended for acoustic voice analyses (Titze and Winholtz 1993; Baken and Orlikoff 2000; Deliyski et al. 2005a) because these properties allow direct focusing on the sound direction of the voice (Švec and Granqvist 2010). The frequency range of the microphones should cover the frequency spectrum of the human voice, i.e., a range of 20–20,000 Hz (Baken and Orlikoff 2000). The frequency response curve of intensity at different frequencies of the microphones should be flat with a maximum deviation of 2 dB, especially between 20–8000 Hz, but ideally up to 20,000 Hz (Švec and Granqvist 2010). Each component of a microphone generates noise, which is described as the equivalent noise level in dB(A) (Švec and Granqvist 2010). The level of self-noise of the microphones should be as low as possible without affecting the voice signal. Therefore, the voice signal must be loud enough to mask the self-noise with a minimum difference of 10 dB (Šrámková et al. 2015). The human voice cannot produce a quieter sound than 35 dB(A) (Šrámková et al. 2015), so the equivalent noise level must be lower than 25 dB(A). The maximum performance of a voice must also be validly measurable (i.e., measured with 3% THD) (Švec and Granqvist 2010). The maximum loudness of the human voice is 124 dB(A) measured at a distance of 30 cm (Boren et al. 2013). Finally, the microphones should have high sensitivity in recording voices to prevent a higher gain level, which thus avoids a higher noise level. Therefore, condenser microphones with a sensitivity of less than 60 dB are not recommended (Titze 1995).

The last aspect of microphone properties concerns differences between head-mounted and hand-mounted microphones. The advantages of head-mounted microphones are a consistent distance to the voice source and a reduction in ambient noise, i.e., noises from technical equipment, environmental sounds, and background noise (Titze and Winholtz 1993; Švec and Granqvist 2010). Overall, more accurate results were observed in various voice quality parameters with head-mounted microphones (Titze and Winholtz 1993). A critical point to note with head-mounted microphones is the so-called "proximity effect," which can lead to an increase in lower frequencies and thus a distortion of acoustic values. However, modern head-mounted microphone types are capable of compensating for an almost flat frequency response at a certain distance (Švec and Granqvist 2010). Handheld microphones are typically used at a distance of 30 cm. The individuals must control the distance, and environmental noises must be taken into account more strongly. Shields or sound absorbers can be helpful in this regard. For head-mounted microphones, a distance of 30 cm is usually also considered during intensity calibration. For the calibration of the measured intensity output of the microphones, dB sound level meters designated as IEC 651 Type II and IEC 61672-1 are recommended as a minimum standard. A description of microphone calibration is provided, for example, by Maryn and Zarowski (2015) or Patel et al. (2018).

Regarding recording systems, there are various options described in the literature, such as personal computers, digital audio tapes, minidisc recorders, hard disk recorders, solid-state recorders, and analog cassette tapes (Vogel and Morgan 2009). It is crucial to standardize modern recording systems and hardware configurations that are suitable and designed for acoustic analyses, so that valid and reliable data can be obtained for clinical and scientific purposes (Deliyski et al. 2005a; Vogel and Maruff 2008; Vogel et al. 2014). Currently, in addition to the precise specific properties of calibrated head-mounted microphones, the preamplifiers to be used and the digitization of the audio signal are also being more closely defined (Patel et al. 2018).

A preamplifier is an electronic device for amplifying a weak audio input signal. The specifications of the preamplifier should (a) have an input impedance that is at least as high as the minimum termination impedance required by the microphone, (b) have a gain that is set so that the levels of the loudest phonations remain slightly below the saturation/clipping level (overdrive), (c) have no equalizers or bass/treble controls (to prevent alteration of the sound spectrum), (d) have no automatic gain control or other signal processing circuits, such as noise suppression, that can alter the original signal of the microphone (Patel et al. 2018).

The conversion of the analog audio input signal of the recording to digital pro cessing can be done with an internal high-quality computer sound card (e.g., for a personal computer) or with an external sound card (often in combination with a microphone preamplifier) that is connected via USB (e.g., for a laptop). External computer hardware is always preferable to internal computer hardware (Patel et al. 2018).

The minimum specifications for digitizing the audio signal include setting a sampling rate of 44.1 kHz, but not lower than 26 kHz (Deliyski et al. 2005b), a minimum resolution of 16 bits (24 bits preferred for an increased dynamic range) (Patel et al. 2018), and an audio file format without compression or a lossless compression format (e.g., the wav format) (Vogel and Morgan 2009).

2.3.2 Other Factors for the Basis of Valid Results in Acoustics

There are various examination conditions that can affect the reliability of objective acoustic analysis. They must be controlled and appropriately considered by the examiners. Overall, there are two main factors that can significantly distort acoustic analysis: a) room acoustics, b) the vocal behavior of the patients during the recording. This chapter also discusses the influence of various mouth-nose coverings based on a meta-analysis, due to the recent COVID-19 pandemic. These three areas are described in more detail in the following sections.

Room Acoustics

Ambient noise is one of the most important external factors that must always be controlled by the investigators when an audio recording takes place; it must always be as low as possible (Carson et al. 2003; Deliyski et al. 2005c, 2006; Vogel and Morgan 2009). This influencing factor is even more significant than the type of microphone (Bottalico et al. 2020).

The control of ambient noise can be evaluated using two different measurement techniques. First, the ambient noise level should be at least 10 dB lower than the sound level of the quietest phonation of the voice signal, which is recommended for acceptable conditions in acoustic voice recordings and analyses (Šrámková et al. 2015). For example, when recording a voice range profile, where the quietest phonation is required, this would mean that ambient noise should be <25 dB(A) or <38 dB(C).

A second measurement technique that is recommended is the examination of the signal-to-noise ratio (SNR) by comparing the intensity levels of the voice signal and the ambient noise sources (Deliyski et al. 2005c,2006). Acceptable SNR values range between 30 and 42 dB(A), preferably the greater than 42 dB(A), the better (Deliyski et al. 2005c). To explain the calculation of the SNR, the following example is provided: If the phonation was measured at 75 dB(A), the noise should not be higher than 45 dB(A) (difference = 30 dB(A)) to still ensure the reliability of the acoustic evaluations of the measurement parameters; however, it would be better if the measured noise level were below 33 dB(A) (difference = 42 dB(A)) to enable the accuracy of the analyses within an error probability of 1%.

In addition to the fact that voice recordings for acoustic analyses should be made in an environment as quiet as possible, a recording environment should also be sought that is as little contaminated by reverberation as possible due to room acoustics. The reverberation time/echo (i.e., the time in which the intensity level decreases by 60 dB) is an important indicator of how much reverberation is actually present in the room. For voice recordings, the reverberation time should not exceed 1.0 seconds (Everest and Pohlmann 2009). Thus, longer reverberation times must be avoided during recording. This can be achieved by using surface materials with relatively high sound absorption (e.g., heavy carpets, fabric ceilings, or curtains) instead of surface materials with relatively low sound absorption (e.g., wooden floors, plaster, and glass windows).

Patient Vocal Behavior

The voice production and characteristics of the patients' voices can also play a crucial role in the acoustic analysis. Tested factors such as loudness, pitch, gender, and vowels were examined for their possible influence on the reliability of the objective acoustic analysis results (Brockmann et al. 2008, 2011). These studies found that loudness has the greatest influence on the acoustic parameters in analyses that evaluate the habitual speaking voice and should be controlled. This control is particularly important for the sustained phonation of vowels, which are part of specific acoustic voice quality analyses. Here, the volume of the sustained phonation of the vowels should be comparable to that of the habitual speaking loudness (e.g., measured by reading a phonetically balanced text). A blanket adjustment of the phonation loudness for all patients during sustained vowels (e.g., 80 dB at a distance of 10 cm) is therefore not recommended, as this could lead to misinterpretations in the results of the objective acoustic analysis. For example, a person with a quieter habitual speaking voice (e.g., 68 dB), measured at a distance of 10 cm, records a slight disturbed anomaly in voice quality (breathiness). If this person is now made to phonate about 12 dB louder to reach 80 dB standard volume for the examination, this automatically results in an improvement in voice quality (reduction of breathiness), which is perceptually and acoustically registered. This phenomenon has been demonstrated in studies (Södersten et al. 1991; Hertegård and Gauffin 1991). Also, when consciously increasing the speaking loudness, other anomalies in voice quality can be measured, such as tense or pressed. Thus, the result of the acoustic analysis also changes significantly (Yanushevskaya et al. 2013; Lebbe et al. 2013).

Influence of Mouth-Nose Masks with Corresponding Hygiene Standards
On the one hand, to ensure high measurement accuracy of the individual measurement methods, but on the other hand, to protect the investigation staff and the patients, appropriate measures must be taken in certain situations regarding hygiene standards. For example, during the coronavirus pandemic from March 11, 2020, until the lifting of the global emergency on May 5, 2023 (WHO 2023), the goal was, among other things, to control and prevent all diseases and deaths related to the coronavirus, particularly through hand hygiene, social behavior, and mouth-nose coverings (e.g., medical face masks or particle-filtering half masks, the so-called FFP masks). At that time, it was particularly important to wear various mouth-nose coverings to avoid potential respiratory droplet infections or airborne viruses, which were widespread in everyday life and clinical settings and are still partially used. The wearing of such masks led to hypotheses, such as that sound transmission could be limited by mouth-nose coverings and act as a low-pass filter, so that sound in the mid and high-frequency range is dampened, affecting speech intelligibility and acoustic voice analyses (Corey et al. 2021; Sönnichsen et al. 2022; Oren et al. 2023). However, a recent meta-analysis could not confirm this for the common clinical acoustic voice parameters of voice quality and habitual loudness (Barsties v. Latoszek et al. 2023a), and thus there is currently no restriction on recordings or analyses compared to wearing a mouth-nose covering (e.g., medical face/surgical masks and FFP2/(K)N95 masks) or none that investigators need to consider. It is merely noted that significant differences in measurement results can arise between the masks. In 4 out of 6 acoustic parameters examined, significant differences were found in the indirect comparison between surgical masks and FFP2/(K)N95 masks. If a mask is worn by patients

for hygiene standards, the same mask type should always be used in clinical routine and not changed, to ensure high comparability and validity of the measurement results.

2.3.3 Software Capabilities

The analysis of voice recordings is evaluated using various computer programs and different acoustic measurement parameters. The following Table 2.2 provides an initial overview of the current diagnostic software capabilities used in research to evaluate acoustic parameters, which are also generally suitable for clinical practice.

2.3.4 Acoustic Assessment Using Multiparametric Indices

Acoustic measurements complement auditory-perceptual assessments, e.g., for voice quality analysis, and increase the validity of voice diagnostics because they are based on objective measurements and are therefore less influenced by subjective factors, such as the evaluator with varying intra- or inter-rater reliability (Barsties and De Bodt 2015).

Although a variety of measurement methods based on acoustic signal processing have been used in the clinical identification and quantification of anomalies in the voice, the validity of these measurements, e.g., in comparison to perceptual aspects of voice quality (e.g., with hoarseness, roughness, and breathiness), was long unclear. A recent analysis showed that only four acoustic single parameters demonstrated highly valid results and a significant distinction to certain voice quality characteristics such as hoarseness vs. breathiness (Barsties v. Latoszek et al. 2023b).

- For the aspect of hoarseness, the Harmonics-to-Noise Ratio (HNR) ($r = -0.71$ and 81.2% ability to discriminate between the determination of hoarseness and normophonia) with a normal value >23.34 dB and the Jitter five point period perturbation quotient (PPQ5) ($r = 0.71$ and 83.3% ability to discriminate between the determination of hoarseness and normophonia) with a normal value <0.29% showed clear significant results compared to breathiness and are therefore suitable for the objective evaluation of hoarseness (Barsties v. Latoszek et al. 2023b).

- For the aspect of breathiness, the Cepstral Peak Prominence smoothed (CPPS) ($r = -0.81$ and 91.5% ability to discriminate between the determination of breathiness and not) with a norm value >14.47 dB and the Glottal-to-Noise Excitation Ratio (GNE) ($r = -0.78$ and 88.6% ability to discriminate between the determination of breathiness and not) with a norm value >0.89 asserted themselves against the voice quality aspect of hoarseness, thus making them clearly suitable for the objective evaluation of breathiness (Barsties v. Latoszek et al. 2023b).

Table 2.2 Overview of acoustic diagnostic software, sorted alphabetically

Name of the Software (Manufacturer)	Source	Measurement Parameters	Application/ Recordings/ Analyses only possible in combination with specific hardware	Access	Reference
ADSV (Kay Pentax)	https://www.pentaxmedical.com/pentax/en/99/1/Analysis-of-Dysphonia-in-Speech-and-Voice-ADSV	CSID, CPP, CPP-SD; CPP-F0; L/H ratio, L/H ratio-SD	No, although Kay Pentax offers its own hardware	Commercial	Murton et al. (2020)
DIVAS (Xion Medical)	https://www.xion-medical.com/de/produkte/software	Jitter, Shimmer, F0, SPL, DSI	Yes	Commercial	Berger et al. (2019; 2022); Aichinger et al. (2012)
Dr. Speech (Tiger DRS, Inc.)	http://www.drspeech.com/product/vocalassessment	Jitter, Shimmer, NNE, SNR, HNR, F0, SPL, F0 tremor, amplitude tremor	No	Commercial	Núñez Batalla et al. (2014)
MDVP (Kay Pentax)	https://www.pentaxmedical.com/pentax/en/99/1/Acoustic	Jitter, Shimmer, vAm, F0, vF0, NHR, NSH, NVB, NUV, DUV, DVB, DSH, VTI, SPI, FTRI, ATRI	No, although Kay Pentax offers its own hardware	Commercial	Nicastri et al. (2004)
Praat (University of Amsterdam)	https://www.fon.hum.uva.nl/praat/	Jitter, Shimmer, HNR, NHR, HNR-D, F0, SPL, F1-F4, H1-H2, Slope, Tilt, Hfno, NVB, NUV, DVB, CPPS, GNE, AVQI, ABI	No	Freeware	Maryn et al. (2009b)

(continued)

Table 2.2 (continued)

Name of the Software (Manufacturer)	Source	Measurement Parameters	Application/ Recordings/ Analyses only possible in combination with specific hardware	Access	Reference
Vox Metria (CTS Informatica)	https://www.ctsinformatica.com.br/english/voxmetria-voxmetria-voice-analysis-and-vocal-quality	Jitter, Shimmer, GNE, F0, F1-F2, SPL, Irregularity, Noise	No	Commercial	Lopes et al. (2017)
VOXplot (Lingphon)	https://voxplot.lingphon.com/de/	Jitter, Shimmer, HNR, HNR-D, CPPS, GNE, F0, H1-H2, Hfno, Slope, Tilt, DVB, AVQI, ABI	No	Freeware	Barsties v. Latoszek et al. (2021a)
Vox Phonetography (Vox Phonetography)	https://voxphonetography.com/	F0, SPL, HNR, CPPS, SPR	No	Plugin – Commercial	Nijkamp and Maryn (2018)
Wevosys (Lingwaves)	https://www.wevosys.de/produkte/lingwaves/lingwaves.html	Jitter, Shimmer, F0, Singer's Formant, SPL, GNE, DSI, Irregularity, Noise, Overall Grade	Yes	Commercial	Aichinger et al. (2012); Hanschmann et al. (2015); Nijkamp and Maryn (2018)

Abbreviations: ATRI = Amplitude Tremor Intensity Index; CSID = Cepstral Spectral Index of Dysphonia; CPP = Cepstral Peak Prominence; CPP-SD = Standard Deviation of CPP; CPP-F0 = Fundamental Tone of the Cepstral Peak, i.e., the strongest harmonic energy in the voice signal; CPPS = Cepstral Peak Prominence Smoothed; DSI = Dysphonia Severity Index; DVB = Degree of Voice Breaks; DSH = Degree of Subharmonics; DUV = Degree of Voiceless; F0 = Fundamental Frequency; F1–F2 = Formant Analysis of F1 and F2; F1–F4 = Formant Analysis of F1 to F4; FTRI = Frequency Tremor Intensity Index; GNE = Glottal-to-Noise Excitation Ratio; H1–H2 = Ratio between the Energies of the First Harmonic Peak to the Second Harmonic Peak; Hfno = High Frequency Noise; HNR = Harmonics-to-Noise Ratio; HNR-D = Harmonics-to-Noise Ratio according to Dejonckere; L/H ratio = Ratio of Low Energy (<4 kHz) to High Energy (>4 kHz) in the Spectrum; L/H ratio-SD = Standard Deviation of the L/H ratio; NHR = Noise-to-Harmonics Ratio; NNE = Normalized Noise Energy; NSH = Number of Sub-Harmonic Segments; NUV = Number of Unvoiced Segments; NVB = Number of Voice Breaks; SNR = Signal-to-Noise Ratio; SPI = Soft Phonation Index; SPL = Sound Pressure Level (Volume/Intensity); SPR = Singing Power Ratio; vAm = Peak-to-Peak Amplitude Variation; vF0 = Fundamental Frequency Variation; VTI = Voice Turbulence Index

It should be noted, however, that the above-mentioned voice quality values for HNR, PPQ5, CPPS, and GNE are only applicable to the vowel phonation of the vowel /a:/ for a duration of 3 seconds with the analysis software VOXplot/Praat. Detailed information on these, additionally traditionally frequently used, and also further discussed acoustic individual parameters in the course of the book, are described in detail in the VOXplot manual by Mayer (2023) and should be referred to if more details and background knowledge are desired. However, the analysis of sustained vowel phonations does not necessarily correspond to the analysis result of continuous speech, which therefore limited and restricted the acoustic analyses to sustained phonations over a long period. However, to apply an analysis of traditionally frequently used acoustic parameters such as jitter, shimmer, and HNR to continuous speech, a special filtering between voiced and voiceless segments is necessary and has been successfully used since 2010 (Maryn 2010; Maryn et al. 2010). Certain spectral or cepstral parameters, however, can be applied directly to continuous speech without such filtering (Awan et al. 2009). When the use of continuous speech in acoustic analyses is utilized, it is imperative to control and evaluate the duration and use of the speech task with a standardized text in the various languages. Voice samples with a longer duration of continuous speech can increase the perceptual severity of the deviation in voice quality, while shorter voice samples have higher rater reliability and also higher correlations with acoustic analyses (Sampaio et al. 2020; Englert et al. 2022a). It has therefore proven useful to match the length of continuous speech to the length of sustained phonation, which is usually 3 seconds without voice onset and offset (Barsties and Maryn 2015). Thus, the voice sample of both speech tasks would be approximately 6 seconds in total.

The choice of the most suitable form of continuous speech task usually depends on the abilities of the individuals being examined. Typically, phonetically balanced texts or individual sentences are read. However, reading a standardized text is not suitable in some clinical settings, e.g., when focusing on pediatric patients or a population segment simply unable to read (illiteracy). These aspects significantly limit the validity of a general recommendation for reading standardized texts or sentences for acoustic analyses of continuous speech (Englert et al. 2019, 2020).

In summary, it becomes clear that for a balanced and ecological validity of a voice quality analysis, both sustained phonation and continuous speech must be used. The duration of the voice sample of both speech tasks and the form of continuous speech must be examined in advance and also adapted to specific cultural populations.

To increase the clinical utility of acoustic measurement methods, it is necessary to improve all the above-mentioned validity characteristics for acoustic voice quality analyses. A significant contribution to these improvements, confirmed in numerous studies, results from a combination of several acoustic parameters, which are summarized in a model or index (Barsties and De Bodt 2015; Barsties v. Latoszek et al. 2021a). The most frequently evaluated acoustic indices described in the literature that meet the above conditions are the Acoustic Voice Quality Index (AVQI), the Cepstral Spectral Index of Dysphonia (CSID), the Acoustic

Breathiness Index (ABI), and the Dysphonia Severity Index (DSI) (Barsties v. Latoszek et al. 2021a; Saeedi et al. 2022).

The CSID is part of the commercial "Analysis of Dysphonia in Speech and Voice" software (by KayPENTAX, Montvale, New Jersey, USA), which is increasingly used in North America. Compared to Europe, it is less widespread. The CSID is a multifactorial index that analyzes the severity of general voice quality deviation when evaluating a sustained vowel or continuous speech (e.g., a phonetically balanced text or sentences of the Consensus Auditory-Perceptual Evaluation of Voice; Kempster et al. 2009) and correlates with perceptual hoarseness. However, the research data on the various characteristics of validity, reliability, and the application spectrum of the CSID are significantly lower than for the other acoustic indices (Barsties v. Latoszek et al. 2021a, Saeedi et al. 2022). For these reasons, the CSID will not be further considered in the following discussion, but only the AVQI, the ABI, and the DSI.

Acoustic Voice Quality Index

The Acoustic Voice Quality Index is a multiparametric, acoustically-based index for the objective voice quality assessment of hoarseness. Using the software Praat and an individually developed script (Barsties and Maryn 2016) or the freeware VOXplot (see Sect. 2.3.3), signal processing, analysis, and evaluation are enabled. The AVQI includes the following six acoustic parameters: Harmonics-to-Noise Ratio, Shimmer in %, Shimmer in dB, general slope of the Long-Term Average Spectrum (Slope), tilt through the Long-Term Average Spectrum (Tilt), and Cepstral Peak Prominence Smoothed (CPPS; which makes the main contribution in this model) (Maryn et al. 2010).

For the AVQI analysis, 3 seconds of a sustained vowel /a:/ without voice onset and offset and a speech sample of continuous speech (usually a passage of a phonetically balanced text) are used and analyzed in a combined form. Both types of voice samples contribute to the final AVQI result, as the assessment of the sustained vowel alone does not have sufficient ecological validity. Since its development in 2010, the AVQI has undergone two important and validated adjustments (Jayakumar and Benoy 2024; Batthyany et al. 2024). First, the structure of the signal processing analysis was fully integrated into Praat (AVQI v.02), instead of using two software programs as before. Second, the two types of speech material were equally weighted, allowing for a more balanced assessment for the final AVQI result (AVQI v.03). The duration of the continuous speech portion of AVQI v.03 has now been standardized to the number of syllables specific to the language. In English, the text with a standardized number of 22 syllables is: *"When the sunlight strikes raindrops in the air, they act as a prism and form a rainbow. The rain"* (Castillo-Allendes et al. 2023), which results in about 3 seconds of voiced segments. The adjusted AVQI v.03 thus avoids over- or underweighting the sustained vowel. This AVQI version is the most current, which, in addition to the aforementioned advantages, is also significantly more accurate in terms of diagnostic validity compared to earlier AVQI versions (Jayakumar and Benoy 2024).

Therefore, this version is also used as the standard when AVQI measurements are discussed.

The AVQI result consists of only one value that users receive, and the assessment scale ranges from 0 to 10 (which can also be undercut or exceeded), with a higher value indicating stronger hoarseness and vice versa. The threshold value varies between the different AVQI versions (Stappenbeck et al. 2020; Batthyany et al. 2024) and languages/cultural backgrounds (Englert et al. 2022b; Batthyany et al. 2024). The AVQI has high clinical utility, and good results have been achieved in meta-analyses regarding diagnostic accuracy, criterion validity for perceptual assessment, and the ability to detect voice changes over time after various voice treatments (Jayakumar and Benoy 2024; Batthyany et al. 2024). The diagnostic accuracy of the AVQI (n = 11,696), the criterion validity to the G of the GRBAS scale (n = 10,683), and the measurements of voice changes (n = 734) were evaluated based on different large numbers of voice samples and are among the largest studies in the field of voice quality analysis to date (Batthyany et al. 2024). The results of this meta-analysis on AVQI by Batthyany et al. (2024) form the basis for assessing AVQI's diagnostic quality, which will be described further. The ability to distinguish between the absence and confirmation of hoarseness with the AVQI showed an agreement of a summarized 93.7%, determined by a statistic of threshold optimization curves. Sufficiently high values of pooled sensitivity of 83% (95% confidence interval (95% CI): 82%–83%), pooled specificity of 89% (95% CI: 88%–90%), a pooled positive likelihood ratio of 7.75 (95% CI: 6.04–9.95), and a pooled negative likelihood ratio of 0.20 (95% CI: 0.17–0.23) were analyzed. High correlations with a weighted mean correlation coefficient of r = 0.838 for criterion validity and change sensitivity after a voice treatment of r = 0.796 were determined for the AVQI.

It is not possible to derive a general AVQI norm value from the data of this meta-analysis, as the summarized sensitivity and specificity have been compiled from all versions and development stages of AVQI. Another meta-analysis on the AVQI with only a part of the data from Batthyany et al. (2024) was analyzed for AVQI v.03 (total n = 4,001; vocally-healthy n = 547; voice-disordered n = 3,454) (Jayakumar and Benoy 2024). From eight studies, an average norm value for normophonia for AVQI v.03 of 2.22 was calculated.

▶ In comparison, the English language has a slightly lower AVQI v.03 norm value of 1.17 (Sensitivity: 62%; Specificity: 95%) (Castillo-Allendes et al. 2023).

To interpret a difference between two AVQI measurements and to assess natural fluctuations in the voice when the same measurement conditions prevail (excluding systematic errors such as measurement apparatus, execution protocol, room, measurement time), a test-retest study was also conducted on vocally-healthy adults (Gierlich and Barsties v. Latoszek in press).

> A difference value of 0.78 to 0.95 between two AVQI measurements is considered a natural voice fluctuation and an insignificant difference in the perceptual hoarseness assessment of AVQI v.03 (Gierlich and Barsties v. Latoszek in press; Hosokawa et al. 2024). Insofar as no systematic error is present, difference values of up to >–0.95 between two AVQI measurements are attributed to a treatment effect (Example: Test value AVQI = 3.10 and retest value AVQI = 2.10 difference of −1.00).

Other aspects that have been investigated in studies on AVQI include, for example, age, which has minimal to no influence on the AVQI value (especially in younger adults), and gender, which has no influence on AVQI results (Barsties v. Latoszek et al. 2019a; Jayakumar et al. 2022).

Acceptable values for AVQI in the assessment of voice within the framework of detecting voice disorders (normal versus organic/functional voice disorders) have been determined (Barsties v. Latoszek et al. 2019b). A moderate to high correlation with standardized questionnaires for assessing voice impairments due to voice problems was also found (Ulozaite-Staniene et al. 2019; Pommée et al. 2020).

The AVQI is also robust against fluctuations in room acoustics, background noise, and microphone quality (Ulozaite-Staniene et al. 2019; Bottalico et al. 2020). Nevertheless, acoustic measurements should be controlled and implemented according to the criteria described above, as described in Sects. 2.3.1. and 2.3.2., to ensure a valid and reliable AVQI analysis.

Although AVQI was developed to depict hoarseness, AVQI analyses take into account voice anomalies regarding the parameter breathiness more strongly than roughness (Barsties v. Latoszek et al. 2023c). Therefore, further research is needed to represent roughness within hoarseness more representatively.

Caution is also advised when using updates of the Praat software, as this can significantly affect the analysis functions of AVQI (Stappenbeck et al. 2020). It is therefore advisable, if a new version of Praat is to be used, to critically test it in advance and compare the AVQI values with existing recordings. An alternative option is the freeware VOXplot (see Sect. 2.3.3). Here, a consistent standard of the Praat version is integrated with high user-friendliness. Additionally, there is a quick & easy application with high control of potential error sources (e.g., stereo recordings, differences in the sampling rate of recordings, ensuring the correct speech material for analysis, adjustable language variability with corresponding norm values, etc.) to further increase reliability in AVQI analyses.

Acoustic Breathiness Index

The Acoustic Breathiness Index is also a multiparametric acoustic index like AVQI, but unlike AVQI, it examines the degree of breathiness as a voice quality parameter. Further interfaces with AVQI and ABI are that (a) the same statistical procedure was used for the development of the index, (b) signal processing, analysis, and evaluation are performed using the software Praat (see Sect. 2.3.3) and an individually developed script or the freeware VOXplot, (c) the same speech tasks of continuous speech and the sustained vowel /a:/ are the subject of the analysis, and (d) the assessment scheme of the index is rated on a scale from 0–10 (the higher the ABI value, the breathier the voice). The combined speech tasks of continuous speech and the sustained vowel /a:/ for ABI are identical in duration and type as in AVQI v.03. Nine individual acoustic measurement parameters are required for quantification. These measurement parameters are: CPPS, Jitter %, Glottal-to-Noise Excitation Ratio with a maximum frequency of 4500 Hz, relative level of high-frequency noise between 0 to 6 kHz and 6 to 10 kHz (Hfno), Harmonics-to-Noise Ratio according to Dejonckere, differences between the amplitudes of the first and second harmonic peaks in the spectrum (H1-H2), Shimmer %, Shimmer dB, and the period standard deviation (Barsties v. Latoszek et al. 2017).

ABI's diagnostic accuracy also has high clinical utility, which was confirmed by a meta-analysis (Barsties v. Latoszek et al. 2021b). More than 3603 voice samples were summarized and evaluated, of which 467 were vocally-healthy and 3136 were voice-disordered. The results of the meta-analysis on ABI serve as a basis for assessing ABI's diagnostic quality, which is described below (Barsties v. Latoszek et al. 2021b). The pooled sensitivity of ABI is 84% (95% CI: 83%–85%) and the pooled specificity is 92% (95% CI: 89%–94%). The ability to distinguish between the absence and confirmation of breathiness by ABI showed an agreement of 94%, determined by a threshold optimization curve statistic. Since comparable standards exist in all included studies of the meta-analysis by Barsties v. Latoszek et al. (2021b), a general, weighted ABI norm value from six languages could be determined:

- ▶ The weighted ABI norm value is 3.40 (pooled sensitivity: 86%, 95% CI: 84%–87%; pooled specificity: 90%, 95% CI: 88%–92%), while an ABI norm value for the English language is 2.35 (sensitivity: 84%; specificity: 81%) (Castillo-Allendes et al. 2023; Barsties v. Latoszek et al. 2021b).

- ▶ An absolute difference value of 0.66 between two ABI measurements is considered a natural voice fluctuation, and insofar as no systematic error is present, difference values of two ABI measurements that are >−0.66 (example: test value ABI = 4.50 and retest value ABI = 3.80 difference of −0.70) can be interpreted as a treatment effect (Gierlich and Barsties v. Latoszek in press).

The criterion validity between ABI and an auditory-perceptual assessment of breathiness ranges from r = 0.746 to r = 0.890 (Barsties v. Latoszek et al. 2021b) and its accuracy on therapy-related changes in voice quality is considered sufficiently sensitive with correlation values from r = 0.71 to r = 0.88 (Barsties v. Latoszek and Lehnert 2018; Hosokawa et al. 2019). Neither age and gender nor the degree of roughness have a significant impact on the ABI assessment, whether based on natural (Hosokawa et al. 2019) or computer-generated/synthetic voices (Barsties v. Latoszek et al. 2023c). Caution is advised, as with AVQI analyses, when using version updates of Praat that have not been critically evaluated beforehand, as the function can be altered by the update (Stappenbeck et al. 2020). However, one can also resort to the freeware VOXplot (see Sect. 2.3.3.) to gain more reliability in ABI analyses and simplified handling for users.

Dysphonia Severity Index

The Dysphonia Severity Index is another multivariable index that includes four individual parameters (Wuyts et al. 2000). There are three acoustic parameters, namely the jitter % (calculated on the sustained vowel /a:/—as with AVQI and ABI), the highest fundamental frequency (VRP- F0-high; from the Voice Range Profile, see Sect. 2.3.5) and the lowest intensity (VRP- I-min; from the Voice Range Profile, see Sect. 2.3.5)—and one aerodynamic parameter, namely the maximum phonation time (MPT) on the vowel /a:/ (see Sect. 2.4). The DSI value is rated on a scale from −5 to +5. The DSI values are calculated using the following formula: $DSI = 0.13 \times MPT + 0.0053 \times VRP\text{-}\ F0\text{-}high - 0.26 \times VRP\text{-}\ I\text{-}min - 1.18 \times Jitter\ \% + 12.4$.

In general, normal and vocally-healthy individuals have a value of +5 (or even beyond) and severely disordered voices have a value of −5 or beyond (Wuyts et al. 2000).

The original purpose of the DSI was to objectively and quantitatively determine the degree of hoarseness based on different sustained phonations on the vowel /a:/. A meta-analysis examined this with regard to the normative DSI value in the relevant literature (Sobol and Sielska-Badurek 2022). These results were summarized based on 1330 vocally-healthy subjects, and they determined a DSI normative value of 3.1 (95% CI: DSI = +2.1–+4.0). However, since most of the measured parameters in the DSI formula (i.e., MPT, VRP- F0-high, and VRP- I-min) do not directly and necessarily correlate with the degree of hoarseness but are aimed at vocal function, it is therefore not surprising that their combination only approximates the auditory-perceptual voice quality ratings to a limited extent (Maryn et al. 2017). This was also confirmed in other studies, e.g., in direct comparison to AVQI (Uloza et al. 2018). AVQI achieved significantly higher values in hoarseness assessment regarding criterion validity and diagnostic accuracy. In measurements that therefore strongly relate to vocal function, it is concluded that the DSI can also evaluate limitations of vocal function and thus can also be used as a general measure of vocal efficiency, vocal performance, or the presence of a voice disorder (Maryn et al. 2017; Barsties v. Latoszek et al. 2019b). The DSI achieved an accuracy of 88% when the criterion was not hoarseness but the presence of a voice disorder for classification, from which the DSI normative value was also determined to be 3.1 (Barsties v. Latoszek et al. 2019b).

▶ Thus, the following DSI classification for grading the severity of dysphonia as in Wuyts et al. (2000) can be maintained, and DSI values >3.1 are classified as normal/no dysphonia, 3.1 to −0.1 as mild, −0.1 to −3.1 as moderate, and <−3.3 as severe.

The DSI was classified as a useful and practical measurement parameter (Wuyts et al. 2000; Hakkesteegt et al. 2008a; Hussein Gaber et al. 2014; Nemr et al. 2016), with an acceptable inter-variability of DSI values between examiners (Hakkesteegt et al. 2008b). It is clinically used as a measurement parameter to evaluate changes after voice therapy, voice training, or phonosurgery (Timmermans et al. 2005; Hakkesteegt et al. 2010; Awan and Ensslen 2010; Van Lierde et al. 2011; Young et al. 2016; Meister et al. 2017; Nusseck et al. 2021). Further studies on the DSI showed that geographical and ethnic differences in DSI values can occur (Jayakumar and Savithri 2012). Differences in the reliability of the DSI between hardware and sofware components are evident (Aichinger et al. 2012). The test and retest variability of the DSI ranges from 1.7 to 2.0 (Awan et al. 2012) and 2.5 (Hakkesteegt et al. 2008b). An influencing factor on the DSI value due to the age of the subjects is possible, but not due to gender (Hakkesteegt et al. 2006a; Goy et al. 2013; Maruthy and Ravibabu 2015; Nemr et al. 2016; Barsties v. Latoszek et al. 2019a). There is a correlation between self-perceived voice problems and DSI values (Wuyts et al. 2000; Hakkesteegt et al. 2010). Due to the differences found by Aichinger et al. (2012) through the use of different hardware and software components in the calculation of the DSI than those originally developed by Kay Pentax (Wuyts et al. 2000), there is currently only one validated adaptation of the formula with the software Praat, which is comparable in DSI results to the originally developed Kay Pentax hardware and software (Maryn et al. 2017): $DSI_{Praat} = 1.127 + 0.164*MPT + 0.0053*\textit{VRP-F0-high}—0.038x\textit{VRP-I-min} -5.3*\textit{PPQ5}$

2.3.5 Acoustic Assessment of Voice Function

The voice range profile (VRP)/voice range profile/voice range profile/singing voice range/phonogram is a method for graphically representing a computer-assisted real-time profile of voice data, which is displayed in a coordinate system (Titze 1992a; Heylen et al. 1996; Ternström et al. 2016). It maps the range of vocal fundamental frequencies (F0), measured in Hertz (Hz) or semitones, on the horizontal axis and the sound intensities, measured as sound pressure level in decibels (dB), on the y-axis (see Fig. 2.3).

The Voice Range Profile (VRP) has—as seen in Fig. 2.3—a characteristic shape despite interindividual variations and variabilities due to, for example, warm-up exercises before the recording, vowel choice, gender, and age of the patients (Titze 1992a; Coleman 1993; Heylen et al. 1996; Ternström et al. 2016). Fluctuations of about 2 dB in consecutive trials between two VRP recordings are within the normal range, and a pitch variation is considered acceptable if it does not deviate more than 3.5% from the previously measured frequency (Printz et al. 2018). The VRP makes it possible to depict a balance between the capacities of a voice and the demands placed on it (Coleman 1993). From a clinical perspective, it is therefore more a reflection of vocal performance capabilities (voice function) than a measurement of actual phonatory functions (Heylen et al. 1996).

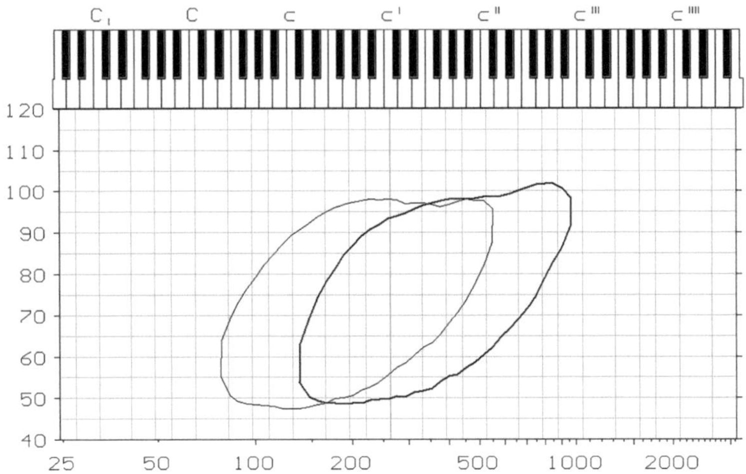

Fig. 2.3 The two plotted voice range profiles (created with the Voice-Range-Profile-Contour software by Pabon et al. 2011) show the normative, averaged minimum and maximum boundary curves (contour) of vocally-healthy women and men, derived from various datasets from up to 11 studies included in the Voice-Range-Profile-Contour software by Pabon et al. (2011): gray line = men, black line = women

The VRP is considered a quantitative measure of voice function to determine the normal ranges for men and women with and without voice disorders, to investigate vocal changes due to vocal strain, to determine pitch range and intensity volume, to record changes after voice treatments, to indicate register size and transitions, and to conduct further objective assessments in the entire VRP range of individual cells in the voice range profile (here not only in the contour) through acoustic parameters to anomalies in voice quality (Heylen et al. 1996; Ikeda et al. 1999).

The characteristics of the VRP can be divided into the following groups: frequency and intensity limits of the minimum and maximum vocal performance, shape and quality of the individual cells that make up the entire voice range profile.

The frequency range of the physiological voice range represents the modal (chest voice) and falsetto register (head voice) or the entire voice category (in classical singing: soprano, mezzo-soprano, alto, tenor, baritone, bass). Most often, only the highest and lowest pitch are indicated/interpreted in examination protocols (Friedrich and Dejonckere 2005). The lowest pitch is achieved through a laryngeal posture with relaxed and short vocal folds as well as moderate transglottal air pressure. The highest pitchis attained with particularly high activity of the cricothyroid muscle, which leads to elongated and tense vocal folds, combined with high subglottic pressure. This also requires great force to hold the vocal folds together (Ternström et al. 2016).

▶ According to the guidelines of the European Laryngological Society, the lowest frequencies (VRP-F0-low) should be <165 Hz for women and about 73 Hz for men; the highest frequencies (VRP-F0-high) should be>659 Hz for women and >294 Hz for men to be considered normal (Friedrich and Dejonckere 2005). The voice range (VRP-semitone range) that results from this is rated as normal for both genders by this guideline with $\geq$24 semitones (Friedrich and Dejonckere 2005).

▶ The intensity values that arise from the VRP are the minimum intensity (VRP-I-min), the maximum intensity (VRP-I-max), and theintensity range (VRP-intensity range), which according to the European Laryngological Society are classified as physiological for both genders if the intensities are >90 dB for I-max, <55 dB for I-min, and theintensity range is >40 dB.

The contour of the VRP sets an upper and a lower volume limit for the frequency range. The lower boundary or lower phonation threshold must be carefully determined and defined by the examiners for each VRP. Accordingly, patients must be stimulated to determine the maximum performance of the quietest volume. Examiners must also audibly and visually assess the extent to which voice control is present during the phonation attempt, as different intensity levels at the beginning and end of the vocalization must be evaluated. The quiet voice is a motor skill that can be improved through training, and the vibration amplitude of the vocal folds can become irregular at low glottal airflow (Ternström et al. 2016). The lower boundaryof the VRP clinically represents the elasticity and flexibility of the vocal folds that enable quiet phonation for a normal voice (Titze 1992b). The height of the upper boundaryindicates the maximum intensity in a loud voice. This limit is determined by the maximum glottal airflow, mouth opening, acoustic resonances of the vocal tract, non-linear maximum vibration amplitude (which leads to clipping in the voice recording), and the voice register (i.e., modal/chest voice vs. falsetto voice) (Ternström et al. 2016). The vocal effort required for the upper boundaryis related to the tension of the thyroarytenoid muscle and the other laryngeal adductors to increase subglottic pressure so that a loud voice can be produced (Ternström et al. 2016). Several peculiarities can be observed in the VRP boundaries of men and women (Ternström et al. 2016):

First, there is a dip in the upper boundary that characterizes the individual vocal performance between modal and falsetto voice.

Secondly, the upper boundary from the low to the mid-range pitches reflects the least susceptible volume fluctuations, which are due to fluctuations in the vocal tract resonances. Since it is not possible to produce a very low and very loud voice, patients are forced to raise the pitch to achieve a louder voice. However, if patients frequently raise the pitch in everyday life to achieve higher voice intensity, voice complaints and vocal fatigue can result (Schutte 1986; Solomon 2008). Additionally, individuals with a flat upper boundary from the low to the mid-range pitches of the VRP are generally limited in their vocal dynamics during everyday phonation (see later for moderately pathological VRPs—discongruity). Especially during prolonged speaking, this requires great effort, e.g., with high professional voice demands, often resulting in voice problems or disorders (Schutte 1986). Even though there are different calculation methods and definitions for the slope of a VRP—which have been investigated in several studies and make it difficult to compare study results—(Heylen et al. 1996), the overall slope of the VRP generally increases with increasing volume by about 8 to 10 dB per octave (Titze and Sundberg 1992), so that the loudest voice at low frequencies usually has a lower intensity level than the quietest voice at the upper end of the frequency range (Ternström et al. 2016). Other acoustic parameters such as jitter, shimmer, crest factor, harmonics-to-noise ratio, singing power ratio, and the cepstral peak prominence smoothed can be visualized over the entire performance of the cells in the VRP (Pabon 1991; Nijkamp 2019; Pabon and Ternström 2020). This application of further acoustic parameters has the potential to investigate phonation strategies and contribute to a better understanding of phonation in general (Ternström et al. 2016).

The result of a VRP for general clinical application in voice diagnostics for the examination of voice function is shown in Fig. 2.4. The four boundary parameters of the VRP and the ranges of semitones and intensity are crucial here. For better orientation, the final VRP is divided into four quadrants, which should also help

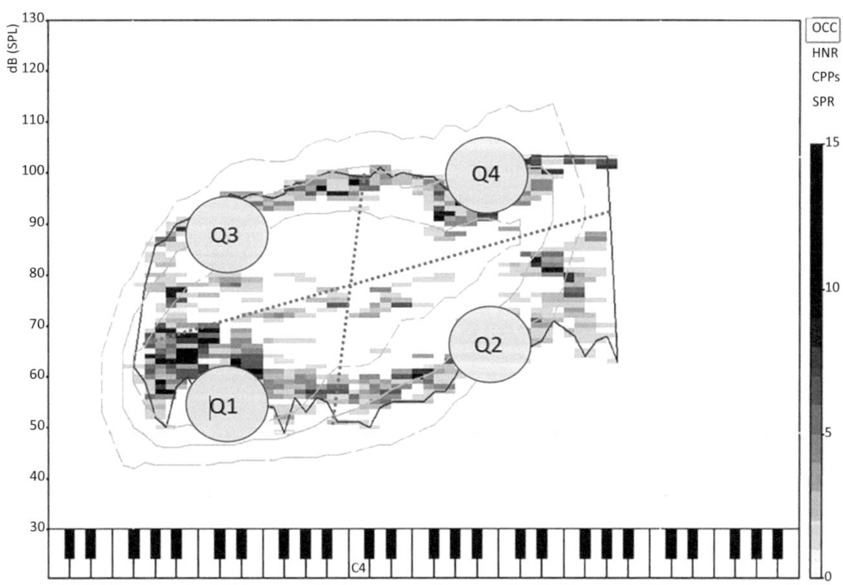

Fig. 2.4 Example of a healthy voice (normal/large voice range) of a 35-year-old male subject, illustrating the general clinical reference points of a VRP and its division into quadrants (Q1–Q4) for orientation during a VRP assessment *Source* SRH University of Applied Sciences Heidelberg, Campus Düsseldorf

with orientation during the assessment (see Sect. 3.1). In Q1, the low and soft phonation is verified (VRP- F0-low and VRP- I-min). Q1 and Q2 represent the piano contour of the voice range profile, where the intensity fluctuation of the piano contour is minimal for a physiological voice. The endpoints of the VRP- F0-high in Q2 and Q4 should be relatively congruent. Q3 represents the loud chest voice (modal forte contour of the voice range profile). In Q4, the other two boundary parameters are usually determined (VRP- F0-high and VRP- I-max) and correspond to the head voice register in the forte contour of the voice range profile. The slope of the forte contour of the voice range profile should also be relatively flat from Q3 to Q4 and not rise too steeply. The (VRP-) semitone range is determined by the difference between VRP- F0-high and VRP- F0-low, and the (VRP-) intensity range by the difference between VRP- I-max and VRP- I-min.

Based on these results, four voice range profile boundaries can be clearly identified according to Schutte (1986): (a) normal/large voice range (physiological), (b) discongruityvoice range (narrow-ascending VRP with normal limits but restrictions in volume at Q2 and Q3), (c) medium-sized voice range (semitone: small semitone range but normal intensity range; intensity: small intensity range but normal semitone range), (d) small voice range (small semitoneand intensity range).

To clinically evaluate the voice range profile boundaries and assess a certain severity of voice function, the following interpretation procedure, which is based on the evaluation of modal and falsetto voice (other registers such as pulse register/glottal fry or whistle register as well as ventricular phonation are excluded here), is helpful:

Interpretation Procedure for Determining the Voice Range Profile Contour

1. *Compare the normal values of the boundary parameters and the two ranges from the European Laryngological Society (ELS) protocol* (Friedrich and Dejonckere 2005). Create a table for better clarity; marking with ***bold-italic*** can help to quickly draw attention to pathological results compared to physiological results.
2. *Apply contour shapes & definitions according to* Schutte (1986) *as the first approach for boundary determination.* Determine the appropriate contour type by the process of elimination. These interpretations can be expanded depending on the measurement outcome, especially in cases of minimal voice abnormalities (e.g., passaggio area, falsetto register or chest register fluctuations in the forte and/or piano contour of the voice range profile boundaries).

For better illustration of the interpretation suggestions and grading of the severity of the VRP's for clinical voice diagnostics, the following examples are referenced.

Case Study: Slightly Pathological VRP = Tendency to Normal
Person: female, 53 years old, teacher—Functional Dysphonia (Fig. 2.5)

VRP Parameter	Results	Normal Values
Softest intensity (VRP- I-min)	50 dB	<55 dB
Loudest intensity (VRP- I-max)	111 dB	>90 dB
Lowest pitch (VRP- F0-low)	103 Hz	F: < 165 Hz
Highest pitch (VRP- F0-high)	818 Hz	F: > 659 Hz
(VRP-) semitone range	36 ST	≥24 ST
(VRP-) Intensity range	61 dB	>40 dB
VRP-boundaries	**Tendency to normal**	large/normal

Conclusion: Contour tendency to normal:

1. The four boundary parameters of the VRP are all within the normal range.
2. The two boundaries are within the normal range.
3. A consistently significant drop relative to I-max in the forte contour: concerning Q3/Q4 from C3-D#5.
4. Significant drops in the piano contour from F3-C#5.
5. No obvious congruence between the piano contour and the forte contour. The piano contour is 5 ST lower in range in the falsetto register than the forte contour.

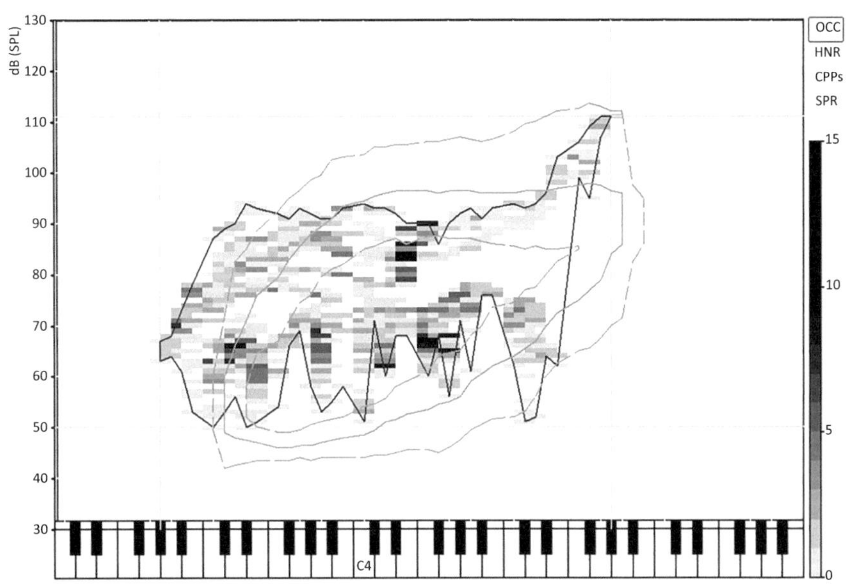

Fig. 2.5 VRP—Tendency to normal *Source* TheVoice Clinic, Böblingen

This example illustrates a few features that can be described as tending towards normal, based on qualitative features in the contour. General features for classifying a VRP as "tending to normal" would be, for example:

- Clear dynamic drops in the piano and/or forte contour relative to the normal voice fields
- Insufficient congruence of the F0-high values in the piano and forte contour
- Insufficient dynamic ratio between chest and head voice in the forte contour, so that it is evident that there is a significant deviation in relation to the two registers as well as to the normal voice fields in relation to the two registers as well as to the normal voice fields

Case study: moderately severe pathological VRPs = discongruity and medium-sized (semitone or intensity)

1. Person: male, 51 years, truck driver—idiopathic vocalis atrophy (Fig. 2.6)

VRP Parameter	Results	Normal values
Softest intensity (VRP- I-min)	51 dB	<55 dB
Loudest intensity (VRP- I-max)	99 dB	>90 dB
Lowest pitch (VRP- F0-low)	105 Hz	F: < 73 Hz
Highest pitch (VRP- F0-high)	513 Hz	F: > 294 Hz

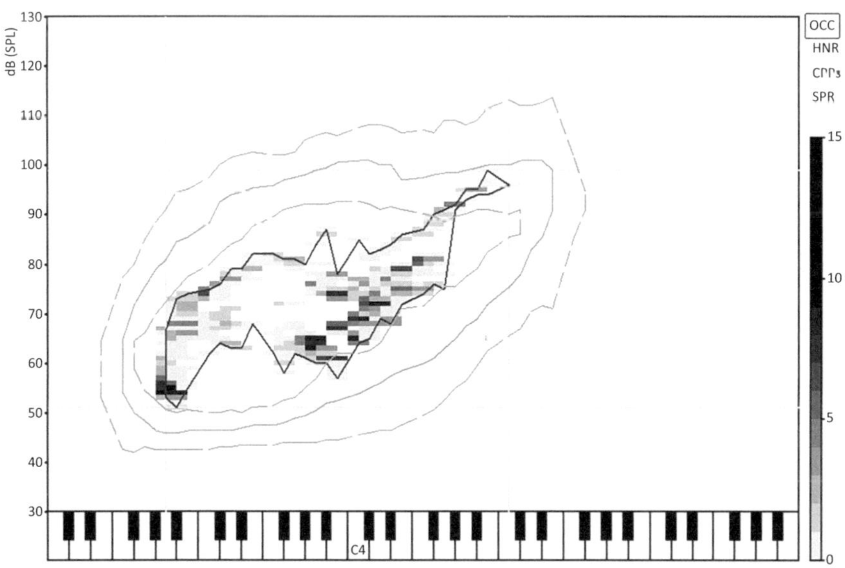

Fig. 2.6 VRP—discongruity *Source* TheVoice Clinic, Böblingen

VRP Parameter	Results	Normal values
(VRP-) semitone range	28 ST	≥24 ST
(VRP-) intensity range	48 dB	>40 dB
VRP-boundaries	**discongruity**	large/normal

Conclusion: Contour discongruity:

1. All boundary parameters of the VRP are within the normal range.
2. Both boundaries are within the normal range.
3. Significant dips in the piano contour from A#2-F#3.
4. Narrowly ascending piano and forte contour (low intensity variety), which according to the definition of Schutte (1986) is to be evaluated as discongruity:
   Forte contour: lower intensity in Q3 compared to Q4
   Piano contour: too high intensity in Q2

2. Person: male, 53 years, restaurant manager—Reinke's edema (Fig. 2.7)

VRP Parameters	Results	Normal Values
Softest intensity (VRP- I-min)	**66 dB**	<55 dB
Loudest intensity (VRP- I-max)	109 dB	>90 dB
Lowest pitch (VRP- F0-low)	66 Hz	F: < 73 Hz
Highest pitch (VRP- F0-high)	**160 Hz**	F: > 294 Hz

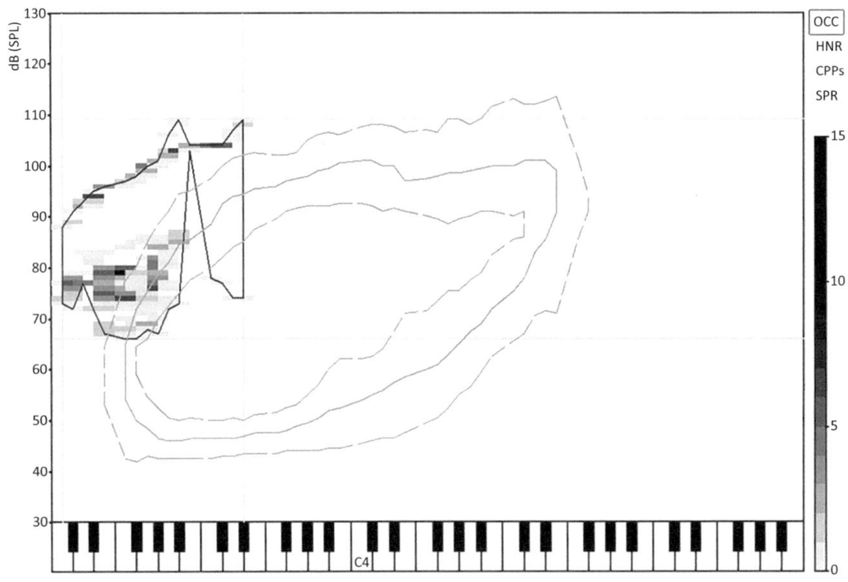

Fig. 2.7 VRP—medium-sized (semitone) *Source* TheVoice Clinic, Böblingen

VRP Parameters	Results	Normal Values
(VRP-) semitone range	**15 ST**	≥24 ST
(VRP-) intensity range	43 dB	>40 dB
VRP-boundaries	**medium-sized (semitone)**	large/normal

Conclusion: Contour medium-sized (semitone):

1. Two out of four boundary parameters of the VRP are not within the normal range, of which only F0-high has an impact on the ranges.
2. The semitone range is pathological, but the intensity range is physiological, which according to the definition of Schutte (1986) defines a medium-sized VRP.
3. A significant dip in the piano contour from A#2-C3 is present.

- A peculiarity of this semitone medium-sized VRP is that hardly any low intensity is possible, but a maximum intensity of >90 dB is possible across the entire semitone range from C#2-D#3.

3. Person: female, 56 years, saleswoman—post leukoplakia 3 months ago without intervention (Fig. 2.8)

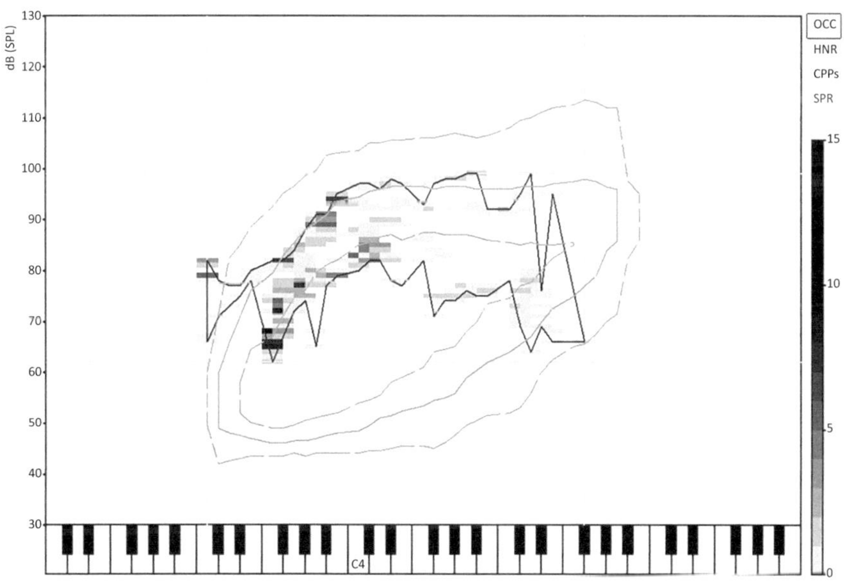

Fig. 2.8 VRP—medium-sized (intensity) *Source* TheVoice Clinic, Böblingen

VRP Parameters	Results	Norm Values
Softest intensity (VRP- I-min)	**62 dB**	<55 dB
Loudest intensity (VRP- I-max)	99 dB	>90 dB
Lowest pitch (VRP- F0-low)	128 Hz	F: < 165 Hz
Highest pitch (VRP- F0-high)	742 Hz	F: > 659 Hz
(VRP-) semitone range	30 ST	≥24 ST
(VRP-) intensity range	**37 dB**	>40 dB
VRP-boundaries	**medium-sized (intensity)**	large/normal

Conclusion: Contour medium-sized (intensity):

1. Three out of four boundary parameters of the VRP are within the normal range, only VRP- I-min is not.
2. The dynamic range is pathological, however, the semitone range is physiological, an addition to the original definition by Schutte (1986).
3. Additionally significant drops in the piano contour: from B3-C5.
4. Significant drops in the forte contour: Q4 from E5-F#5.

Severely pathological VRP = small
Person: female, 54 years, clerk (not a professional speaker)—unilateral recurrent nerve paresis (right) after cervical spine surgery (Fig. 2.9)

VRP Parameters	Results	Norm Values
Softest intensity (VRP- I-min)	46 dB	<55 dB
Loudest intensity (VRP- I-max)	**79 dB**	>90 dB
Lowest pitch (VRP- F0-low)	134 Hz	F: < 165 Hz
Highest pitch (VRP- F0-high)	**434 Hz**	F: > 659 Hz
(VRP-) semitone range	**21 ST**	≥24 ST
(VRP-) intensity range	**33 dB**	>40 dB
VRP-boundaries	**small**	large/normal

Conclusion: Contour small:

1. Two out of four boundary parameters of the VRP are not within the normal range, both of which (I-max & F0-high) have a significant influence on the fact that both ranges are not within the normal range.
2. Both ranges are not within the normal range; thus, according to the definition of Schutte (1986), a small VRP is given.

Due to the shape of the VRP (visual assessment), a chest and head voice is present, which can be detected in the piano and forte contour.

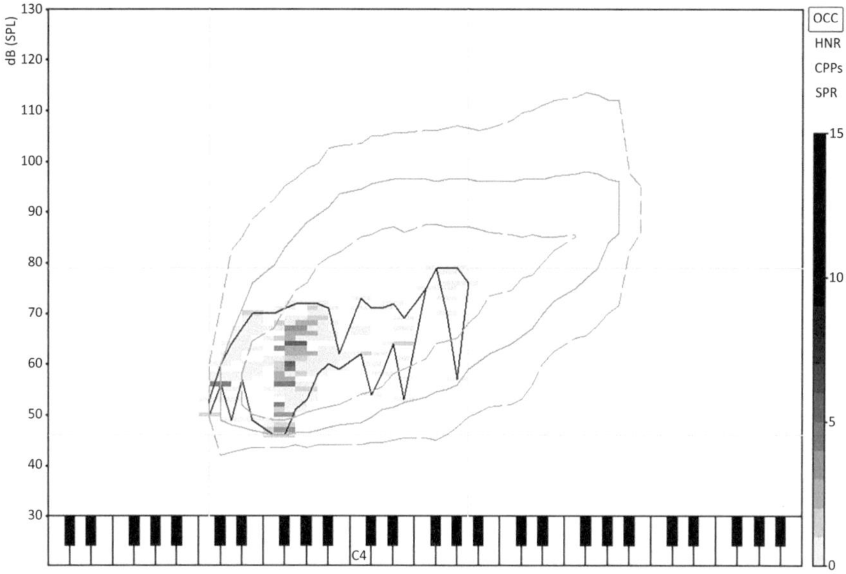

Fig. 2.9 VRP—small *Source* SRH Waldklinik Gera

Examples of special forms:

Ventricular phonation

Person: female, 20 years old, speech therapy student (Fig. 2.10)

VRP Parameters	Results
Softest intensity (VRP- I-min)	48 dB
Loudest intensity (VRP- I-max)	84 dB
Lowest pitch (VRP- F0-low)	65 Hz
Highest pitch (VRP- F0-high)	128 Hz
(VRP-) semitone range	11 ST
(VRP-) intensity range	52 dB

- No further interpretation possible, as only the pulsation register is present.

Combination of medium-sized and discongruity voice range profile contour

Person: female, 75 years, retiree—post phonosurgery of a ventricular cyst (Fig. 2.11)

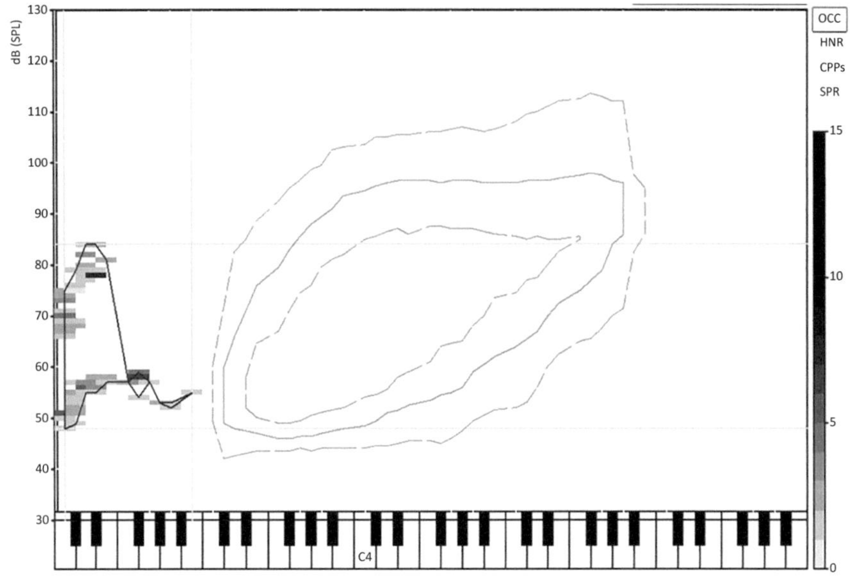

Fig. 2.10 VRP—use of ventricular phonation *Source* SRH University of Applied Sciences Heidelberg, Campus Düsseldorf

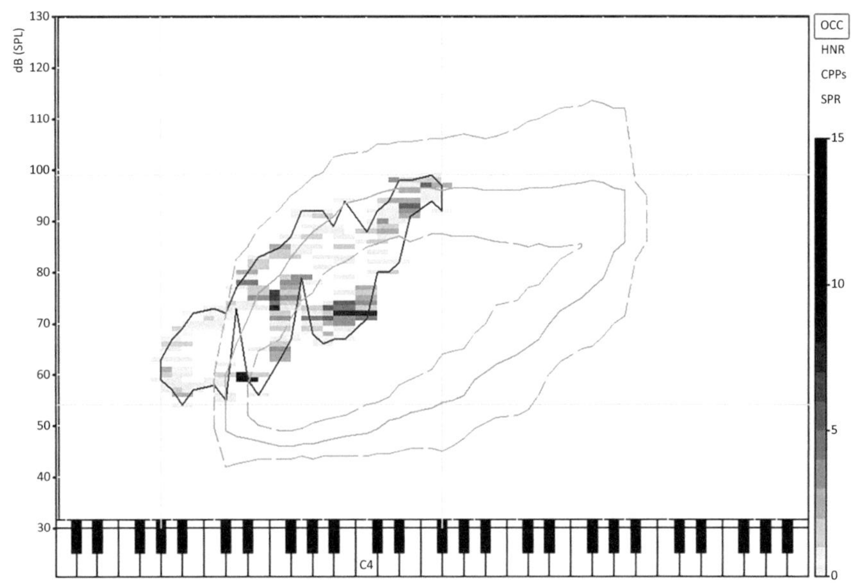

Fig. 2.11 VRP—medium-sized and discongruity *Source* TheVoice Clinic, Böblingen

VRP Parameters	Results	Norm Values
Softest intensity (VRP- I-min)	54 dB	<55 dB
Loudest intensity (VRP- I-max)	99 dB	>90 dB
Lowest pitch (VRP- F0-low)	106 Hz	F: < 165 Hz
Highest pitch (VRP- F0-high)	**371 Hz**	F: > 659 Hz
(VRP-) semitone range	**22 ST**	≥24 ST
(VRP-) intensity range	45 dB	>40 dB
VRP-boundaries	**medium-sized & discongruity**	large/normal

Conclusion: Contour corresponds to a combination of medium-sized & discongruity:

1. Three out of four boundary parameters of the VRP are within the normal range, only VRP- F0-high is not, which has a significant impact on the semitone range.
2. The semitone range is pathological, but the intensity range is physiological, according to the definition by Schutte (1986), this corresponds to a medium-sized voice range profile contour.
3. Narrow ascending piano and forte contour, which according to the definition by Schutte (1986) is also considered discongruity: *Forte contour:* low volume in Q3 relative to Q4
   Piano contour: too high volume in Q2

The examples and interpretations presented above are only applicable to adults. For children between 6–11 years, the following boundary values from Table 2.3 can be used as an initial guide for interpretation.

▶ In addition to the VRP, the Speech Range Profile (SRP) is also used for acoustic voice function testing to analyze the speaking voice.

The SRP also consists of F0 (measured in Hz) and its intensity values (measured in dB). As with the VRP, computer-assisted phonetography should be preferred when taking an SRP to create a speech profile in real-time (Sanchez et al. 2014). From the semitone and intensity "speech cloud" of a habitual speaking voice from the SRP, the average values of pitch and loudness, which are described

Table 2.3 VRP boundary parameters for boys and girls between 6–11 years (Wuyts et al. 2002)

VRP parameters	Boys	Girls
Softest intensity (VRP- I-min)	<56 dB	<54 dB
Loudest intensity (VRP- I-max)	>87 dB	>83 dB
Lowest pitch (VRP- F0-low)	<210 Hz	<220 Hz
Highest pitch (F0-high)	>680 Hz	>750 Hz

as the average speaking pitch in Hz and average speaking loudness in dB, are derived (see Fig. 2.12). For economical voice production, the average speaking pitch should lie in the neutral pitch (frequency range of individual speakers with the least phonation effort). A crucial factor for the optimal regulation of effort is the subglottic pressure (Titze 1989). This speaking pitch is usually located in the lower third of the semitone range of the VRP.

Various factors influence the results of the SRP. On the one hand, the result of the average speaking pitch is influenced by various factors such as gender (Berg et al. 2017; Spazzapan et al. 2022), different levels of intensity (Berg et al. 2017), speech tasks for analysis (Barsties 2013), medications (Sataloff et al. 2005), pathologies/syndromes (such as voice disorders (Verdolini et al. 2006), hemodialysis in renal failure (Sagiroglu and Doganer 2018), trisomy 21 (Lee et al. 2009), smoking (Byeon and Cha 2020; Ma et al. 2023), languages (Altenberg and Ferrand 2006; Scharff-Rethfeldt et al. 2008; Nevo et al. 2015) and age (Berg et al. 2017; Spazzapan et al. 2022) as well as other aspects such as relatively conditioned by body size (Barsties et al. 2016) and voice training (Siupsinskiene 2003). In the case of aging, for example, no changes in the average speaking pitch are observed in women despite advancing age due to hormone therapy because of menopause (Lin and Wang 2020).

Differences in the average speaking pitch can also be detected in the classification of singing categories of soprano/alto (female) and tenor/baritone/bass (male).

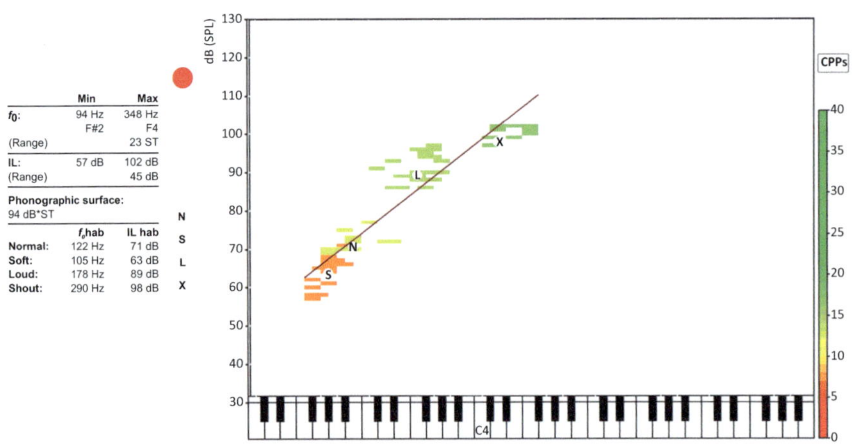

Fig. 2.12 Example of a healthy voice of a 35-year-old male subject, with four different levels of SRPs at different volumes (S = soft—quiet speaking voice, N = normal—habitual speaking voice, L = loud—loud speaking voice, X = shout—calling voice). The points S, N, L, and X mark the corresponding mean values of F0 and intensity in the graph. For the SRP analysis from quiet to loud, the text from "The North Wind and the Sun" (text length identical as for the AVQI and ABI examinationin German language (Barsties v. Latoszek et al. 2020a) and for the calling voice the words "Hello Anton" were used *Source* SRH University of Applied Sciences Heidelberg, Campus Düsseldorf

Soprano and tenor singers achieve higher values in the average speaking pitch compared to the other categories within the gender group (Morris et al. 1995).

The measurements of the intensity results from the SRP, on the other hand, vary due to the distance of the calibrated sound level meters and their general accuracy/deviation (type class), measurement speed settings, background noise, and calibration procedures for microphones (Švec and Granqvist 2010).

Furthermore, habitual loudness can change with different speaking tasks, with serial speaking being significantly softer than reading aloud or spontaneous storytelling (Zraick et al. 2004). The intensity at different levels of volume (i.e., quiet, normal, and loud) varies between men and women (Berg et al. 2017), with intensity generally increasing over a lifetime at normal loudness (Stathopoulos et al. 2011).

▶ The standard values for the SRP are based on measurements with the calibrated software Vox Phonetography and considering the proven factors described above that can influence the speaking voice, so the standard values for speaking pitches and speaking loudness from the various speaking situations can be found at the example of German speakers in the following Tables 2.4 & 2.5.

Further reference values of SRPs for individuals under 18 years old are shown by the results of, for example, Berger et al. (2019). In this study, 1564 German-Speaking children and adolescents aged 5.5 to 17.5 years were recruited, and the SRP measurements were documented in four levels of intensity as in Table 2.6, but now with means and standard deviations.

Table 2.4 Standard values of the different SRPs for men (vocally-healthy and non-smokers) with the software Vox Phonetography according to Lübke et al. (in press)

Measurement values	Situations	18–44 years		45–60 years		>60 years	
		Lower limit	Upper limit	Lower limit	Upper limit	Lower limit	Upper limit
Frequency (Hz)	1	92 Hz	106 Hz	83 Hz	109 Hz	96 Hz	127 Hz
	2	97 Hz	113 Hz	91 Hz	120 Hz	113 Hz	138 Hz
	3	151 Hz	199 Hz	148 Hz	191 Hz	163 Hz	202 Hz
	4	257 Hz	319 Hz	252 Hz	312 Hz	235 Hz	305 Hz
Loudness (dB)	1	62 dB	67 dB	59 dB	68 dB	67 dB	70 dB
	2	71 dB	74 dB	70 dB	76 dB	74 dB	77 dB
	3	82 dB	91 dB	82 dB	91 dB	83 dB	89 dB
	4	96 dB	101 dB	95 dB	101 dB	94 dB	100 dB

Calibration using a dB meter at a distance of 30 cm and 90° with a microphone distance of 5–10 cm (45°) as well as calibration in dB(C) according to Maryn and Zarowski (2015);
Situations using the "North Wind and the Sun" text passage as in the German version of AVQI and ABI (Barsties v. Latoszek et al. 2020a): (1) soft speaking voice, (2) habitual speaking voice, (3) loud voice as in a classroom, and (4) shouting voice determined by the shout of "Hello Anton"

Table 2.5 Standard values of the different SRPs for women (vocally-healthy, no hormone therapy, and non-smokers) with the software Vox Phonetography according to Lübke et al. (in press)

Measurement values	Situations	18–44 years		45–60 years		>60 years	
		Lower limit	Upper limit	Lower limit	Upper limit	Lower limit	Upper limit
Frequency (Hz)	1	183 Hz	216 Hz	152 Hz	175 Hz	146 Hz	183 Hz
	2	193 Hz	216 Hz	173 Hz	192 Hz	154 Hz	190 Hz
	3	271 Hz	305 Hz	232 Hz	301 Hz	234 Hz	323 Hz
	4	365 Hz	433 Hz	360 Hz	444 Hz	351 Hz	452 Hz
Loudness (dB)	1	63 dB	67 dB	64 dB	68 dB	64 dB	71 dB
	2	71 dB	73 dB	72 dB	76 dB	72 dB	77 dB
	3	81 dB	88 dB	83 dB	87 dB	82 dB	87 dB
	4	91 dB	100 dB	92 dB	98 dB	92 dB	96 dB

Calibration using a dB meter at a distance of 30 cm and 90° with a microphone distance of 5–10 cm (45°) as well as calibration in dB(C) according to Maryn and Zarowski (2015);
Situations using the "North Wind and the Sun" text passage as in the German version of AVQI and ABI (Barsties v. Latoszek et al. 2020a): (1) soft speaking voice, (2) habitual speaking voice, (3) loud voice as in the classroom, and (4) calling voice determined by the shout of "Hello Anton"

In conclusion, the different volume levels in relation to the pitch increase in the SRP can be summarized by two parameters (SRP-Slope and SRP-Interdependence), which are gender-independent (Lübke et al. in press). They define the physiological increase in pitch with a simultaneous increase in loudness, both of which are strongly influenced by subglottic pressure, such as a doubling of subglottic pressure with a 10 dB increase in the middle range of the intensity range, or a pitch increase of up to 6 Hz with +1 cm H_2O of subglottic pressure (Debruyne and Buekers 1998). Thus, the SRP interdependence parameters between pitch and loudness can be useful in evaluating voice disorders, as an excessive increase in pitch and loudness indicates vocal abuse or vocal incapacity, suggesting that the voice is being used in an ineffective manner, especially if the vocal possibilities of a lower-louder voice are present in the VRP (Debruyne and Buekers 1998). It becomes more problematic and treatment-intensive if the vocal possibilities to use a lower-louder voice are not present even in the VRP, as is the case with a discongruity VRP.

▶ The SRP-Slope parameter describes the increase in loudness and pitch of all four intensity levels (from soft to calling voice) in decibels (dB) per octave (Oct) and is given with a standard value of >18.61 dB/Oct (between 18–44 years), >16.94 dB/Oct (between 45–60 years), and >15.33 dB/Oct (>60 years) (Lübke et al. in press). The SRP interdependence voice parameter also complements the measurement of the slope ratio of pitch and loudness and is expressed in semitones (ST) per decibel (dB). A standard value here corresponds to <0.696 ST/dB (between 18–44 years), <0.721 ST/dB (between 45–60 years), and <0.819 ST/dB (>60 years) (Lübke et al. in press).

Table 2.6 Reference values for different SRPs for German-Speaking children and adolescents according to Berger et al. (2019)

Measurements	Situations	5.5–10.5 years		10.5–14.5 years		14.5–17.5 years	
		Mean	Standard deviation	Mean	Standard deviation	Mean	Standard deviation
Male							
Frequency (Hz)	1	197.03 Hz	39.23 Hz	171.80 Hz	40.03 Hz	122.20 Hz	24.11 Hz
	2	223.29 Hz	34.75 Hz	187.30 Hz	40.72 Hz	122.27 Hz	25.83 Hz
	3	253.73 Hz	34.38 Hz	208.90 Hz	45.40 Hz	134.48 Hz	28.09 Hz
	4	311.80 Hz	44.96 Hz	287.22 Hz	58.74 Hz	207.51 Hz	48.74 Hz
Loudness (dB)	1	52.12 dB	3.09 dB	51.34 dB	3.19 dB	50.02 dB	3.19 dB
	2	59.34 dB	3.30 dB	59.10 dB	3.31 dB	58.11 dB	3.58 dB
	3	66.77 dB	4.29 dB	66.09 dB	4.10 dB	65.23 dB	4.21 dB
	4	82.51 dB	6.46 dB	83.45 dB	6.05 dB	82.72 dB	6.54 dB
Female							
Frequency (Hz)	1	204.47 Hz	41.46 Hz	195.54 Hz	38.03 Hz	194.05 Hz	32.14 Hz
	2	223.27 Hz	34.19 Hz	213.53 Hz	31.33 Hz	205.77 Hz	27.67 Hz
	3	250.30 Hz	34.68 Hz	232.99 Hz	30.55 Hz	222.54 Hz	26.27 Hz
	4	315.65 Hz	42.59 Hz	307.76 Hz	44.39 Hz	302.92 Hz	44.35 Hz
Loudness (dB)	1	51.77 dB	2.99 dB	51.42 dB	2.98 dB	51.10 dB	3.30 dB
	2	58.62 dB	3.27 dB	59.13 dB	3.20 dB	58.58 dB	3.11 dB
	3	65.54 dB	4.17 dB	65.42 dB	3.80 dB	64.85 dB	3.76 dB
	4	79.78 dB	5.59 dB	80.73 dB	5.38 dB	80.55 dB	5.52 dB

Recording system: DiVAS software (XION Medical, Berlin) with a self-calibrated USB microphone headset, positioned at a distance of 30 cm from the mouth

Ambient noise: <40 dB(A); calibration in dB(A)

Situations by counting in automatic speech from 21 to 30: (1) soft speaking voice, (2) habitual speaking voice, (3) loud voice as in a classroom, and (4) calling voice

2.4 Voice Assessment through Aerodynamics

In aerodynamics, the interaction of air pressure and airflow influences vocal fold vibration. Aerodynamic measurements of airflow, air pressure, and air volume thus reflect the efficient use of laryngeal structures. Compared to acoustic analyses, aerodynamic measurements are closely linked to the theoretical understanding of vocal fold structure, movement, and laryngeal activity (Bless 1991). They indicate changes in voice function and are useful tools in the assessment of dysphonia (Bless 1991; Yiu et al. 2004; Ketelslagers et al. 2007).

The clinical application of aerodynamic measurements such as mean airflow, subglottal pressure, and temporal phonation measurements (e.g., maximum phonation time) is supported by a high EBM level. Aerodynamic parameters provide valuable information about the interaction between inspiratory and phonatory mechanisms of speech and offer a detailed insight into the underlying physiology of phonation, the degree of effort on voice production, and the compensatory behaviors used by patients with voice disorders (Awan et al. 2013).

Recommended aerodynamic measurement procedures—according to the protocol of the American Speech-Language Hearing Association—include the average glottal airflow rate (l/sec or ml/sec), the average subglottic air pressure (cm of water or kPa), and measurements of vocal loudness and pitch (Patel et al. 2018). All these measurement procedures are recorded using a pneumotachograph. Patients are instructed to produce short utterances through a face mask, each consisting of at least five syllables /p+vowel/ at a rate of about 1.5–2 syllables per second, to capture and analyze oral airflow and air volume (Patel et al. 2018). The acquisition of this measurement technology is costly and therefore not widespread in clinical practice.

Another reliable measurement parameter frequently used in clinical practice and research is, for example, the maximum phonation time (MPT) (Friedrich and Dejonckere 2005; Speyer et al. 2010; Barsties v. Latoszek et al. 2023d). The MPT is a measurement parameter that is often used to assess vocal functions due to its non-invasiveness, quick execution, and low cost (Speyer et al. 2010). The MPT is considered an aerodynamic assessment that measures glottal efficiency by determining the ability to control the pulmonary aerodynamic and myoelastic forces of the larynx (Solomon et al. 2000). MPT measurements are determined by the maximum possible duration of phonation at habitual speaking pitch and loudness of a vowel (e.g., /a:/) after maximum inhalation, with the total duration of phonation measured in seconds. This measurement procedure can derive the efficiency of the phonation-breathing mechanism (Speyer et al. 2010). To sustain a steady tone over a long period, healthy lung function with sufficient lung capacity and airflow rate is a prerequisite (Solomon et al. 2000). The alignment of subglottic pressure and glottal resistance is also crucial for sustained phonation over a longer period. If the MPT duration is low, it is assumed that the dosage of breathing is difficult or that the glottal resistance, depending on the voice pathology, is too low, and that this low vocal performance would also result in noticeable voice quality (e.g., a breathy voice, see also Table 4.1 in Sect. 4.2) (Barsties and De Bodt 2015).

The MPT is determined through multiple trials and compared with normative data (Baken and Orlikoff 2000). According to Baken and Orlikoff (2000), men achieve higher MPT values than women (approx. 24 sec vs. 19 sec). Interindividual variability and influencing factors such as the number of trials, loudness during execution, vocal condition, body weight, and age also affect the result (Schmidt et al. 1988; Lee et al. 1999; Baken and Orlikoff 2000; Maslan et al. 2011; Barsties et al. 2013; Johnson and Goldfine 2016; Cunha et al. 2019). However, posture (standing or sitting) and inspiratory breathing type (such as thoracic, clavicular, costo-abdominal, and paradoxical) do not influence the MPT result (Cunha et al. 2019; Siegburg 2024).

> An MPT result >15 sec is considered physiological for both genders according to the European Laryngological Society (ELS) protocol of 2001 (Friedrich and Dejonckere 2005).

The test-retest reliability of the MPT is acceptable, with a significant extension of the MPT duration from 1.01 seconds to be expected in vocally-healthy subjects (Awan et al. 2013). Voice therapy is considered effective if the MPT duration after treatment is at least 1.41 seconds longer than the MPT value before treatment (Rodríguez-Parra et al. 2009). Thus, the MPT can be used as a clinically significant measurement parameter for the effectiveness of voice therapy with 1.01–1.41 seconds for pre- and post-treatment comparisons. The information about the aerodynamic function during phonation provided by the MPT is closely related to the laryngeal airway resistance (Solomon et al. 2000).

2.5 Voice Assessment through Self-Perception

The patient's self-assessment, such as the quantification of self perceived vocal limitations, is a highly recommended voice measurement in a voice diagnostic battery (Dejonckere et al. 2001; Rodríguez-Parra et al. 2009; Boominathan et al. 2014).

For every person, the constant availability of their own voice, whether for private or professional use, is of essential importance, without any limitation of physical, functional, or emotional functions, according to the International Classification of Functioning (for more information see Sect. 3.2; Ma et al. 2007).

To measure the extent of activity and participation limitations, self-report questionnaires are used to quantify the impact of the voice disorder on daily life, which can affect voice quality and/or voice function. In recent decades, various questionnaires with different psychometric properties have been developed (Franic et al. 2005).

The Voice Handicap Index (VHI) is a standardized questionnaire, in its original form using 30 statements, to determine self-perceived vocal impairments (Jacobson et al. 1997; see Sect. 3.1). It has subscales with statements on physical, functional, and emotional categories. Each category includes 10 statements, which are rated on a five-point equal appearing interval scale. The VHI total score or total value (VHI-T) ranges from 0 to 120 points. The VHI is a popular clinical tool to quantify the impact of a voice disorder on daily voice-related activities and to assess changes after voice treatment from the patient's perspective. The VHI has been examined in numerous validation studies in various languages and is one of the most widely used measurement methods in voice diagnostics (Herbst et al. 2015; Barsties v. Latoszek et al. 2020b). Voice treatment is considered effective if the VHI score after treatment is at least 13 points lower than the score before treatment. The required improvement of 13 points is based on the average test-retest value for the VHI from various treatment studies, with the range of the underlying individual studies between 8 and 18 points (Hakkesteegt et al. 2006b; Van Gogh et al. 2007; Niebudek-Bogusz et al. 2011; Herbst et al. 2015). Further studies on the VHI examined, for example, the validity of the VHI by reducing statements to a total of 9, 10, or 18 (Rosen et al. 2004; Nawka et al. 2009; Feige et al. 2020), the targeted application in various voice pathologies (Moerman et al. 2004; Wingate et al. 2005; Evans et al. 2009; Schindler et al. 2009; Sanuki et al. 2014; Karlsen et al. 2015; Kovatch et al. 2019; Crawley et al. 2018; Tafiadis et al. 2020), the connection to objective measurements (Schindler et al. 2009; Pommée et al. 2020; Zhao et al. 2020; Valentino et al. 2021) and its applicability as a screening tool for voice disorders (Niebudek-Bogusz et al. 2011). Furthermore, additional variants based on the VHI have been developed, for example, to examine the singing voice (see here examples of German validation studies by Lorenz et al. 2013; Barsties et al. 2015) or to make an adaptation for the pediatric patient group (Zur et al. 2007).

Due to its sensitivity to changes after voice treatment, the VHI has established itself as a useful tool for evaluating the voice (Rosen et al. 2000; Hengen et al. 2017; Moore et al. 2017; Joshi et al. 2017).

▶ For classifying the gradation of the severity of the perceptible impairment of voice problems for VHI patients in the German-speaking area, it was shown that the VHI-T is classified as normal between 0 to 14, mild between 15 to 28, moderate between 29 to 50, and severe between 51 to 120 (Nawka et al. 2003).

In addition to querying a self-report of the individual impacts of voice problems, other aspects are also important, such as the symptoms of vocal fatigue or laryngeal discomfort.

Vocal fatigue is a natural reaction to increased vocal demands in vocally-healthy individuals; however, vocal fatigue is also associated with (primary or secondary) functional dysphonia and must therefore be differentiated from pathological vocal fatigue (Stappenbeck et al. 2022). Vocal fatigue is a multifactorial conglomerate that includes subjectively perceived vocal complaints as well as possible physiological deficits and can manifest symptomatically through increased subjectively perceived vocal effort in patients or through neuromuscular deficits (Hunter et al. 2020). Since the current state of research on capturing the symptom of vocal fatigue is still heterogeneous, vocal fatigue is primarily diagnosed based on patient assessments (Stappenbeck et al. 2022), e.g., with the Vocal Fatigue Index (VFI) questionnaire.

Regarding laryngeal discomfort, it is important to specify these from pain in general. Pain is classified by the *International Association for the Study of Pain* as an unpleasant sensory and emotional experience associated with actual or potential tissue damage (Mathieson et al. 2009). The quantification of frequency and severity of various laryngeal discomfort showed reliable results through the subjective assessment of patients (Lukaschyk et al. 2017 , 2021).

At present, the symptoms of vocal fatigue or laryngeal discomfort can only be validly assessed through questionnaires.

For this purpose, two additional standardized and validated questionnaires are presented, which can validly capture these two symptoms.

First, the Vocal Fatigue Index (VFI) contains 19 items, which in their original form are distributed across three areas (i.e., #1 = fatigue and avoidance of voice use, #2 = physical discomfort when using the voice, #3 = improvement of symptoms or their absence with voice rest) to quantify the extent of vocal fatigue (Nanjundeswaran et al. 2015; Barsties v. Latoszek et al. 2021c). The VFI is rated on a five-point scale (0 = never, 1 = almost never, 2 = sometimes, 3 = almost always, 4 = always). The statements of the VFI are negatively formulated for areas #1 and #2. The higher the score on the scale of these two areas, the greater the vocal fatigue. Area #3 of the VFI is positively formulated, i.e., a lower score corresponds to greater vocal fatigue. The VFI has no overall score, and the calculation of the VFI is based on intermediate scores for the three areas. However, recent developments in the VFI recommend only two areas. Areas #1 and #2 of the original VFI version are to be combined, as there is no conceptual difference between #1 and #2, and the order of the questions is to be statistically reorganized (Nanjundeswaran et al. 2019). Nanjundeswaran et al. (2019) applied a statistical method of Mokken scaling, in which the structures of #1 and #2 were restructured into a single cluster 1 (Part 1), and cluster 2 (Part 2) remained unchanged and corresponded to #3. Both parts of the VFI are good predictors for diagnosing vocal fatigue (Nanjundeswaran et al. 2019; Barsties v. Latoszek et al. 2023e). This adaptation of the VFI has also been validated for example in the German language (Barsties v. Latoszek et al. 2023e) and is considered the final version of the VFI (see Sect. 3.1).

▶ Vocal fatigue is considered proven in the VFI if $\geq$ 18 points in cluster 1 and $\leq$ 8 points in cluster 2 are determined in the patient self-evaluation (Barsties v. Latoszek et al. 2023e).

Secondly, the Vocal Tract Discomfort Scale captures the frequency and severity of certain laryngeal discomfort in the vocal tract (see Sect. 3.1.). The laryngeal discomfort to be assessed is: burning, tightness, dryness, pain, tickling, soreness, irritation, and lump sensation (Mathieson et al. 2009; Lukaschyk et al. 2017). They are rated on a six-point equal appearing interval scale (frequency from never to always and severity from none to extreme).

▶ The classification of the validated VTD in German is derived from the sum of the values for frequency and severity as follows: no laryngeal discomfort between 0 to 13 points; mild between 14 to 26 points; moderate between 27 to 40 points; severe between 41 to 96 (Lukaschyk et al. 2021).

References

Aichinger P, Feichter F, Aichstill B, Bigenzahn W, Schneider-Stickler B (2012) Inter-device reliability of DSI measurement. Logoped Phoniatr Vocol 37(4):167–173. https://doi.org/10.3109/14015439.2012.687761

Altenberg EP, Ferrand CT (2006) Fundamental frequency in monolingual English, bilingual English/Russian, and bilingual English/Cantonese young adult women. J Voice 20(1):89–96. https://doi.org/10.1016/j.jvoice.2005.01.005

Awan SN, Roy N, Dromey C (2009) Estimating dysphonia severity in continuous speech: application of a multi-parameter spectral/cepstral model. Clin Linguist Phon 23(11):825–841. https://doi.org/10.3109/02699200903242988

Awan SN, Ensslen AJ (2010) A comparison of trained and untrained vocalists on the Dysphonia Severity Index. J Voice 24(6):661–666. https://doi.org/10.1016/j.jvoice.2009.04.001

Awan SN, Miesemer SA, Nicolia TA (2012) An examination of intrasubject variability on the Dysphonia Severity Index. J Voice 26(6):814.e21–5. https://doi.org/10.1016/j.jvoice.2012.04.004

Awan SN, Novaleski CK, Yingling JR (2013) Test-retest reliability for aerodynamic measures of voice. J Voice 27(6):674–684. https://doi.org/10.1016/j.jvoice.2013.07.002

Bargar I. (2024). [Die Reliabilität und Validität eines Palpationstools zur statischen laryngealen Untersuchung]. Unpublished Bachelorthesis, SRH University of Applied Sciences Heidelberg, Düsseldorf

Baken RJ, Orlikoff RF (2000) Clinical measurement of speech and voice, 2. Aufl. Singular Thomson Learning, San Diego, CA, USA

Barsties B (2013) [Effects of different tasks on determination of the speaking fundamental frequency]. HNO 61(7):609–616. https://doi.org/10.1007/s00106-012-2665-0

Barsties B, Verfaillie R, Roy N, Maryn Y (2013) Do body mass index and fat volume influence vocal quality, phonatory range, and aerodynamics in females? Codas. 25(4):310–318. https://doi.org/10.1590/s2317-17822013000400003

Barsties B, De Bodt M (2015) Assessment of voice quality: Current state-of-the-art. Auris Nasus Larynx 42(3):183–188. https://doi.org/10.1016/j.anl.2014.11.001

Barsties B, Maryn Y (2015) The improvement of internal consistency of the Acoustic Voice Quality Index. Am J Otolaryngol 36(5):647–656. https://doi.org/10.1016/j.amjoto.2015.04.012

Barsties B, Kropp J, Dicks P, Grzondziel V, Morsomme D (2015) [Reliability and validity of the "Voice Handicap Index (VHI) adapted to the singing voice"]. Laryngorhinootologie 94(7):441–446. https://doi.org/10.1055/s-0034-1387765

Barsties B, Verfaillie R, Dicks P, Maryn Y (2016) Is the speaking fundamental frequency in females related to body height? Logoped Phoniatr Vocol 41(1):27–32. https://doi.org/10.3109/14015439.2014.941928

Barsties B, Maryn Y (2016) External Validation of the Acoustic Voice Quality Index Version 03.01 With Extended Representativity. Ann Otol Rhinol Laryngol 125(7):571–83. https://doi.org/10.1177/0003489416636131

Barsties B, Thede T (2016) Evaluation of laryngeal palpation methods. IN: M. De Bodt, & Y. Maryn. Spanning in en rond de larynx: stand van zaken 3:32–47

Barsties v. Latoszek B, Maryn Y, Gerrits E, De Bodt M (2017) The Acoustic Breathiness Index (ABI): a multivariate acoustic model for breathiness. J Voice 31(4):511.e11–511.e27. https://doi.org/10.1016/j.jvoice.2016.11.017

Barsties v. Latoszek B, Lehnert B (2018) [Internal validation of the Acoustic Voice Quality Index version 03.01 and Acoustic Breathiness Index]. Laryngorhinootologie 97(9):630–635. https://doi.org/10.1055/a-0596-7819

Barsties v. Latoszek B, Maryn Y, Gerrits E, De Bodt M (2018) A meta-analysis: acoustic measurement of roughness and breathiness. J Speech Lang Hear Res 61(2):298–323. https://doi.org/10.1044/2017_JSLHR-S-16-0188

Barsties v. Latoszek B, Ulozaitė-Stanienė N, Maryn Y, Petrauskas T, Uloza V (2019a) The influence of gender and age on the Acoustic Voice Quality Index and Dysphonia Severity Index: a normative study. J Voice 33(3):340–345. https://doi.org/10.1016/j.jvoice.2017.11.011

Barsties v. Latoszek B, Ulozaitė-Stanienė N, Petrauskas T, Uloza V, Maryn Y (2019b) Diagnostic accuracy of dysphonia classification of DSI and AVQI. Laryngoscope 129(3):692–698. https://doi.org/10.1002/lary.27350

Barsties v. Latoszek B, Lehnert B, Janotte B (2020a) Validation of the Acoustic Voice Quality Index Version 03.01 and Acoustic Breathiness Index in German. J Voice 34(1):157.e17–157.e25. https://doi.org/10.1016/j.jvoice.2018.07.026

Barsties v. Latoszek B, Watts CR, Neumann K. (2020b) The effectiveness of voice therapy on voice-related handicap: A network meta-analysis. Clin Otolaryngol 45(5):796–804. https://doi.org/10.1111/coa.13596

Barsties v. Latoszek B, Mathmann P, Neumann K (2021a) The cepstral spectral index of dysphonia, the acoustic voice quality index and the acoustic breathiness index as novel multiparametric indices for acoustic assessment of voice quality. Curr Opin Otolaryngol Head Neck Surg 29(6):451–457. https://doi.org/10.1097/MOO.0000000000000743

Barsties v. Latoszek B, Kim GH, Delgado Hernández J, Hosokawa K, Englert M, Neumann K, Hetjens S (2021b) The validity of the Acoustic Breathiness Index in the evaluation of breathy voice quality: a meta-analysis. Clin Otolaryngol 46(1):31–40. https://doi.org/10.1111/coa.13629

Barsties v. Latoszek B, Auner M, Graf S (2021c) Cross-cultural adaption and validation of the Vocal Fatigue Index in German. J Voice 35(1):161.e1–161.e13. https://doi.org/10.1016/j.jvoice.2019.08.003

Barsties v. Latoszek B, Jansen V, Watts CR, Hetjens S (2023a) The impact of protective face coverings on acoustic markers in voice: a systematic review and meta-analysis. J Clin Med 12(18):5922. https://doi.org/10.3390/jcm12185922

Barsties v. Latoszek B, Mayer J, Watts CR, Lehnert B (2023b) Advances in clinical voice quality analysis with VOXplot. J Clin Med 12(14):4644. https://doi.org/10.3390/jcm12144644

Barsties v. Latoszek B, Englert M, Lucero JC, Behlau M (2023c) The performance of the Acoustic Voice Quality Index and Acoustic Breathiness Index in synthesized voices. J Voice 37(5):804.e21–804.e28. https://doi.org/10.1016/j.jvoice.2021.05.005

Barsties v. Latoszek B, Watts CR, Schwan K, Hetjens S (2023d) The maximum phonation time as marker for voice treatment efficacy: a network meta-analysis. Clin Otolaryngol 48(2):130–138. https://doi.org/10.1111/coa.14019

Barsties v. Latoszek B, Göllner M, Mathmann P, Neumann K (2023e) The German restructured Vocal Fatigue Index and characteristics of dysphonic and vocally healthy populations. J Voice 37(3):469.e11–469.e18. https://doi.org/10.1016/j.jvoice.2021.01.024

Batthyany C, Barsties v. Latoszek B, Maryn Y. (2024) Meta-analysis on the validity of the Acoustic Voice Quality Index. J Voice 38(6):1527.e1-1527.e19. https://doi.org/10.1016/j.jvoice.2022.04.022

Bele IV (2005) Reliability in perceptual analysis of voice quality. J Voice 19(4):555–573. https://doi.org/10.1016/j.jvoice.2004.08.008

Berg M, Fuchs M, Wirkner K, Loeffler M, Engel C, Berger T (2017) The speaking voice in the general population: normative data and associations to sociodemographic and lifestyle factors. J Voice 31(2):257.e13–257.e24. https://doi.org/10.1016/j.jvoice.2016.06.001

Berger T, Peschel T, Vogel M, Pietzner D, Poulain T, Jurkutat A, Meuret S, Engel C, Kiess W, Fuchs M (2019) Speaking voice in children and adolescents: normative data and associations with BMI, tanner stage, and singing activity. J Voice 33(4):580.e21–580.e30. https://doi.org/10.1016/j.jvoice.2018.01.006

Berger T, Fuchs M, Dippold S, Meuret S, Zebralla V, Yahiaoui-Doktor M, Wirkner K, Loeffler M, Engel C (2022) Standardization and feasibility of voice range profile measurements in epidemiological studies. J Voice 36(1):142.e9–142.e20. https://doi.org/10.1016/j.jvoice.2020.04.014

Bless DM (1991) Assessment of laryngeal function. In: Ford CN, Bless DM (Ed) Phonosurgery: assessment and surgical management of voice disorders. Raven Press Ltd, NY, USA, S 95–122

Boles RW, Gao WZ, Johns MM, Daniero JJ, Grant NN, Rubin AD, Bhatt NK, Hapner ER, O'Dell K (2023) Flexible versus rigid laryngoscopy: a prospective, blinded comparison of image quality. J Voice 37(3):440–443. https://doi.org/10.1016/j.jvoice.2021.02.010

Boominathan P, Samuel J, Arunachalam R, Nagarajan R, Mahalingam S (2014) Multi parametric voice assessment: Sri Ramachandra University protocol. Indian J Otolaryngol Head Neck Surg. 66(Suppl 1):246–251. https://doi.org/10.1007/s12070-011-0460-y

Boren B, Roginska A, Gill BP (2013) Maximum Averaged and Peak Levels of Vocal Sound Pressure. [Conference Paper] presented at the 135th Convention of the Audio Engineering Society; 2013 October 17–20 New York, USA

Bottalico P, Codino J, Cantor-Cutiva LC, Marks K, Nudelman CJ, Skeffington J, Shrivastav R, Jackson-Menaldi MC, Hunter EJ, Rubin AD (2020) Reproducibility of voice parameters: the effect of room acoustics and microphones. J Voice 34(3):320–334. https://doi.org/10.1016/j.jvoice.2018.10.016

Brockmann M, Storck C, Carding PN, Drinnan MJ (2008) Voice loudness and gender effects on jitter and shimmer in healthy adults. J Speech Lang Hear Res 51(5):1152–1160. https://doi.org/10.1044/1092-4388(2008/06-0208)

Brockmann M, Drinnan MJ, Storck C, Carding PN (2011) Reliable jitter and shimmer measurements in voice clinics: the relevance of vowel, gender, vocal intensity, and fundamental frequency effects in a typical clinical task. J Voice 25(1):44–53. https://doi.org/10.1016/j.jvoice.2009.07.002

Buder EH (2000) Acoustic analysis of voice quality: a tabulation of algorithms 1902–1990. In: Kent RD, Ball MJ (Ed) Voice quality measurement. Singular Publishing Group, San Diego, CA, S 119–244

Byeon H, Cha S (2020) Evaluating the effects of smoking on the voice and subjective voice problems using a meta-analysis approach. Sci Rep 10(1):4720. https://doi.org/10.1038/s41598-020-61565-3

Carding P, Carlson E, Epstein R, Mathieson L, Shewell C (2000) Formal perceptual evaluation of voice quality in the United Kingdom. Logoped Phoniatr Vocol 25(3):133–138. https://doi.org/10.1080/14015430050175860

Carson CP, Ingrisano DR, Eggleston KD (2003) The effect of noise on computer-aided measures of voice: a comparison of CSpeechSP and the Multi-Dimensional Voice Program software using the CSL 4300B module and multi-speech for Windows. J Voice 17(1):12–20. https://doi.org/10.1016/s0892-1997(03)00031-6

Castillo-Allendes A, Codino J, Cantor-Cutiva LC, Nudelman CJ, Rubin AD, Barsties v. Latoszek B, Hunter EJ (2023) Clinical utilityand validation of the Acoustic Voice Quality and Acoustic Breathiness Indexes for voice disorder assessment in Englishspeakers. J Clin Med 12(24):7679. https://doi.org/10.3390/jcm12247679

Coleman RF (1993) Sources of variation in phonetograms. J Voice 7(1):1–14. https://doi.org/10.1016/s0892-1997(05)80107-9

Corey RM, Jones U, Singer AC (2021) Comparison of the acoustic effects of face masks on speech. Hear J 74(1):36–39. https://doi.org/10.1097/01.HJ.0000725092.55506.7e

Crawley BK, Dehom S, Thiel C, Yang J, Cragoe A, Mousselli I, Krishna P, Murry T (2018) Assessment of clinical and social characteristics that distinguish presbylaryngis from pathologic presbyphonia in elderly individuals. JAMA Otolaryngol Head Neck Surg 144(7):566–571. https://doi.org/10.1001/jamaoto.2018.0409

Cunha LJ, Pereira EC, Ribeiro VV, Dassie-Leite AP (2019) Influence of the body position and emission number in the results of the maximum phonation times of adults without vocal complaints. J Voice 33(6):831–837. https://doi.org/10.1016/j.jvoice.2018.05.010

Davaris N, Voigt-Zimmermann S, Roessner A, Arens C (2017) [Narrow band imaging for evaluation of laryngeal mucosal lesions]. HNO 65(6):527–542. https://doi.org/10.1007/s00106-017-0336-x

De Bodt MS, Van de Heyning PH, Wuyts FL, Lambrechts L (1996) The perceptual evaluation of voice disorders. Acta Otorhinolaryngol Belg 50(4):283–291

Debruyne F, Buekers R (1998) Interdependency between intensity and pitch in the normal speaking voice. Acta Otorhinolaryngol Belg 52(3):201–205

Dejonckere PH, Bradley P, Clemente P, Cornut G, Crevier-Buchman L, Friedrich G, Van De Heyning P, Remacle M, Woisard V (2001) Committee on Phoniatrics of the European Laryngological Society (ELS). A basic protocol for functional assessment of voice pathology, especially for investigating the efficacy of (phonosurgical) treatments and evaluating new assessment techniques. Guideline elaborated by the Committee on Phoniatrics of the European Laryngological Society (ELS). Eur Arch Otorhinolaryngol 258(2):77–82. https://doi.org/10.1007/s004050000299

Dejonckere PH, Crevier-Buchman L, Marie JP, Moerman M, Remacle M, Woisard V (2003) European Research Group on the Larynx. Implementation of the European Laryngological Society (ELS) basic protocol for assessing voice treatment effect. Rev Laryngol Otol Rhinol (Bord) 124(5):279–283

Deliyski DD, Evans MK, Shaw HS (2005a) Influence of data acquisition environment on accuracy of acoustic voice quality measurements. J Voice 19(2):176–186. https://doi.org/10.1016/j.jvoice.2004.07.012

Deliyski DD, Shaw HS, Evans MK (2005b) Influence of sampling rate on accuracy and reliability of acoustic voice analysis. Logoped Phoniatr Vocol 30(2):55–62. https://doi.org/10.1080/1401543051006721

Deliyski DD, Shaw HS, Evans MK (2005c) Adverse effects of environmental noise on acoustic voice quality measurements. J Voice 19(1):15–28. https://doi.org/10.1016/j.jvoice.2004.07.003

Deliyski DD, Shaw HS, Evans MK, Vesselinov R (2006) Regression tree approach to studying factors influencing acoustic voice analysis. Folia Phoniatr Logop 58(4):274–288. https://doi.org/10.1159/000093184

DGHNO-KHC. (2023). [Aufbereitung von starren und flexiblen Optiken in der HNO-Praxis – Gemeinsame Stellungnahme der AG HNO-Infektiologie und Hygiene und der AG Endoskopie der DGHNO-KHC und des BVHNO]. https://cdn.hno.org/media/Anlagen_News/SN_DGHNO-KHC_BVHNO_Aufbereitung_Optiken_6-23.pdf. Accessed: 1. November 2023

Englert M, Lima L, Constantini AC, Barsties v. Latoszek B, Maryn Y, Behlau M (2019) Acoustic Voice Quality Index – AVQI for brazilian portuguese speakers: analysis of different speech material. Codas 31(1):e20180082. https://doi.org/10.1590/2317-1782/20182018082

Englert M, Lima L, Behlau M (2020) Acoustic Voice Quality Index and Acoustic Breathiness Index: analysis with different speech material in the Brazilian Portuguese. J Voice 34(5):810.e11–810.e17. https://doi.org/10.1016/j.jvoice.2019.03.015

Englert M, Lima L, Barsties v. Latoszek B, Behlau M (2022a) Influence of the voice sample length in perceptual and Acoustic Voice Quality Analysis. J Voice 36(4):582.e23–582.e32. https://doi.org/10.1016/j.jvoice.2020.07.010

Englert M, Barsties v. Latoszek B, Behlau M (2022b) The impact of languages and cultural backgrounds on voice quality analyses. *Folia Phoniatr Logop.* ; 74(2):141–152. https://doi.org/10.1159/000518206

Evans E, Carding P, Drinnan M (2009) The voice handicap index with post-laryngectomy male voices. Int J Lang Commun Disord 44(5):575–586. https://doi.org/10.1080/13682820902928729

Everest FA, Pohlmann K (2009) Master Handbook of Acoustics. US: McGraw-Hill/TAB Electronics

Feige K, Strauss A, Strauss G (2020) Voice Handicap Index-18 as an instrument for assessing subjective voice impairment between voice pre- and post-treatment. J Voice 34(5):810.e1–810.e10. https://doi.org/10.1016/j.jvoice.2019.04.005
Fleischer S (2020) [Tipps und Tricks für die Laryngoskopie]. HNO Nachrichten. 50(2):30–37
Franic DM, Bramlett RE, Bothe AC (2005) Psychometric evaluation of disease specific quality of life instruments in voice disorders. J Voice 19(2):300–315. https://doi.org/10.1016/j.jvoice.2004.03.003
Friedrich G, Dejonckere PH (2005) [The voice evaluation protocol of the European Laryngological Society (ELS) -- first results of a multicenter study]. Laryngorhinootologie 84(10):744–752. https://doi.org/10.1055/s-2005-861450
Gierlich J, Barsties v. Latoszek B (in press) Test-retest reliability of the Acoustic Voice Quality Index and the Acoustic Breathiness Index. J Voice https://doi.org/10.1016/j.jvoice.2023.07.013
Goy H, Fernandes DN, Pichora-Fuller MK, van Lieshout P (2013) Normative voice data for younger and older adults. J Voice 27(5):545–555. https://doi.org/10.1016/j.jvoice.2013.03.002
Hakkesteegt MM, Brocaar MP, Wieringa MH, Feenstra L (2006a) Influence of age and gender on the dysphonia severity index. A study of normative values. Folia Phoniatr Logop 58(4):264–73. https://doi.org/10.1159/000093183
Hakkesteegt MM, Wieringa MH, Gerritsma EJ, Feenstra L (2006b) Reproducibility of the Dutch version of the Voice Handicap Index. Folia Phoniatr Logop 58(2):132–138. https://doi.org/10.1159/000089613
Hakkesteegt MM, Brocaar MP, Wieringa MH, Feenstra L (2008a) The relationship between perceptual evaluation and objective multiparametric evaluation of dysphonia severity. J Voice 22(2):138–145. https://doi.org/10.1016/j.jvoice.2006.09.010
Hakkesteegt MM, Wieringa MH, Brocaar MP, Mulder PG, Feenstra L (2008b) The interobserver and test-retest variability of the dysphonia severity index. Folia Phoniatr Logop 60(2):86–90. https://doi.org/10.1159/000114650
Hakkesteegt MM, Brocaar MP, Wieringa MH (2010) The applicability of the dysphonia severity index and the voice handicap index in evaluating effects of voice therapy and phonosurgery. J Voice 24(2):199–205. https://doi.org/10.1016/j.jvoice.2008.06.007
Hanschmann H, Gärtner S, Berger R (2015) Comparability of computer-supported concurrent voice analysis. Folia Phoniatr Logop 67(1):8–14. https://doi.org/10.1159/000381094
Hengen J, Peterson M, McAllister A (2017) Patient characteristics and intervention effect as measured by Voice Handicap Index. Logoped Phoniatr Vocol 42(2):93–98. https://doi.org/10.1080/14015439.2016.1219387
Herbst CT, Oh J, Vydrová J, Švec JG (2015) DigitalVHI–a freeware open-source software application to capture the Voice Handicap Index and other questionnaire data in various languages. Logoped Phoniatr Vocol 40(2):72–76. https://doi.org/10.3109/14015439.2013.830769
Herbst CT (2020) Electroglottography – an update. J Voice 34(4):503–526. https://doi.org/10.1016/j.jvoice.2018.12.014
Hertegård S, Gauffin J (1991) Insufficient vocal fold closure as studied by inverse filtering. In: Gauffin J, Hammarberg B (Ed) Vocal fold physiology: acoustic, perceptual, and physiological aspects of voice mechanisms. Whurr Publishers, London, S 243–250
Heylen LG, Wuyts FL, Mertens FW, Pattyn JE (1996) Phonetography in voice diagnoses. Acta Otorhinolaryngol Belg 50(4):299–308
Heylen L, Wuyts FL, Mertens F, De Bodt M, Van de Heyning PH (2002) Normative voice range profiles of male and female professional voice users. J Voice 16(1):1–7. https://doi.org/10.1016/s0892-1997(02)00065-6
Hirano M (1981) Psycho-acoustic evaluation of voice. In G.E. Arnold, F. Winckel, B D. Wyke (Ed) Disorders of human communication 5. Clinical examination of voice. Vienna, Austria: Springer-Verlag; S 81–84
Hopkins HH (1959) Optical system having cylindrical rod-like lenses, U. States, Editor. Watson W and Sons Ltd: GB

Hosokawa K, Barsties v. Latoszek B, Ferrer-Riesgo CA, Iwahashi T, Iwahashi M, Iwaki S, Kato C, Yoshida M, Umatani M, Miyauchi A, Matsushiro N, Inohara H, Ogawa M, Maryn Y (2019) Acoustic Breathiness Index for the Japanese-Speaking Population: validation study and exploration of affecting factors. J Speech Lang Hear Res 62(8):2617–2631. https://doi.org/10.1044/2019_JSLHR-S-19-0077

Hosokawa K, Iwahashi T, Iwahashi M, Iwaki S, Yoshida M, Kitayama I, Miyauchi A, Ogawa M, Inohara H (2024) The minimal important difference of Acoustic Voice Quality Index in the treatment of voice disorders. 134(6):2805–2811. https://doi.org/10.1002/lary.31230 Laryngoscope

Hunter EJ, Cantor-Cutiva LC, van Leer E, van Mersbergen M, Nanjundeswaran CD, Bottalico P, Sandage MJ, Whitling S (2020) Toward a consensus description of vocal effort, vocal load, vocal loading, and vocal fatigue. J Speech Lang Hear Res 63(2):509–532. https://doi.org/10.1044/2019_JSLHR-19-00057

Hussein Gaber AG, Liang FY, Yang JS, Wang YJ, Zheng YQ (2014) Correlation among the dysphonia severity index (DSI), the RBH voice perceptual evaluation, and minimum glottal area in female patients with vocal fold nodules. J Voice 28(1):20–23. https://doi.org/10.1016/j.jvoice.2013.08.002

Ikeda Y, Masuda T, Manako H, Yamashita H, Yamamoto T, Komiyama S (1999) Quantitative evaluation of the voice range profile in patients with voice disorder. Eur Arch Otorhinolaryngol 256(Suppl 1):S51–S55. https://doi.org/10.1007/pl00014154

Ippers M (2024) [Die Reliabilität und Validität eines Palpationstools zur dynamischen laryngealen Untersuchung]. Unpublished Bachelorthesis, SRH University of Applied Sciences Heidelberg, Düsseldorf

Jacobson BH, Johnson A, Grywalski C, Silbergleit A, Jacobson G (1997) The Voice Handicap Index (VHI): development and validation. Am J Speech Lang Pathol 6(3):66–70

Jayakumar T, Savithri SR (2012) Effect of geographical and ethnic variation on Dysphonia Severity Index: a study of Indian population. J Voice 26(1):e11–e16. https://doi.org/10.1016/j.jvoice.2010.05.008

Jayakumar T, Benoy JJ, Yasin HM (2022) Effect of age and gender on Acoustic Voice Quality Index across lifespan: a cross-sectional study in Indian Population. J Voice 36(3):436.e1–436.e8. https://doi.org/10.1016/j.jvoice.2020.05.025

Jayakumar T, Benoy JJ (2024) Acoustic Voice Quality Index (AVQI) in the measurement of voice quality: a systematic review and meta-analysis. J Voice 38(5):1055-1069. https://doi.org/10.1016/j.jvoice.2022.03.018

Johnson AM, Goldfine A (2016) Intrasubject reliability of maximum phonation time. J Voice 30(6):775.e1–775.e4. https://doi.org/10.1016/j.jvoice.2015.11.019

Joshi A, Dave VJ, Bradoo R, Sapkale D (2017) Evaluation of validity of Voice Handicap Index among Indian Population. Int J Phonosurg Laryngol. 7(2):59–62

Karlsen T, Heimdal JH, Grieg AR, Aarstad HJ (2015) The Norwegian Voice Handicap Index (VHI-N) patient scores are dependent on voice-related disease group. Eur Arch Otorhinolaryngol 272(10):2897–2905. https://doi.org/10.1007/s00405-015-3659-9

Kempster GB, Gerratt BR, Verdolini Abbott K, Barkmeier-Kraemer J, Hillman RE (2009) Consensus auditory-perceptual evaluation of voice: development of a standardized clinical protocol. Am J Speech Lang Pathol 18(2):124–132. https://doi.org/10.1044/1058-0360(2008/08-0017)

Ketelslagers K, De Bodt MS, Wuyts FL, Van de Heyning P (2007) Relevance of subglottic pressure in normal and dysphonic subjects. Eur Arch Otorhinolaryngol 264(5):519–523. https://doi.org/10.1007/s00405-006-0212-x

Klinge K, Müller A (2013) Ultrasound as a useful diagnostic tool in the follow-up of laryngeal carcinoma. Int J Otorhinolaryngol Clin. 5(3):154–156

Khoddami SM, Ansari NN, Jalaie S (2015) Review on laryngeal palpation methods in muscle tension dysphonia: validity and reliability sssues. J Voice 29(4):459–468. https://doi.org/10.1016/j.jvoice.2014.09.023

Kovatch KJ, Reyes-Gastelum D, Hughes DT, Hamilton AS, Ward KC, Haymart MR (2019) Assessment of voice outcomes following surgery for thyroid cancer. JAMA Otolaryngol Head Neck Surg 145(9):823–829. https://doi.org/10.1001/jamaoto.2019.1737

Kreiman J, Gerratt BR, Kempster GB, Erman A, Berke GS (1993) Perceptual evaluation of voice quality: review, tutorial, and a framework for future research. J Speech Hear Res 36(1):21–40. https://doi.org/10.1044/jshr.3601.21

Kreiman J, Gerratt BR (2011) Perceptual assessment of voice quality: past, present, and future. In: Ma EPM, Yiu EML (Ed) Handbook of voice assessments. Singular Publishing Group, San Diego, S 291–304

Lebbe E, Verstraete J, Deklerck J, Maryn Y (2013) [De invloed van intensiteit op akoestische stemkwaliteitsmetingen]. Stem- Spraak- en Taalpathologie 18:1–8

Lechien JR, Geneid A, Bohlender JE, Cantarella G, Avellaneda JC, Desuter G, Sjogren EV, Finck C, Hans S, Hess M, Oguz H, Remacle MJ, Schneider-Stickler B, Tedla M, Schindler A, Vilaseca I, Zabrodsky M, Dikkers FG, Crevier-Buchman L (2023) Consensus for voice quality assessment in clinical practice: guidelines of the European Laryngological Society and Union of the European Phoniatricians. Eur Arch Otorhinolaryngol 280(12):5459–5473. https://doi.org/10.1007/s00405-023-08211-6

Lee L, Stemple JC, Kizer M (1999) Consistency of acoustic and aerodynamic measures of voice production over 28 days under various testing conditions. J Voice 13(4):477–483. https://doi.org/10.1016/s0892-1997(99)80003-4

Lee MT, Thorpe J, Verhoeven J (2009) Intonation and phonation in young adults with Down syndrome. J Voice 23(1):82–87. https://doi.org/10.1016/j.jvoice.2007.04.006

Lieberman J (1998) Principles and techniques of manual therapy: application in the management of dysphonia. In: Harris TM, Harris S, Rubin JS, Howard DM (Ed) The Voice Clinical Handbook. Whurr Publishers, London, S 91–138

Lin RJ, Wang T (2020) Comparison of fundamental frequency in postmenopausal women who are treated with hormone replacement therapy vs those who are not: a systematic review and meta-analysis. JAMA Otolaryngol Head Neck Surg 146(11):1045–1053. https://doi.org/10.1001/jamaoto.2020.2174

Lopes LW, da Silva KE, da Silva ED, Almeida AA, Silva POC, Lucero J, Behlau M (2017) Performance of phonatory deviation diagrams in synthesized voice analysis. Folia Phoniatr Logop 69(5–6):246–260. https://doi.org/10.1159/000487941

Lorenz A, Kleber B, Büttner M, Fuchs M, Mürbe D, Richter B, Sandel M, Nawka T (2013) [Validation of the German version of the Singing Voice Handicap Index]. HNO 61(8):699–706. https://doi.org/10.1007/s00106-013-2721-4

Lübbers W, Lübbers C (2016) [Namensgeber historischer Instrumente der Hals-Nasen-Ohrenheilkunde]. Endo Press GmbH, Tuttlingen

Lübke CS, Binkofski F, Barsties v. Latoszek B (in press) Speech Range Profile data in German-Speaking adults with Vox Phonetography. J Voice. https://doi.org/10.1016/j.jvoice.2025.02.002

Lukaschyk J, Brockmann-Bauser M, Beushausen U (2017) Transcultural adaptation and validation of the German Version of the Vocal Tract Discomfort Scale. J Voice 31(2):261.e1–261.e8. https://doi.org/10.1016/j.jvoice.2016.05.006

Lukaschyk J, Abel J, Brockmann-Bauser M, Keilmann A, Braun A, Rohlfs AK (2021) Cross-validation and normative values for the German Vocal Tract Discomfort Scale. J Speech Lang Hear Res 64(6):1855–1868. https://doi.org/10.1044/2021_JSLHR-20-00462

Ma EP, Yiu EM, Abbott KV (2007) Application of the ICF in voice disorders. Semin Speech Lang 28(4):343–350. https://doi.org/10.1055/s-2007-986531

Ma Z, Bullen C, Chu JTW, Wang R, Wang Y, Singh S (2023) Towards the objective speech assessment of smoking status based on voice features: a review of the literature. J Voice 37(2):300.e11–300.e20. https://doi.org/10.1016/j.jvoice.2020.12.014

Maruthy S, Ravibabu P (2015) Comparison of dysphonia severity index between younger and older carnatic classical singers and nonsingers. J Voice 29(1):65–70. https://doi.org/10.1016/j.jvoice.2014.05.001
Maryn Y, Roy N, De Bodt M, Van Cauwenberge P, Corthals P (2009a) Acoustic measurement of overall voice quality: a meta-analysis. J Acoust Soc Am 126(5):2619–2634. https://doi.org/10.1121/1.3224706
Maryn Y, Corthals P, De Bodt M, Van Cauwenberge P, Deliyski D (2009b) Perturbation measures of voice: a comparative study between Multi-Dimensional Voice Program and Praat. Folia Phoniatr Logop 61(4):217–226. https://doi.org/10.1159/000227999
Maryn Y (2010) Acoustic measurement of overall voice quality in sustained vowels and continuous speech. Unveröffentlichte Doktorarbeit, University of Ghent, Ghent, Belgium
Maryn Y, Corthals P, Van Cauwenberge P, Roy N, De Bodt M (2010) Toward improved ecological validity in the acoustic measurement of overall voice quality: combining continuous speech and sustained vowels. J Voice 24(5):540–555. https://doi.org/10.1016/j.jvoice.2008.12.014
Maryn Y, Roy N (2012) Sustained vowels and continuous speech in the auditory-perceptual evaluation of dysphonia severity. J Soc Bras Fonoaudiol. 24(2):107–112. https://doi.org/10.1590/s2179-64912012000200003
Maryn Y, Zarowski A (2015) Calibration of clinical audio recording and analysis systems for sound intensity measurement. Am J Speech Lang Pathol 24(4):608–618. https://doi.org/10.1044/2015_AJSLP-14-0082
Maryn Y, Morsomme D, De Bodt M (2017) Measuring the Dysphonia Severity Index (DSI) in the program Praat. J Voice 31(5):644.e29–644.e40. https://doi.org/10.1016/j.jvoice.2017.01.002
Maslan J, Leng X, Rees C, Blalock D, Butler SG (2011) Maximum phonation time in healthy older adults. J Voice 25(6):709–713. https://doi.org/10.1016/j.jvoice.2010.10.002
Mathieson L, Hirani SP, Epstein R, Baken RJ, Wood G, Rubin JS (2009) Laryngeal manual therapy: a preliminary study to examine its treatment effects in the management of muscle tension dysphonia. J Voice 23(3):353–366. https://doi.org/10.1016/j.jvoice.2007
Mayer J (2023) VOXplot: Manual. https://voxplot.lingphon.com/en/support/. Accessed: 1. October 2023
Meister J, Hagen R, Shehata-Dieler W, Kühn H, Kraus F, Kleinsasser N (2017) Pitch Elevation in male-to-female transgender persons-the Würzburg approach. J Voice 31(2):244.e7–244.e15. https://doi.org/10.1016/j.jvoice.2016.07.018
Moerman M, Martens JP, Dejonckere P (2004) Application of the Voice Handicap Index in 45 patients with substitution voicing after total laryngectomy. Eur Arch Otorhinolaryngol 261(8):423–428. https://doi.org/10.1007/s00405-003-0683-y
Moore J, Greenberg C, Thibeault SL (2017) Predictors of six-month change in the Voice Handicap Index in a treatment-seeking population. J Voice 31(1):41–47. https://doi.org/10.1016/j.jvoice.2016.02.004
Morris RJ, Brown WS Jr, Hicks DM, Howell E (1995) Phonational profiles of male trained singers and nonsingers. J Voice 9(2):142–148. https://doi.org/10.1016/s0892-1997(05)80247-4
Murton O, Hillman R, Mehta D (2020) Cepstral peak prominence values for clinical voice evaluation. Am J Speech Lang Pathol 29(3):1596–1607. https://doi.org/10.1044/2020_AJSLP-20-00001
Nanjundeswaran C, Jacobson BH, Gartner-Schmidt J, Verdolini AK (2015) Vocal Fatigue Index (VFI): development and validation. J Voice 29(4):433–440. https://doi.org/10.1016/j.jvoice.2014.09.012
Nanjundeswaran C, van Mersbergen M, Morgan K (2019) Restructuring the Vocal Fatigue Index using Mokken Scaling: insights into the complex nature of vocal fatigue. J Voice 33(1):110–114. https://doi.org/10.1016/j.jvoice.2017.09.008
Nawka T, Wiesmann U, Gonnermann U (2003) [Validation of the German version of the Voice Handicap Index]. HNO 51(11):921–930. https://doi.org/10.1007/s00106-003-0909-8

Nawka T, Verdonck-de Leeuw IM, De Bodt M, Guimaraes I, Holmberg EB, Rosen CA, Schindler A, Woisard V, Whurr R, Konerding U (2009) Item reduction of the voice handicap index based on the original version and on European translations. Folia Phoniatr Logop 61(1):37–48. https://doi.org/10.1159/000200767

Nemr K, Simões-Zenari M, de Souza GS, Hachiya A, Tsuji DH (2016) Correlation of the Dysphonia Severity Index (DSI), consensus auditory-perceptual evaluation of voice (CAPE-V), and gender in Brazilians with and without voice disorders. J Voice 30(6):765.e7–765.e11. https://doi.org/10.1016/j.jvoice.2015.10.013

Nevo L, Nevo C, Oliveira G (2015) A comparison of vocal parameters in adult bilingual Hebrew-English speakers. Codas. 27(5):483–491. https://doi.org/10.1590/2317-1782/20152015096

Nicastri M, Chiarella G, Gallo LV, Catalano M, Cassandro E (2004) Multidimensional Voice Program (MDVP) and amplitude variation parameters in euphonic adult subjects. Normative study. *Acta Otorhinolaryngol Ital.* 24(6):337–341

Niebudek-Bogusz E, Kuzańska A, Woznicka E, Sliwinska-Kowalska M (2011) Assessment of the voice handicap index as a screening tool in dysphonic patients. Folia Phoniatr Logop 63(5):269–272. https://doi.org/10.1159/000324214

Nijkamp M, Maryn Y (2018) Comparing the accuracy of two phonetography systems. In: The Fall Voice Conference. Motif, Seattle, Washington

Nijkamp M (2019) Vox Phonetography v.1.2: Modern Praat based phonetography for the clinical voice pathologist. [Software Manual]. https://voxphonetography.com/. Accessed: 9. January 2023

Núñez Batalla F, González Márquez R, Peláez González MB, González Laborda I, Fernández Fernández M, Morato GM (2014) Acoustic voice analysis using the Praat program: comparative study with the Dr. Speech program. *Acta Otorrinolaringol Esp.* 65(3):170–176. https://doi.org/10.1016/j.otorri.2013.12.004

Nusseck M, Immerz A, Spahn C, Echternach M, Richter B (2021) Long-term effects of a voice training program for teachers on vocal and mental health. J Voice 35(3):438–446. https://doi.org/10.1016/j.jvoice.2019.11.016

Ongkasuwan J, Ocampo E, Tran B (2017a) Laryngeal ultrasound and vocal fold movement in the pediatric cardiovascular intensive care unit. Laryngoscope 127(1):167–172. https://doi.org/10.1002/lary.26051

Ongkasuwan J, Devore D, Hollas S, Jones J, Tran B (2017b) Laryngeal ultrasound and pediatric vocal fold nodules. Laryngoscope 127(3):676–678. https://doi.org/10.1002/lary.26209

Oren L, Rollins M, Gutmark E, Howell R (2023) How face masks affect acoustic and auditory perceptual characteristics of the singing voice. J Voice 37(4):515–521. https://doi.org/10.1016/j.jvoice.2021.02.028

Pabon JPH (1991) Objective voice-quality parameters in the computer phonetogram. J Voice 5(3):203–216. https://doi.org/10.1016/S0892-1997(05)80188-2

Pabon P, Ternström S, Lamarche A (2011) Fourier descriptor analysis and unification of voice range profile contours: method and applications. J Speech Lang Hear Res 54(3):755–776. https://doi.org/10.1044/1092-4388(2010/08-0222)

Pabon P, Ternström S (2020) Feature maps of the acoustic spectrum of the voice. J Voice 34(1):161.e1–161.e26. https://doi.org/10.1016/j.jvoice.2018.08.014

Patel RR, Awan SN, Barkmeier-Kraemer J, Courey M, Deliyski D, Eadie T, Paul D, Švec JG, Hillman R (2018) Recommended protocols for instrumental assessment of voice: American Speech-Language-Hearing Association expert panel to develop a protocol for instrumental assessment of vocal function. Am J Speech Lang Pathol 27(3):887–905. https://doi.org/10.1044/2018_AJSLP-17-0009

Pommée T, Maryn Y, Finck C, Morsomme D (2020) The Acoustic Voice Quality Index, version 03.01, in French and the Voice Handicap Index. J Voice 34(4):646.e1–646.e10. https://doi.org/10.1016/j.jvoice.2018.11.017

Printz T, Sorensen JR, Godballe C, Grøntved ÅM (2018) Test-retest reliability of the dual-microphone voice range profile. J Voice 32(1):32–37. https://doi.org/10.1016/j.jvoice.2017.03.019

Ricci-Maccarini A, Bergamini G, Fustos R (2018) Proposal of a form for the collection of videolaryngostroboscopy basic findings. Eur Arch Otorhinolaryngol 275(7):1927–1933. https://doi.org/10.1007/s00405-018-4991-7

Rodríguez-Parra MJ, Adrián JA, Casado JC (2009) Voice therapy used to test a basic protocol for multidimensional assessment of dysphonia. J Voice 23(3):304–318. https://doi.org/10.1016/j.jvoice.2007.05.001

Rosen CA, Murry T, Zinn A, Zullo T, Sonbolian M (2000) Voice handicap index change following treatment of voice disorders. J Voice 14(4):619–623. https://doi.org/10.1016/s0892-1997(00)80017-x

Rosen CA, Lee AS, Osborne J, Zullo T, Murry T (2004) Development and validation of the voice handicap index-10. Laryngoscope 114(9):1549–1556. https://doi.org/10.1097/00005537-200409000-00009

Rothenberg M (1980) Acoustic interaction between the glottal source and the vocal tract. In: Hirano KN, Stevens M (Ed) Vocal fold physiology. University of Tokyo Press, S 305–328

Roy N, Barkmeier-Kraemer J, Eadie T, Sivasankar MP, Mehta D, Paul D, Hillman R (2013) Evidence-based clinical voice assessment: a systematic review. Am J Speech Lang Pathol 22(2):212–226. https://doi.org/10.1044/1058-0360(2012/12-0014)

Saeedi S, Aghajanzade M, Khatoonabadi AR (2022) A literature review of voice indices available for voice assessment. JRSR. 9(4):151–155. https://doi.org/10.30476/jrsr.2022.93362.1235

Saindani S, Gandhi S, Bhatta S, Bhola G (2023) A prospective observational study to determine the added clinical value of videokymography to videostroboscopy in patients with change in voice. Indian J Otolaryngol Head Neck Surg. 75(2):934–946. https://doi.org/10.1007/s12070-022-03164-4

Sagiroglu S, Doganer A (2018) The effect of electrolyte balance on the voice in hemodialysis patients. Eur Arch Otorhinolaryngol 275(11):2755–2761. https://doi.org/10.1007/s00405-018-5098-x

Sampaio M, Vaz Masson ML, de Paula Soares MF, Bohlender JE, Brockmann-Bauser M (2020) Effects of fundamental frequency, vocal intensity, sample duration, and vowel context in cepstral and spectral measures of dysphonic voices. J Speech Lang Hear Res 22;63(5):1326–1339. https://doi.org/10.1044/2020_JSLHR-19-00049

Sanuki T, Yumoto E, Kodama N, Minoda R, Kumai Y (2014) Long-term Voice Handicap Index after type II thyroplasty using titanium bridges for adductor spasmodic dysphonia. Auris Nasus Larynx 41(3):285–289. https://doi.org/10.1016/j.anl.2013.11.001

Sanchez K, Oates J, Dacakis G, Holmberg EB (2014) Speech and voice range profiles of adults with untrained normal voices: methodological implications. Logoped Phoniatr Vocol 39(2):62–71. https://doi.org/10.3109/14015439.2013.777109

Sataloff RT, Hawkshaw MJ, Anticaglia J (2005) Medications and the voice. In: Sataloff RT (Ed) Professional Voice: The Science and Art of Clinical Care. Plural Publishing, San Diego

Scharff-Rethfeldt W, Miller N, Mennen I (2008) [Speaking Fundamental Frequency differences in highly proficient bilinguals of German/English]. Sprache-Stimme-Gehör. 32(3):123–128. https://doi.org/10.1055/s-0028-1083799

Schindler A, Mozzanica F, Vedrody M, Maruzzi P, Ottaviani F (2009) Correlation between the Voice Handicap Index and voice measurements in four groups of patients with dysphonia. Otolaryngol Head Neck Surg 141(6):762–769. https://doi.org/10.1016/j.otohns.2009.08.021

Schmidt P, Klingholz F, Martin F (1988) Influence of pitch, voice sound pressure, and vowel quality on the maximum phonation time. J Voice 2(3):245–249. https://doi.org/10.1016/S0892-1997(88)80082-1

Schutte HK (1986) [Belastbaarheid van de stem en het fonetogram]. Logopedie en Foniatrie. 58:140–144

Shrivastav R (2011) Evaluating voice quality. In: Ma EPM, Yiu EML (Ed) Handbook of voice assessments. Singular Publishing Group, San Diego, S 305–318

Siegburg JC (2024) [Erforschung zum Durchführungsablauf zur maximalen Tonhaltedauer: Prospektive Querschnittstudie zum Vergleich von diagnostischen Werten zur maximalen

Tonhaltedauer in Abhängigkeit vom Atemtypus]. Unpublished Bachelorthesis, SRH University of Applied Sciences Heidelberg, Bonn

Siupsinskiene N (2003) Quantitative analysis of professionally trained versus untrained voices. Medicina (Kaunas) 39(1):36–46

Sobol M, Sielska-Badurek EM (2022) The Dysphonia Severity Index (DSI)-normative values. Systematic review and meta-analysis. *J Voice*. 36(1):143.e9–143.e13. https://doi.org/10.1016/j.jvoice.2020.04.010

Södersten M, Lindestad PA, Hammarberg B (1991) Vocal fold closure, perceived breathiness, and acoustic characteristics in normal adult speakers. In: Gauffin J, Hammarberg B (Ed) Vocal fold physiology: acoustic, perceptual, and physiological aspects of voice mechanisms. Whurr Publishers, London, S 217–224

Solomon NP, Garlitz SJ, Milbrath RL (2000) Respiratory and laryngeal contributions to maximum phonation duration. J Voice 14(3):331–340. https://doi.org/10.1016/s0892-1997(00)80079-x

Solomon NP (2008) Vocal fatigue and its relation to vocal hyperfunction. Int J Speech Lang Pathol 10(4):254–266. https://doi.org/10.1080/14417040701730990

Sönnichsen R, Llorach Tó G, Hochmuth S, Hohmann V, Radeloff A (2022) How face masks interfere with speech understanding of normal-hearing individuals: vision makes the difference. Otol Neurotol 43(3):282–288. https://doi.org/10.1097/MAO.0000000000003458

Spazzapan EA, Fabron EMG, Berti LC, Chagas EFB, Marino VCC (2022) Acoustic characteristics of the voice for Brazilian Portuguese speakers across the life span. J Voice 36(6):876.e17–876.e26. https://doi.org/10.1016/j.jvoice.2020.09.019

Speyer R, Bogaardt HC, Passos VL, Roodenburg NP, Zumach A, Heijnen MA, Baijens LW, Fleskens SJ, Brunings JW (2010) Maximum phonation time: variability and reliability. J Voice 24(3):281–284. https://doi.org/10.1016/j.jvoice.2008.10.004

Šrámková H, Granqvist S, Herbst CT, Švec JG (2015) The softest sound levels of the human voice in normal subjects. J Acoust Soc Am 137(1):407–418. https://doi.org/10.1121/1.4904538

Stappenbeck L, Barsties v. Latoszek B, Janotte B, Lehnert B (2020) Acoustic Voice Quality Index and Acoustic Breathiness Index as two examples for strengths and weaknesses of free software in medicine. Biomed Signal Process Control 59(5):101938. https://doi.org/10.1016/j.bspc.2020.101938

Stappenbeck LE, Bartel S, Brockmann-Bauser M (2022) [Vocal fatigue as an indicator of complex voice disorders-a diagnostic and therapeutic challenge]. HNO 70(11):837–841. https://doi.org/10.1007/s00106-022-01186-6

Stathopoulos ET, Huber JE, Sussman JE (2011) Changes in acoustic characteristics of the voice across the life span: measures from individuals 4–93 years of age. J Speech Lang Hear Res 54(4):1011–1021. https://doi.org/10.1044/1092-4388(2010/10-0036)

Švec JG, Granqvist S (2010) Guidelines for selecting microphones for human voice production research. Am J Speech Lang Pathol 19(4):356–368. https://doi.org/10.1044/1058-0360(2010/09-0091)

Tafiadis D, Helidoni ME, Chronopoulos SK, Kosma EI, Alexandropoulou A, Ziavra N, Velegrakis GA (2020) The Hellenic Voice Handicap Index of different laryngeal mass lesions: a receiver-operating characteristic analysis. J Voice 34(6):966.e1–966.e10. https://doi.org/10.1016/j.jvoice.2019.06.016

Ternström S, Pabon P, Södersten M (2016) The voice range profile: its function, applications, pitfalls and potential. Acta Acust United Acust. 102(2):268–283

Timmermans B, De Bodt MS, Wuyts FL, Van de Heyning PH (2005) Analysis and evaluation of a voice-training program in future professional voice users. J Voice 19(2):202–210. https://doi.org/10.1016/j.jvoice.2004.04.009

Titze IR (1980) Comments on the myoelastic – aerodynamic theory of phonation. J Speech Hear Res 23(3):495–510. https://doi.org/10.1044/jshr.2303.495

Titze IR (1989) On the relation between subglottal pressure and fundamental frequency in phonation. J Acoust Soc Am 85(2):901–906. https://doi.org/10.1121/1.397562

Titze IR (1992a) Acoustic interpretation of the voice range profile (phonetogram). J Speech Hear Res 35(1):21–34. https://doi.org/10.1044/jshr.3501.21

Titze IR (1992b) Phonation threshold pressure: a missing link in glottal aerodynamics. J Acoust Soc Am 91(5):2926–2935. https://doi.org/10.1121/1.402928

Titze IR, Sundberg J (1992) Vocal intensity in speakers and singers. J Acoust Soc Am 91(5):2936–2946. https://doi.org/10.1121/1.402929

Titze IR, Winholtz WS (1993) Effect of microphone type and placement on voice perturbation measurements. J Speech Hear Res 36(6):1177–1190. https://doi.org/10.1044/jshr.3606.1177

Titze IR (1995) Workshop on acoustic voice analysis: summary statement. NCVS, Iowa City

Tsuji DH, Hachiya A, Dajer ME, Ishikawa CC, Takahashi MT, Montagnoli AN (2014) Improvement of vocal pathologies diagnosis using high-speed videolaryngoscopy. Int Arch Otorhinolaryngol. 18(3):294–302. https://doi.org/10.1055/s-0034-1372512

Uloza V, Barsties v. Latoszek B, Ulozaite-Staniene N, Petrauskas T, Maryn Y (2018) A comparison of Dysphonia Severity Index and Acoustic Voice Quality Index measures in differentiating normal and dysphonic voices. Eur Arch Otorhinolaryngol 275(4):949–958. https://doi.org/10.1007/s00405-018-4903-x

Ulozaite-Staniene N, Petrauskas T, Šaferis V, Uloza V (2019) Exploring the feasibility of the combination of acoustic voice quality index and glottal function index for voice pathology screening. Eur Arch Otorhinolaryngol 276(6):1737–1745. https://doi.org/10.1007/s00405-019-05433-5

Valentino WL, Park J, Alnouri G, Gracely EJ, Tami A, Vance D, Palmer J, Sataloff RT (2021) Diagnostic value of acoustic and aerodynamic measurements in vocal fold movement disorders and their correlation with laryngeal electromyography and Voice Handicap Index. J Voice 35(3):497.e1–497.e4. https://doi.org/10.1016/j.jvoice.2019.10.008

Van Lierde KM, D'haeseleer E, Baudonck N, Claeys S, De Bodt M, Behlau M (2011) The impact of vocal warm-up exercises on the objective vocal quality in female students training to be speech language pathologists. J Voice 25(3):e115–21. https://doi.org/10.1016/j.jvoice.2009.11.004

Van Gogh CD, Mahieu HF, Kuik DJ, Rinkel RN, Langendijk JA, Verdonck-de Leeuw IM (2007) Voice in early glottic cancer compared to benign voice pathology. Eur Arch Otorhinolaryngol 264(9):1033–1038. https://doi.org/10.1007/s00405-007-0313-1

Verdolini K, Rosen CA, Branski RC (2006) Classification manual for voice disorders-I. Special interest division 3, voice and voice disorders, American Speech-Language-Hearing Association. Lawrence Erlbaum Associates, Inc., Mahwah

Vogel AP, Maruff P (2008) Comparison of voice acquisition methodologies in speech research. Behav Res Methods 40(4):982–987. https://doi.org/10.3758/BRM.40.4.982

Vogel AP, Morgan AT (2009) Factors affecting the quality of sound recording for speech and voice analysis. Int J Speech Lang Pathol 11(6):431–437. https://doi.org/10.3109/17549500902822189

Vogel AP, Rosen KM, Morgan AT, Reilly S (2014) Comparability of modern recording devices for speech analysis: smartphone, landline, laptop, and hard disc recorder. Folia Phoniatr Logop 66(6):244–250. https://doi.org/10.1159/000368227

Wingate JM, Ruddy BH, Lundy DS, Lehman J, Casiano R, Collins SP, Woodson GE, Sapienza C (2005) Voice Handicap Index results for older patients with adductor spasmodic dysphonia. J Voice 19(1):124–131. https://doi.org/10.1016/j.jvoice.2004.03.006

WHO (2023) Coronavirus disease (COVID-19) pandemic. https://www.who.int/europe/emergencies/situations/covid-19. Accessed: 5. August 2023

Wuyts FL, De Bodt MS, Molenberghs G, Remacle M, Heylen L, Millet B, Van Lierde K, Raes J, Van de Heyning PH (2000) The Dysphonia Severity Index: an objective measure of vocal quality based on a multiparameter approach. J Speech Lang Hear Res 43(3):796–809. https://doi.org/10.1044/jslhr.4303.796

Wuyts FL, Heylen L, Mertens F, De Bodt M, Van de Heyning PH (2002) Normative voice range profiles of untrained boys and girls. J Voice 16(4):460–465. https://doi.org/10.1016/s0892-1997(02)00120-0

Yanushevskaya I, Gobl C, Ní CA (2013) Voice quality in affect cueing: does loudness matter? Front Psychol 4:335. https://doi.org/10.3389/fpsyg.2013.00335
Yiu EM, Yuen YM, Whitehill T, Winkworth A (2004) Reliability and applicability of aerodynamic measures in dysphonia assessment. Clin Linguist Phon 18(6–8):463–478. https://doi.org/10.1080/02699200410001703592
Young WG, Hoffman MR, Koszewski IJ, Whited CW, Ruel BN, Dailey SH (2016) Voice outcomes following a single office-based steroid injection for vocal fold scar. Otolaryngol Head Neck Surg 155(5):820–828. https://doi.org/10.1177/0194599816654899
Zhao EE, Nguyen SA, Salvador CD, O'Rourke AK (2020) A meta-analysis of the association between the Voice Handicap Index and objective voice analysis. J Speech Lang Hear Res 63(10):3461–3471. https://doi.org/10.1044/2020_JSLHR-20-00209
Zraick RI, Marshall W, Smith-Olinde L, Montague JC (2004) The effect of task on determination of habitual loudness. J Voice 18(2):176–182. https://doi.org/10.1016/j.jvoice.2003.09.005
Zraick RI, Wendel K, Smith-Olinde L (2005) The effect of speaking task on perceptual judgment of the severity of dysphonic voice. J Voice 19(4):574–581. https://doi.org/10.1016/j.jvoice.2004.08.009
Zraick RI, Kempster GB, Connor NP, Thibeault S, Klaben BK, Bursac Z, Thrush CR, Glaze LE (2011) Establishing validity of the Consensus Auditory-Perceptual Evaluation of Voice (CAPE-V). Am J Speech Lang Pathol 20(1):14–22. https://doi.org/10.1044/1058-0360(2010/09-0105)
Zur KB, Cotton S, Kelchner L, Baker S, Weinrich B, Lee L (2007) Pediatric Voice Handicap Index (pVHI): a new tool for evaluating pediatric dysphonia. Int J Pediatr Otorhinolaryngol 71(1):77–82. https://doi.org/10.1016/j.ijporl.2006.09.004

Documentation and Objective Setting

3

The documentation and the resulting objectives for treatment are based on voice diagnostics. Therefore, all necessary measurement parameters, which can be classified under the independent 5-pillar system, should be considered. As a minimum standard for the documentation and interpretation of the examination results, Table 3.1 is recommended (this table can also be found as online material for download). This voice examination protocol is a systematic protocol that contains only evidence-based, quantifiable, and valid measurement parameters with thresholds for physiological and pathological assessment according to the current state of research. Each included measurement parameter should also have the potential to specifically evaluate the success of a voice treatment for the individual voice patient (primary critical measurement parameter). The determination of these primary critical measurement parameters is determined according to certain criteria (see Sect. 4.2).

The measurement parameters in this voice examination protocol are imaging techniques of stroboscopy (amplitude, mucosal wave, symmetry & regularity of the phonatory pattern, glottal closure & supraglottic compensation during phonation), perception (GRB and palpation), acoustics (AVQI, ABI, GNE, CPPS, HNR, PPQ5, DSI, VRP and SRP), aerodynamics (MPT) and self-evaluation (VHI, VFI and VTD) (see Chap. 2).

In addition to listing and structuring the measurement parameters, Table 3.1. provides an overview of the standard values, a broad grouping into which category the respective measurement parameter can be counted (voice quality, voice function or both) and, if known, a grading of the severity from slight to severe. All details and sources of the measurement parameters from Table 3.1. can be found in

---

Supplementary Information The electronic version of this chapter contains supplementary material, which can be accessed via the following link https://doi.org/10.1007/978-3-662-68958-5_3. The videos can be played by clicking the DOI link in the legend of a corresponding figure, or by scanning this link with the SN More Media app.

B. Barsties v. Latoszek et al., *Diagnostic and Treatment in Voice Therapy*,
https://doi.org/10.1007/978-3-662-70162-1_3

Table 3.1 Proposal of a multidimensional examination protocol as a minimum standard (own representation)

Pillars of the multidimensional examination	Measurement parameters	Score interpretation/norm values	Result	Physiological (Phy) vs. Pathological (Pat)	Severity (normal, slight, moderate, severe)	Aspect of the voice: Voice Quality (VQ), Voice Function (VF) or Combination (VQ & VF)
Visual analysis	Amplitude	0: normal wide (approx. 1/3 of the visible vocal fold width) + 1: slightly extended ± 1: slightly shortened + 2: moderately extended ± 2: moderately shortened + 3: resounding ± 3: canceled (phonatory stop)			normal, slight, moderate, severe	VQ & VF
	Mucosal wave	0: normal (at least 1/2 of the visible vocal fold width) 1: slightly reduced 2: moderately reduced 3: canceled (phonatory stop)			normal, slight, moderate, severe	VQ & VF
	Symmetry of the phonatory pattern	0: normal (symmetrical oscillations according location and phase) 1: slightly asymmetrical vibration pattern 2: moderately asymmetrical vibration pattern 3: severly asymmetrical vibration pattern			normal, slight, moderate, severe	VQ & VF

(continued)

Table 3.1 (continued)

Pillars of the multidimensional examination	Measurement parameters	Score interpretation/norm values	Result	Physiological (Phy) vs. Pathological (Pat)	Severity (normal, slight, moderate, severe)	Aspect of the voice: Voice Quality (VQ), Voice Function (VF) or Combination (VQ & VF)
	Regularity of the phonatory pattern	0: regular vibration pattern 1: slightly irregular vibration pattern 2: moderately irregular vibration pattern 3: severly irregular vibration pattern			normal, slight, moderate, severe	VQ & VF
	Glottal closure (*Variants*: longitudinalgap, bowing, posterior gap, hourglass-shaped, anterior gap)	0: complete glottal closure 1: slightly incomplete glottal closure 2: moderately incomplete glottal closure 3: severely incomplete glottal closure			normal, slight, moderate, severe	SQ & SF
	Supraglottic compensation during phonation	0: no supraglottic contractions 1: slightly supraglottic contractions 2: moderately supraglottic contractions 3: supraglottic closure			normal, slight, moderate, severe	SQ & SF

(continued)

Table 3.1 (continued)

Pillars of the multidimensional examination	Measurement parameters	Score interpretation/norm values	Result	Physiological (Phy) vs. Pathological (Pat)	Severity (normal, slight, moderate, severe)	Aspect of the voice: Voice Quality (VQ), Voice Function (VF) or Combination (VQ & VF)
Perception	GRB – Grade/ Hoarseness	0 = normal 1 = slightly deviating 2 = moderately deviating 3 = severely deviating			normal, slight, moderate, severe	SQ
	GRB – Roughness	0 = normal 1 = slightly deviating 2 = moderately deviating 3 = severely deviating			normal, slight, moderate, severe	SQ
	GRB – Breathiness	0 = normal 1 = slightly deviating 2 = moderately deviating 3 = severely deviating			normal, slight, moderate, severe	SQ
	Palpation – Total score (static)	< 1.25			–	SQ & SF
	Palpation – Total score (dynamic)	< 1.75			–	SQ & SF
Acoustics	DSI	> 3.1 normal/no dysphonia 3.1 to -0.1 slight −0.1 to −3.3 moderate < −3.3 severe			normal, slight, moderate, severe	SQ & SF
	AVQI - ENG version	< 1.17			–	SQ
	ABI - ENG version	< 2.35			–	SQ

(continued)

Table 3.1 (continued)

Pillars of the multidimensional examination	Measurement parameters	Score interpretation/norm values	Result	Physiological (Phy) vs. Pathological (Pat)	Severity (normal, slight, moderate, severe)	Aspect of the voice: Voice Quality (VQ), Voice Function (VF) or Combination (VQ & VF)
	GNE	> 0.89			–	SQ
	CPPS	> 14.47 dB			–	SQ
	HNR	> 23.34 dB			–	SQ
	PPQ5	< 0.29 %			–	SQ
	SRP- F0	Young (18–44 years) ♀ = 193 Hz to 216 Hz ♂ = 97 Hz to 113 Hz Middle (45–60 years) ♀ = 173 Hz to 192 Hz ♂ = 91 Hz to 120 Hz Older (>60 years) ♀ = 154 Hz to 190 Hz ♂ = 113 Hz to 138 Hz			–	SF
	SRP- I	Young (18–44 years) ♀ = 71 dB to 73 dB ♂ = 71 dB to 74 dB Middle (45–60 years) ♀ = 72 dB to 76 dB ♂ = 70 dB to 76 dB Older (>60 years) ♀ = 72 dB to 77 dB ♂ = 74 dB to 77 dB			–	SF
	SRP- Slope	Young (18–44 years) > 18.61 dB/Oct Middle (45–60 years) > 16.94 dB/Oct Older (>60 years) > 15.33 dB/Oct			–	SF

(continued)

Table 3.1 (continued)

Pillars of the multidimensional examination	Measurement parameters	Score interpretation/norm values	Result	Physiological (Phy) vs. Pathological (Pat)	Severity (normal, slight, moderate, severe)	Aspect of the voice: Voice Quality (VQ), Voice Function (VF) or Combination (VQ & VF)
	SRP-Interdependence	Young (18–44 years) < 0.696 ST/dB Middle (45–60 years) < 0.721 ST/dB Older (>60 years) < 0.819 ST/dB			–	SF
	VRP- F0-high	♀ > 659 Hz ♂ > 294 Hz			–	SF
	VRP- F0-low	♀ < 165 Hz ♂ < 73 Hz			–	SF
	VRP- semitone range	♀ ♂ ≥ 24 ST			–	SF
	VRP- I-max	♀ ♂ > 90 dB			–	SF
	VRP- I-min	♀ ♂ < 55 dB			–	SF
	VRP- intensity range	♀ ♂ > 40 dB			–	SF
	VRP- boundaries	Large = normal Tendency to normal = slight Discongruity = moderate Medium-sized = moderate Small = severe			normal, slight, moderate, severe	SF
Aerodynamics	MPT	> 15 sec			–	SF

(continued)

Table 3.1 (continued)

Pillars of the multidimensional examination	Measurement parameters	Score interpretation/norm values	Result	Physiological (Phy) vs. Pathological (Pat)	Severity (normal, slight, moderate, severe)	Aspect of the voice: Voice Quality (VQ), Voice Function (VF) or Combination (VQ & VF)
Self-evaluation	VHI-T	0 to 14 normal 15 to 28 slight 29 to 50 moderate 51 to 120 severe			normal, slight, moderate, severe	SQ & SF
	VFI- cluster 1	0 to 18			–	SQ & SF
	VFI- cluster 2	8 to 12			–	SQ & SF
	VTD- T	0 to 13 normal 14 to 26 slight 27 to 40 moderate 41 to 96 severe			normal, slight, moderate, severe	SQ & SF
Sum			Number Phy: ______ % Number Pat-SQ: ____ % Number Pat-SF: ____ % Number Pat-SQ & SF: ____ %			Number normal: Number slight: Number moderate: Number severe: Average (Σ /13):

Chap. 2. The results obtained from the voice examination protocol serve as a basis for determining the severity of dysphonia (see Sect. 3.3).

In order to fill out Table 3.1. accordingly for voice patients, Sect. 3.1. presents a procedure for voice diagnostics to efficiently obtain all these measurement parameters in eight steps. The interpretation of the obtained voice diagnostic data for a resulting voice treatment is complex. However, from Sects. 3.2 to 4.2, a red thread is followed and a justification for the path to effective and efficient primary treatment (medical or therapeutic) is created, based on the principles of an ICF-oriented goal setting of functional primary goals, derivation of the severity of dysphonia, scientific clinical reasoning, weighting in the orientation of pathological measurement parameters (voice quality vs. voice function) and derivation of the correlations between the five pillars of voice diagnostics using a correlation matrix.

3.1 Procedure for Voice Diagnostics

The procedure for voice diagnostics of 34 measurement parameters is divided into eight steps (see Table 3.2):

For clinical implementation, videos for the book are also provided as streaming for demonstration purposes, which depict most steps of the examination with a simulation patient.

The following sequence is thus suggested for the clinical examination:

Table 3.2 Representation of the voice parameters to be obtained from Table 3.1 from the course of the voice examination in 8 steps (own representation)

Process of the voice examination in 8 steps	Obtaining the following parameters from the voice examination protocol of Table 3.1
1. Stroboscopy	Amplitude, mucosal wave, symmetry of the phonatory pattern, regularity of the phonatory pattern, glottal closure, and supraglottic compensation during phonation
2. Reading text	GRB, AVQI (Part 1), and ABI (Part 1)
3. Sustained phonation for acoustic voice quality analysis	DSI (Part 1), AVQI (Part 2), ABI (Part 2), GNE, CPPS, HNR, and PPQ5
4. Maximum phonation time	DSI (Part 2), MPT
5. Speech Range Profile (SRP)	SRP-F0, SRP-I, SRP-Slope, SRP-Interdependence
6. Voice Range Profile (VRP)	DSI (Part 3), VRP-F0-high, VRP-F0-low, VRP-semitone range, VRP-I-max, VRP-I-min, VRP-intensity range, VRP-boundaries
7. Palpation	Total value of the static and dynamic evaluation
8. Self-evaluation	Questionnaires: VHI (VHI-T), VFI (VFI-cluster 1 and 2), and VTD (VTD-T)

1. Stroboscopy
The stroboscopy is performed transorally and/or transnasally as described in Sect. 2.1.1.

Transoral stroboscopy generally allows a better assessment of the vocal fold surface than transnasal stroboscopy regarding mucosal wave and motility. However, it requires experience and sufficient practice. For the correct execution of laryngeal examination using stroboscopy of the vocal folds with a rigid endoscope, centering the endoscope is recommended. Alternatively, lateral execution is often helpful for patients with a strong gag reflex. The gag reflex can additionally be reduced by the patient applying acupressure to the chin (labiomental groove) or by using local anesthetic sprays, e.g., Xylocaine or Tetracaine (Vachiramon and Wang 2002; Chan et al. 2010). If the gag reflex is intensified by the anesthetic, it is recommended to wait with the examination until the anesthetic wears off.

Transnasal stroboscopy, on the other hand, is easier to handle and additionally offers a good assessment of the supra- and subglottal areas. It is thus recommended to go close to the glottis with the endoscope and examine regions such as the sinus morgagni, and the subglottic area. The combination of both methods is recommended to obtain a 3D representation of the movement, contact zones, and anatomical as well as physiological features of the vocal folds.

For both procedures, it applies that after successfully reaching the larynx and the vocal folds, the focus of the endoscope must be repeatedly adjusted, as it changes depending on the pitch during phonation. The phoniatric assessment should be standardized with /i:/ in habitual pitch, in low pitch, and in high pitch, as well as the examination of inspiratory phonation and the assessment of the extensibility of the lamina propria. A formation of retrograde mucosal wave is possible here and can additionally be documented.

2. Reading text: Have the text for example "The Rainbow Passage" read aloud (GRB/Part 1 of AVQI/ABI)
As a basis for the assessment of GRB (see Sect. 2.2.1 and Fig. 3.1) and Part 1 for the AVQI & ABI analyses (see Sect. 2.3.4 and Fig. 3.2), the reading aloud of a text is used. The AVQI and ABI analyses are based in English on the first 22 syllables of the text "*The Rainbow Passage*" (see Fig. 3.3). Currently, 11 languages are included in VOXplot to assess AVQI and ABI based on validated text lengths of specific texts available for reading during recording in VOXplot, as well as validated thresholds for both indices (Mayer 2023). These languages are German, Japanese, Korean, Dutch, Spanish, Brazilian-Portuguese, Malayalam, Kannada, Italian, Persian (Farsi), and Finnish next to English. The sound recording is carried out with a suitable acoustic measurement system, as described in Sect. 2.3.1 and 2.3.2. For the English version, the patients should read aloud the phonetically balanced text "The Rainbow Passage" in habitual pitch and loudness:

> "When the sunlight strikes raindrops in the air, they act as a prism and form a rainbow. The rainbow is a division of white light into many beautiful colors. These take the shape of a long round arch, with its path high above, and its two ends apparently beyond the

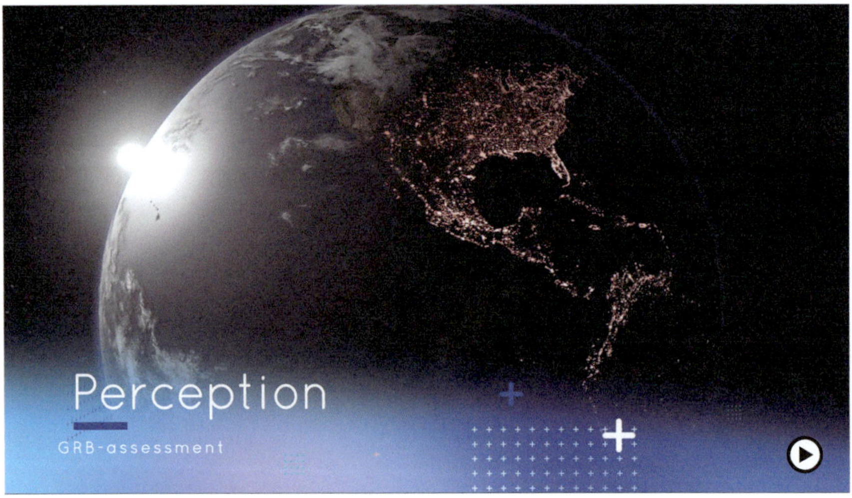

Fig. 3.1 Video for the assessment of GRB (▸ https://doi.org/10.1007/000-dwp)

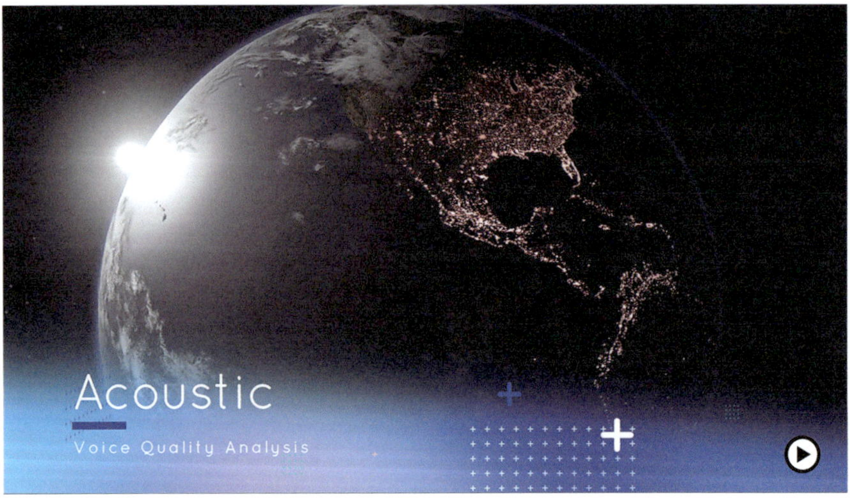

Fig. 3.2 Video for the assessment of the measurement of objective acoustic voice quality with the software VOXplot (▸ https://doi.org/10.1007/000-dwm)

horizon. There is , according to legend, a boiling pot of gold at one end. People look, but no one ever finds it. When a man looks for something beyond his reach, his friends say he is looking for the pot of gold at the end of the rainbow. Throughout the centuries people have explained the rainbow in various ways. Some have accepted it as a miracle without physical explanation. To the Hebrews it was a token that there would be no more universal floods. The Greeks used to imagine that it was a sign from the gods to foretell war or heavy rain. The Norsemen considered the rainbow as a bridge over which the gods

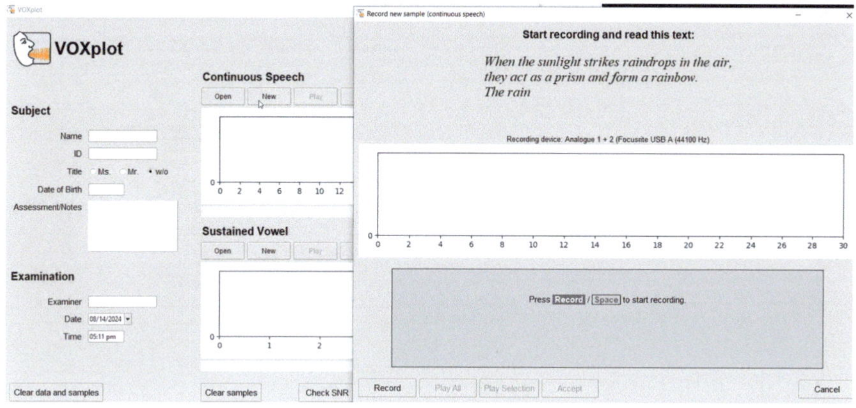

Fig. 3.3 Representation of the software VOXplot v.2.0 (Mayer 2023) with the main menu on the left and the recording window for text reading in English on the right

> passed from earth to their home in the sky. Others have tried to explain the phenomenon physically. Aristotle thought that the rainbow was caused by reflection of the sun's rays by the rain. Since then physicists have found that it is not reflection, but refraction by the raindrops which causes the rainbows. Many complicated ideas about the rainbow have been formed. The difference in the rainbow depends considerably upon the size of the drops, and the width of the colored band increases as the size of the drops increases. The actual primary rainbow observed is said to be the effect of super-imposition of a number of bows. If the red of the second bow falls upon the green of the first, the result is to give a bow with an abnormally wide yellow band, since red and green light when mixed form yellow. This is a very common type of bow, one showing mainly red and yellow, with little or no green or blue." (Fairbanks 1960).

3. Sustained Phonation for Acoustic Voice Quality Analysis

In the third section of the study, the sustained phonation on the vowel /a:/ is performed at habitual pitch and loudness. It is important to select 3 seconds from the recording (preferably without the attack and decay phases) (see Fig. 3.4). This recording is needed for the second part of the AVQI & ABI analyses (see Sect. 2.3.4), as well as the 4 individual parameters for voice quality (CPPS, GNE, HNR, and PPQ5), with PPQ5 also being used for the DSI (see Fig. 3.2).

4. Sustained Phonation regarding the Maximum Phonation Time

To examine the maximum phonation time, the habitual phonation of the vowel /a:/ after maximum inspiration should now be sustained for as long as possible (see Sect. 2.4). The max. phonation time can be measured with a stopwatch or with acoustic analysis programs that can display the duration, for example, in oscillograms and/or spectrograms. The maximum phonation time is also used for the DSI (see Sect. 2.3.4; Fig. 3.5).

5. Speech Range Profile (SRP)

This section of the examination includes the documentation of the speech range profile. The most important parameters in the SRP are the SRP-F0 and SRP-I of

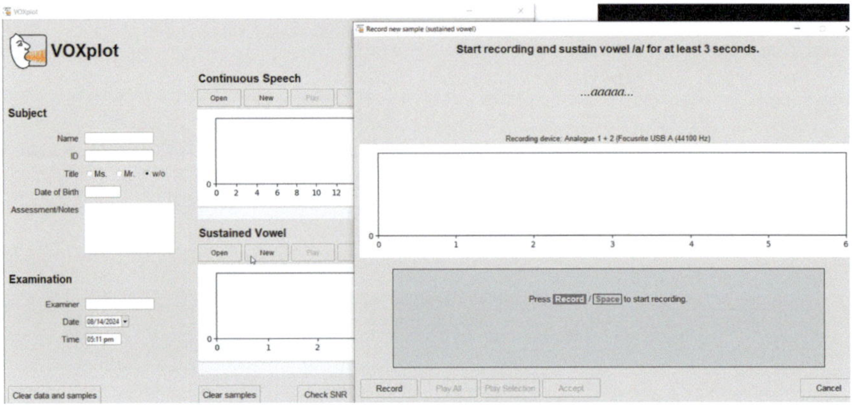

Fig. 3.4 Representation of the VOXplot v.2.0 software (Mayer 2023) with the main menu on the left and the recording window for the sustained phonation of the vowel /a:/ on the right

the habitual speaking voice, which are determined for example over the first 27 syllables of the German version of the text “The North Wind and the Sun” – as well as for the AVQI & ABI analyses in German (see Fig. 2.4; Fig. 3.6). The examination of the SRP can be extended depending on the software. As described in Sect. 2.3.5, these can be parameters that examine the relationship of three additional intensity levels (soft, loud, and calling voice) of the speaking voice, such as the parameters SRP-Slope and SRP-Interdependence.

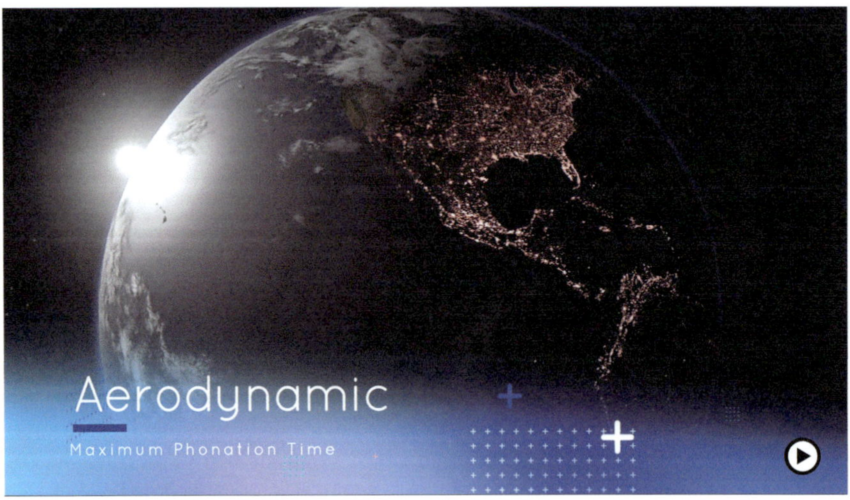

Fig. 3.5 Video on the measurement of objective acoustic voice quality using the VOXplot software (▶ https://doi.org/10.1007/000-dwn)

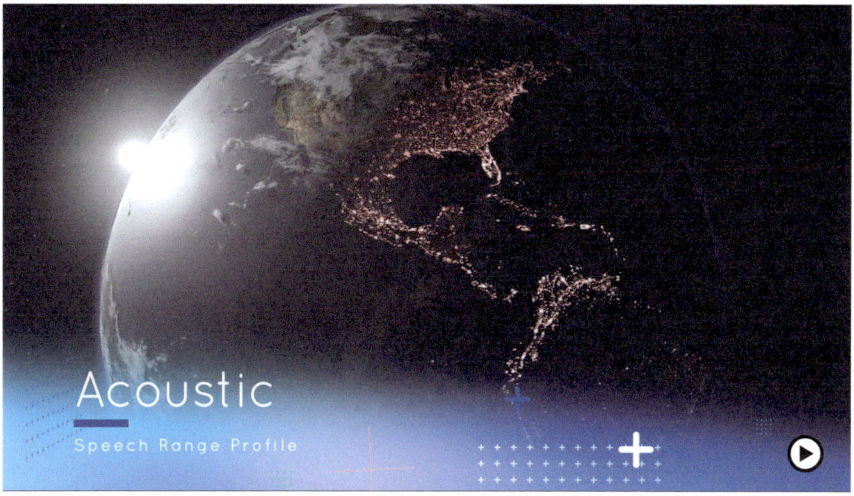

Fig. 3.6 Video on the measurement of an SRP (▸ https://doi.org/10.1007/000-dwk)

6. Voice Range Profile (VRP)
In this section of the examination, the VRP is addressed, and again the vowel /a:/ is used to check the individual parameters of as soft, as loud, as low, and as high as possible, as well as to graphically determine the VRP boundaries (see Sect. 2.3.5; Fig. 3.7). Finally, two parameters from the VRP (VRP-F0-high & VRP-I-min) are used to complete the DSI (see Sect. 2.3.4).

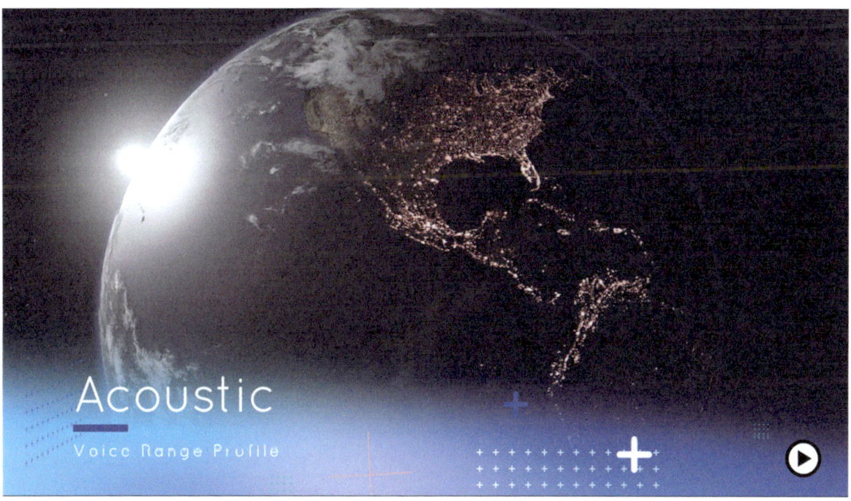

Fig. 3.7 Video on the measurement of a VRP (▸ https://doi.org/10.1007/000-dwq)

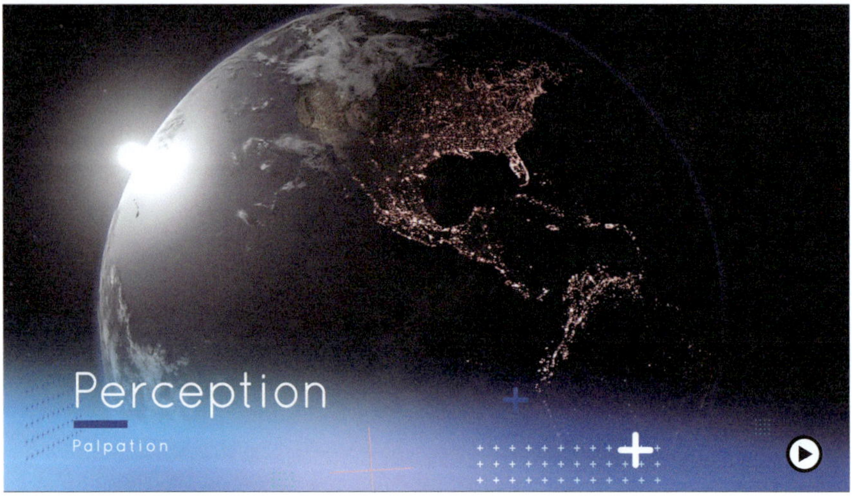

Fig. 3.8 Video on the measurement of palpation (▸ https://doi.org/10.1007/000-dwr)

7. Palpation

As the penultimate examination unit, palpation follows to determine the laryngeal muscle tone, which is examined at rest and during habitual phonation on the vowel /a:/ phonation (see Sect. 2.2.2; Fig. 3.8). In both cases, three areas are assessed for mobility/motility, the thyroid space, and the cricothyroid space, as well as whether pain occurred during the examination. Below is the palpation assessment sheet form by Barsties and Thede (2016) (see Table 3.3), which is used for clinical implementation.

(B) Laryngeal Palpation during Phonation (dynamic assessment)

Areas	Parameters	Value	Intermediate value from the areas	Total value of the dynamic assessment
Position of the larynx/hyoid bone	Remains in the same position	0	0–2	0–9
	Laryngeal elevation	1		
	Laryngeal lowering	1		
Thyrohyoid space	Space remains comparable to the static assessment	0	0–2	
	Space smaller than in the static assessment (unilateral)	1		
	Space smaller than in the static assessment (bilateral)	2		

Areas	Parameters	Value	Intermediate value from the areas	Total value of the dynamic assessment
Cricothyroid space	Space remains palpable	0	0–2	
	Space not palpable (structures are too close together)	1		
	Space smaller than at rest	2		
Pain (inquiry with the patient during the execution of the upper 3 areas)	No pain	0	0–3	
	Pain during palpation for positioning of the larynx/hyoid bone	1		
	Pain during palpation of the thyrohyoid space	1		
	Pain during palpation of the cricothyroid space	1		

Table 3.3 Palpation assessment sheet divided into (A) static assessment and (B) dynamic assessment
(A) Laryngeal palpation at rest (static assessment) (Barsties and Thede 2016)

Areas	Parameter	Value	Intermediate value from the areas	Total value of the static assessment
Laryngeal lateral mobility	No resistance	0	0–2	0–8
	Minimal resistance towards the end of the movement	1		
	High lateral resistance	2		
Thyrohyoid spacc	Space bilaterally equal	0	0–2	
	Space bilaterally unequal	1		
	Space not palpable (structures too close together)	2		
Cricothyroid space	Space palpable	0	0–1	
	Space not palpable (structures too close together)	1		
Pain (inquiry with patient during thc execution of the upper 3 areas)	No pain	0	0–3	
	Pain during laryngeal lateral mobility	1		
	Pain when palpating the thyrohyoid space	1		
	Pain when palpating the cricothyroid space	1		

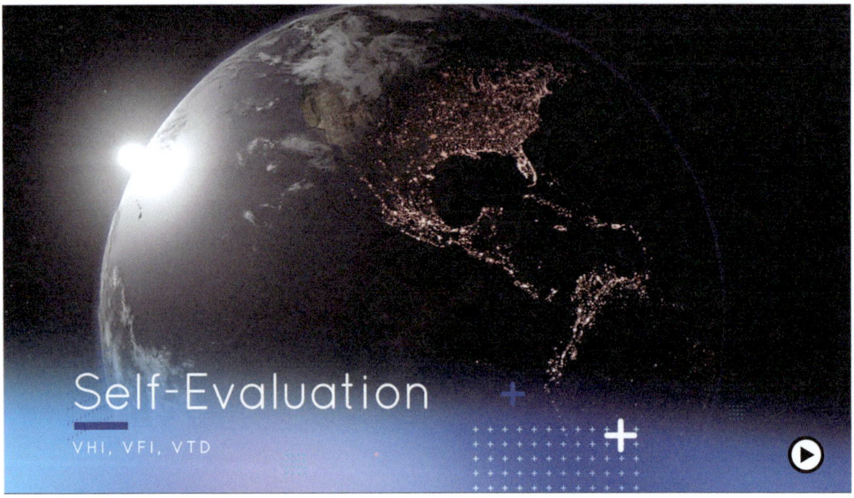

Fig. 3.9 Video on the measurement of questionnaires (▸ https://doi.org/10.1007/000-dws)

8. Self-assessment (VHI, VFI, and VTD)
Patients should complete three questionnaires and provide their current self-assessment for each item/question (see Fig. 3.9). All three questionnaires examine different aspects of voice perception. The VHI checks the perception of the voice disorder on quality of life, the VFI focuses on the symptom of vocal fatigue, and the VTD analyzes symptoms of laryngeal discomfort (see Sect. 2.5). These three questionnaires have been validated with norm values among other things in the German language and are included in full version in the publications by Nawka et al. (2003), Barsties v. Latoszek et al. (2023) and Lukaschyk et al. (2017).

3.2 ICF Model in Voice Disorders

The International Classification of Functioning, Disability and Health (ICF) assesses the human health condition in terms of its functionality and participation in social life as a resource-oriented biopsychosocial model. From the perspective of the ICF, the health condition and its impairments result from a dynamic interaction (see Fig. 3.10) between a patient's health problems (underlying diseases) and various personal and environmental factors,including the context in which problems are highlighted (WHO 2001). Thus, it is essential to determine the severity of a health disorder or disease, which incorporates a broader context of information for the health problem. In the ICF, these are the areas of functionality/disability (components such as body functions and structures, as well as activities and participation) and contextual factors (components such as environmental factors and

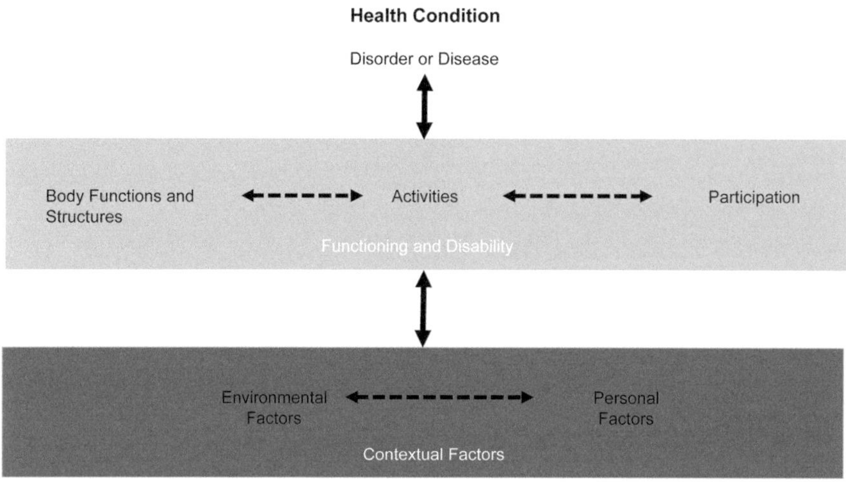

Fig. 3.10 The interaction of the various aspects of the health condition integrated into the ICF model (WHO 2001)

personal factors). Voice disorders in the individual components of the ICF model can be categorized in the area of health disorder (laryngeal pathologies and symptoms of dysphonia such as voice quality or voice function impairments), body functions (e.g., breathing, phonation, and resonance), body structures (anatomical properties of the larynx and vocal tract), activities (e.g., conversations, telephoning, singing, and acting), participation (e.g., familial, social, and professional relationships), environmental factors (reactions of family, friends, colleagues, and society to dysphonia as well as opportunities for the use of aids or support from medical-therapeutic assistance), and personal factors (e.g., coping with illness through various emotions, consideration of the environment through one's own communication style) (see Tab. 3.4).

Treatments specifically applied to one of the aspects to minimize or eliminate the health problem can have interactions with other areas. Thus, one or more disorders can lead to limitations in functionality, which in turn also restricts participation more strongly. On the other hand, body function problems can also have an impact on the health disorder.

In voice disorders, the ICF provides a framework for the investigation and treatment of this health impairment. Additionally, it enables the functionality of patients with voice disorders to be objectified, to use the various components of the ICF, and to create an individual and appropriate treatment program to improve the quality of life.

Tab. 3.4 Overview of ICF components with codes and descriptions (Ma et al. 2007)

ICF Components	Code	Description
Body Functions	B126	Temperament and Personality Functions
	B152	Emotional Functions
	B310	Voice Function
	B3100	Production of Voice
	B3101	Voice Quality
Body Structures	S110	Body Structures of the Brain
	S1106	Body Structures of the Cranial Nerves
	S340	Body Structures of the Larynx
	S3400	Body structures of the Vocal Folds
Activity and Participation	D330	Speaking
	D350	Conversing
	D360	Use of Communication Devices and Techniques
	D3600	Use of Telecommunication Devices
	D845	Acquiring, Keeping, and Terminating Employment
	D850	Remunerative Employment
	D920	Recreation and Leisure
	D9204	Hobbies
	D9205	Social Activities
Environmental Factors	E125	Products and Technology for Communication Purposes
	E225	Climate
	E2250	Temperature
	E2251	Humidity
	E250	Ambient Noise
	E2500	Intensity of Noise
	E2501	Quality of Noise
	E260	Air Quality
	E310–e399	Support and Relationships
	E410–e499	Attitudes
	E515	Architecture and Construction Services, Systems, and Policies
	E580	Health Services, Systems, and Policies

(continued)

Tab. 3.4 (continued)

ICF Components	Code	Description
Personal Factors	Pf1	Sociodemographic Factors/General Personal Data
	Pf2	Body Functions and Structures
	Pf3	Personal Factors related to the Illness
	Pf4	Mental Personal Factors
	Pf5	Events
	Pf6	Lifestyle
	Pf7	Work-related Personal Factors
	Pf8	Other Personal Factors

3.3 Derivation of the Severity of a Voice Disorder

Determining the dysphonia severity degree is complex, and a standardized approach is not uniformly established nationally or internationally. Various experts, associations, and organizations only conditionally make suggestions. One of the beginnings is based on the Dysphonia Index by the phoniatrist Prof. Friedrich (1998, cited in Schneider and Bigenzahn 2007, p. 148). For this, four different measurement methods from four different pillars of voice diagnostics were evaluated in a 4-point equal appearing interval system. The weighting of the individual measurement methods was simply weighted. Based on mean value calculations, the severity could be determined between normal and severe. For the index, perceptual hoarseness (G from GRB), the intensity and semitone voice range from the VRP, the max. phonation time, and the communicative impairment of the patients were considered. A corresponding evidence base for this index is not known. Another approach showed a result from the collaboration of the Brazilian-Belgian cooperation of voice experts, who presented the GALP assessment system to determine the severity of voice problems (Englert et al. 2020). For this, four measurement methods are brought into line with the ICF model and the protocol of the European Laryngological Society (ELS) with a special focus on voice quality in the assessment of severity. The G of the GRB scale, the AVQI, the endoscopic findings, and the VHI are used. In GALP, various scenarios are considered, which are to be associated with all four measurement methods to obtain seven different assessment criteria, from normal to severe, not further specified in case of inappropriate information, or not applicable if information on all four measurement methods is missing. Associations such as the European Laryngological Society, the American Speech-Language Hearing Association, or the Association of the Scientific Medical Societies in Germany (AWMF) do not publish suggestions for determining the dysphonia severity degree (Dejonckere et al. 2001; Patel et al. 2018; DGPP 2023, Lechien et al. 2023).

Since there is no uniform definition or basis for determining the dysphonia severity degree, this book adopts the basic idea of Friedrich (1998) to equally weight the assessment of the severity of a voice disorder through designated measurement parameters (classification from normal=0 to severe=3) and to determine the severity of dysphonia by calculating the mean value. In the protocol of Table 3.1, 13 measurement parameters for the dysphonia severity degree can be considered. These come from the visual analysis (amplitude, mucosal wave, symmetry & regularity of the phonatory pattern, glottal closure, and supraglottic compensation during phonation), perception (GRB), acoustics (DSI and VRP boundaries), and self-perception (VHI-T and VTD-T). The calculation for the dysphonia severity degree thus results from the average of the sum of the 13 measurement parameters, e.g., number normal (0) = 2, number mild (1) = 5, number moderate (2) = 5, number severe (3) = 1; thus (0 + 0 + 1 + 1 + 1 + 1 + 1 + 2 + 2 + 2 + 2 + 2 + 3)/13 = 1.39 → rounded = (1) slight severity of dysphonia. Determining the dysphonia severity degree reflects the averaged extent of the voice disorder and provides an initial indication for a later follow-up examination. It can then be determined whether the chosen voice treatment has brought about a significant improvement and whether the severity of dysphonia has been reduced.

3.4 Therapeutic Goal Setting Based on Evidence-Based Voice Diagnostics

Evidence-based voice diagnostics are the prerequisite for the therapeutic goal setting of a treatment. The requirement for voice diagnostics shows that the smallest common denominator between different voice protocols of the associations (such as the European Laryngological Society, the American Speech-Language Hearing Association, or the German Society for Phoniatrics & Pediatric Audiology for a guideline of the Association of the Scientific Medical Societies) is a multidimensional quantifiable voice diagnostic (Dejonckere et al. 2001; Patel et al. 2018; DGPP 2023, Lechien et al. 2023). This basic idea was adopted for the proposal of voice diagnostics in this book (see Chap. 2). Furthermore, the selection for a minimal standard of the measurement parameters presented here for clinically active physicians or voice therapists in practice or clinic is implementable from an economic, evidence-based, practical, and clinically tested perspective in everyday practice and can help to clearly evaluate treatment effects. The findings obtained in the diagnostics are aligned with the specific functional primary goals, thus using the ICF model as a guide to apply EBM-based treatment methods for voice disorders more precisely. For the determination of the goal setting, information about the disorder and the multidimensional quantifiable voice diagnostics (health disorder as well as body functions and structures) primarily flow in. Personal factors from the medical history (e.g., age, gender, lifestyle, habits, motivation) or environmental factors are not further explained in this book, as the focus is on EBM-supported quantifiable diagnostics using scientific reasoning (see Sect. 4.1). The resulting medical or voice therapeutic treatment approach is determined exclusively based on this form of diagnostics as the primary treatment focus (i.e., the start in the manner of treatment and choice of method in the field of medicine or voice therapy). This proposal for physicians and voice therapists is the basis of an EBM-supported treatment focus for voice disorders, as it addresses specific fundamental pillars in the ICF model and can positively influence the overall context of the health problem of voice patients. This presented approach to the functional impairment of the primary treatment focus is attributed great potential to enable effective and efficient results in the initial phase of voice treatment, based on the current state of research.

The following are possible functional primary goals for voice treatment in primary/secondary functional or organic voice disorders, based on voice diagnostics and their dysphonia severity degree in the examination protocol of Table 3.1:

1. Reduction of general voice disorder signs:
   - Critical parameters of stroboscopy, VHI, DSI
2. Improvement of voice quality in glottal closure insufficiency:
   - Critical parameters are the glottal closure in stroboscopy, B of GRB, ABI, GNE, CPPS, MPT
3. Improvement of *voice quality* and/or *voice condition* and/or *discomfort in the throat,* caused by an *irregular vocal fold vibration* and/or *inappropriate ventricular phonation* and/or *supralaryngeal constriction,* through passive and active exercises for laryngeal muscle tone regulation:
   - Critical parameters of voice quality: regularity/symmetry of stroboscopy, R of GRB, AVQI (e.g., with simultaneously lower or normal ABI value), dynamic evaluation of palpation
   - Critical parameters of voice condition: VRP parameters, MPT, VFI cluster 1
   - Critical parameters of paresthesia in the throat: VTD-T
4. Improvement of phonation duration in glottal closure insufficiency:
   - Critical parameters: glottal closure in stroboscopy, MPT, VRP- intensity range, VRP- semitone range, VRP- boundaries
5. Improvement of *speaking pitch* and/or *speaking loudness (intelligibility):*
   - Critical parameters for speaking pitch: SRP-F0, VRP- semitone range, VRP-F0-min
   - Critical parameters for speaking loudness (intelligibility): SRP-I, VRP-intensity range

References

Barsties B, Thede T (2016) Evaluation of laryngeal palpation methods. In: De Bodt M, Maryn Y (Ed) Spanning in en rond de larynx: stand van zaken 3:32–47

Barsties v. Latoszek B, Göllner M, Mathmann P, Neumann K (2023) The German restructured Vocal Fatigue Index and characteristics of dysphonic and vocally healthy populations. J Voice 37(3):469.e11–469.e18. https://doi.org/10.1016/j.jvoice.2021.01.024

Chan CK, Fok KL, Poon CM (2010) Flavored anesthetic lozenge versus Xylocaine spray used as topical pharyngeal anesthesia for unsedated esophagogastroduodenoscopy: a

randomized placebo-controlled trial. Surg Endosc 24(4):897–901. https://doi.org/10.1007/s00464-009-0687-9
Englert M, Mendoza V, Behlau M, De Bodt M (2020) GALP qualifier scale: initial considerations to classify a voice problem. Folia Phoniatr Logop 72(5):402–410. https://doi.org/10.1159/000502772
Dejonckere PH, Bradley P, Clemente P, Cornut G, Crevier-Buchman L, Friedrich G, Van De Heyning P, Remacle M, Woisard V (2001) Committee on Phoniatrics of the European Laryngological Society (ELS). A basic protocol for functional assessment of voice pathology, especially for investigating the efficacy of (phonosurgical) treatments and evaluating new assessment techniques. Guideline elaborated by the Committee on Phoniatrics of the European Laryngological Society (ELS). Eur Arch Otorhinolaryngol. 258(2):77–82. https://doi.org/10.1007/s004050000299
DGPP (2023) [2k-Leitlinie Diagnostik und Therapie von Störungen der Stimmfunktion (Dysphonien) – Langfassung], 1. Edition, Version 4. https://register.awmf.org/assets/guidelines/049-0081_S2k_Diagnostik-Therapie-Stoerungen-der-Stimmfunktion-Dysphonien_2023-01.pdf. Accessed: 31. January 2023
Fairbanks G (1960) Voice and articulation drillbook, 2nd edn. Harper & Row, New York. S 124–139
Lechien JR, Geneid A, Bohlender JE, Cantarella G, Avellaneda JC, Desuter G, Sjogren EV, Finck C, Hans S, Hess M, Oguz H, Remacle MJ, Schneider-Stickler B, Tedla M, Schindler A, Vilaseca I, Zabrodsky M, Dikkers FG, Crevier-Buchman L (2023) Consensus for voice quality assessment in clinical practice: guidelines of the European Laryngological Society and Union of the European Phoniatricians. Eur Arch Otorhinolaryngol 280(12):5459–5473. https://doi.org/10.1007/s00405-023-08211-6
Lukaschyk J, Brockmann-Bauser M, Beushausen U (2017) Transcultural adaptation and validation of the German version of the vocal tract discomfort scale. J Voice 31(2):261.e1–261.e8. https://doi.org/10.1016/j.jvoice.2016.05.006
Ma EP, Yiu EM, Abbott KV (2007) Application of the ICF in voice disorders. Semin Speech Lang 28(4):343–350. https://doi.org/10.1055/s-2007-986531
Mayer J (2023) VOXplot: Software. https://voxplot.lingphon.com/en/. Accessed: 1. Oktober 2023
Nawka T, Wiesmann U, Gonnermann U (2003) [Validation of the German version of the Voice Handicap Index] . HNO 51(11):921–930. https://doi.org/10.1007/s00106-003-0909-8
Patel RR, Awan SN, Barkmeier-Kraemer J, Courey M, Deliyski D, Eadie T, Paul D, Švec JG, Hillman R (2018) Recommended protocols for instrumental assessment of voice: American Speech-Language-Hearing Association expert panel to develop a protocol for instrumental assessment of vocal function. Am J Speech Lang Pathol 27(3):887–905. https://doi.org/10.1044/2018_AJSLP-17-0009
Schneider B, Bigenzahn W (2007) [Stimmdiagnostik: ein Leitfaden für die Praxis]. Springer, Wien
Vachiramon A, Wang WC (2002) Acupressure technique to control gag reflex during maxillary impression procedures. J Prosthet Dent 88(2):236. https://doi.org/10.1067/mpr.2002.127952
WHO (2001) International classification of functioning, disability and health (ICF). WHO, Genève

4 Clinical Reasoning: The Path to Effective and Efficient Primary Treatment

4.1 Clinical Reasoning in Voice Therapy

Clinical reasoning refers to the thought and decision-making processes involved in the identification and diagnosis of diseases and disorders, which are based on a series of logical conclusions during the examination process, the analysis of findings, and the summarization of results (Wan and Zeng 2020).

The thought processes in decision-making can be roughly divided into four sections: abstraction, abduction, deduction, and induction (Patel et al. 2005). In *abstraction*, a conclusion is drawn from a result in a generalization process (e.g., a patient has a VHI-T = 33, which classifies a moderately impaired voice problem and indicates the presence of a voice disorder).

Abduction is a backward reasoning process to explain why this patient from the abstraction example should have a voice disorder. The term "abductive reasoning" was first coined in the 19th century to describe a general process when a surprising observation leads to a hypothesis (everyday example: "The lawn is wet! Ergo, it probably rained."; voice example: "A patient is hoarse! Ergo, the patient might have developed a functional voice disorder."), which is based on knowledge of possible causes and needs to be tested (continuation of the everyday example: "but it could also have been the neighbor's sprinkler"; voice example: "but it could also be a primarily organic voice disorder.") (ten Cate and Durning 2018). Abduction is considered a primary means of generating new ideas in clinical thinking (Bolton 2015).

Deduction is the process of testing the hypothesis (e.g., a voice disorder) by confirming other findings: If conditions *X* and *Y* are met, the conclusion *Z* must be true (ten Cate and Durning 2018).

Induction is the process of generalizing from multiple cases and is more commonly found in research than in individual patient care. If several patients exhibit similar signs and symptoms, general rules can be established based on significant

B. Barsties v. Latoszek et al., *Diagnostic and Treatment in Voice Therapy*, https://doi.org/10.1007/978-3-662-70162-1_4

and repeatedly tested results to tend to explain new cases (ten Cate and Durning 2018). Part of this process is prospective reasoning (hypothesis formation through data), and another part involves retrospective thinking (hypothesis testing) (Patel et al. 2005).

In clinical reasoning, the diverse medical and/or therapeutic processes are used to structure the meaning, goals, and strategies of therapy on which the decisions made are based—i.e., the collection and analysis of clinical data, the patient's perspective, and the professional assessment by the physician/therapist, as well as their knowledge of internal (individual clinical expertise—EBM Level 5) and external evidence (results from systematic research, from study knowledge—EBM Level 1 to 4) (Higgs and Jones 2000; Scherfer 2006). Thus, clinical reasoning is a tool for clinicians to choose the "best possible action" for the individual patient (Higgs and Jones 2000).

Due to the various aspects to be considered in patient care, different forms of clinical reasoning (e.g., scientific, conditional, ethical, pragmatic, interactive, and narrative reasoning) must also be employed, but clinicians often prefer individually different ways of thinking (Klemme and Siegmann 2006). This book primarily focuses on scientific reasoning (synonyms: procedural or predictive reasoning; Klemme and Siegmann 2006), which centers on determining the correct medical and therapeutic diagnosis (Rogers and Holm 1991). This process is mainly characterized by the three aspects of *diagnosis, prognosis, and treatment,* which are determined by analyzing various signs and symptoms, and is thus considered a classic problem-solving process (Klemme and Siegmann 2006). The central starting point here is to find out which key problem is responsible for the patient's complaints or symptoms (recognition, identification, and definition of the problem), so that solution hypotheses can be developed and tested on this basis (Klemme and Siegmann 2006). Finally, it is examined whether the initially established solution hypothesis is verified or falsified. In the case of falsification, new solution hypotheses must be developed (Klemme and Siegmann 2006).

> ▶ The goal of clinical reasoning for voice practice should be significant improvements in the voice problem, which trigger an avalanche effect through targeted treatment (i.e., minimal stimulus with exponential effect). The treatment is largely based on the findings of voice diagnostics.

Furthermore, general, hierarchically organized treatment principles can be used in voice therapy to achieve medically/therapeutically controlled voice changes in the patient (Mathieson 2001). This treatment principle is particularly applicable in cases of aphonia, so in most cases, the therapy is initially focused on improving the voice components of the vocal sound and thus stabilizing/extending the voice component. Once phonation is present, strategies to stabilize the voice can be introduced before addressing pitch, loudness, and vocal endurance.

For voice therapy, this means that particularly noticeable individual measurement parameters can be specifically improved through certain intervention principles and methods, thus creating a positive interaction effect on other pathological results, even if they were not specifically treated. This leverage effect of the avalanche effect based on the diagnostic findings must also be aligned with conditions such as the dependence on signs or symptoms originating from the voice disorder (see e.g., Sect. 5.1) and other factors such as body structures, environmental factors, and personal factors.

> A minimal standard for clinical reasoning in voice therapy is detecting the (high-ranking) top-3 intra-individual sensitive measurement parameters that best characterize the individual voice disorder.

A challenge in the entire clinical reasoning process is reflection in and on action. Acting in routine actions may not require much effort. However, non-routine tasks often require immediate adaptive action when problems or questions arise. But professionals with non-routine tasks often face problems or questions that require immediate adaptive action (ten Cate and Durning 2018). Therefore, the reflection in action of learners who are becoming professionals must be practiced (Schön 1983). This learning process can be initiated and learned through structured reflection to improve the diagnostic thinking of students (Mamede et al. 2010, 2014). In doing so, the detailed insight into the signs and symptoms of patients should be compared with already existing medical records to identify similarities and discrepancies. Therefore, it is recommended to use conscious reflection as a tool for learning clinical reasoning (Schmidt and Mamede 2015).

Finally, the quality of clinical reasoning is often measured by how few mistakes clinicians make (ten Cate and Durning 2018). Frequently occurring errors are due to various sources of bias.

An initial overview of typical biases in clinical reasoning can be described as follows (Kempainen et al. 2003):

- *Availability bias:* A differential diagnosis is influenced by what is easily retrievable, creating a false sense of prevalence.
- *Representative bias (or judging by similarity):* The clinical suspicion is influenced solely by signs and symptoms, thus neglecting the prevalence of competing diagnoses. This bias can occur if there is no comprehensive multidimensional examination.
- *Confirmation bias (or pseudo-diagnosis):* Additional tests in one direction confirm the suspected diagnosis but fail to test competing hypotheses.
- *Bias due to limited rationality (or search saturation):* Clinicians stop searching for additional diagnoses after the expected diagnosis is made, leading to a premature end of the thought process. Therefore, a comprehensive multidimensional examination should always be conducted.
- *Outcome bias:* A clinical decision is judged based on the outcome rather than the logic and evidence supporting the decision.

A limitation of this approach is when reasoning is considered successful, but the bias is generally not recognized. Only in retrospect can many errors be easily classified as caused by "bias" (Gigerenzer and Gaissmaier 2011). However, most errors seem to be rooted in a limited knowledge base of the clinician (Norman et al. 2017). Finally, so-called biases can indeed serve as heuristics to guide successful behavior (Gigerenzer and Gaissmaier 2011). A preliminary conclusion is that interventions based on error reduction through the identification of heuristics and biases have no impact on diagnostic errors.

4.2 The Systematic Path to the Appropriate Intervention in Three Steps

The first step in Clinical Reasoning consists of evaluating the collected quantified measurement parameters (physiological vs. pathological) from the analyzed voice examination protocol (see Table 3.1 and the Excel macro document for download from Chap. 3). Pathological results are weighted according to the majority principle of the sums in percentage (number of pathological-VQ; number of pathological-VF and number of pathological-VQ & VF) and whether primarily the primary voice quality (VQ—i.e., a change in voice sound) or primarily the primary voice function (VF—i.e., a change in the performance of the voice) is affected in the examined patients, regardless of the voice pathology. Additionally, the proportion of physiological features from the examination protocol is also output in percentage. Some voice parameters consist of a combination of both factors (VQ & VF). They are thus not attributable to a clear weighting and reflect a characteristic feature of a specific voice disorder when occurring pathologically, or this combination only serves to determine the dysphonia severity degree in the further course if a grading from normal to severe is available for this parameter.

Thus, in the first step, the majority of percentage pathological voice parameters can be determined and assigned to a primary voice quality problem or a primary voice function problem. This assignment is a first guide for a treatment approach based on corresponding critical conspicuous voice parameters from this voice area.

The second step and the core of Clinical Reasoning for voice practice highlights correlations from the individual measurement parameters with pathological results. Here, Table 4.1 is intended to help gain an initial guideline for deriving the correlations between the five pillars of voice diagnostics using a correlation matrix. These examples from the correlation matrix are based on the previous results of EBM-supported literature. Therefore, these contents do not have to be comprehensive and complete, as they are subject to the current state of scientific knowledge.

> ▶ Additionally, in the Excel voice examination protocol from Chap. 3 there is also an automatic ranking assessment based on Table 4.1, which considers potential primary critical voice parameters for treatment (evaluation of

Table 4.1 EBM examples from the literature for deriving Clinical Reasoning from the areas of voice diagnostics into a correlation matrix

Focus of the patho-logical diagnostic parameter	Correlation parameter	Ratio and interpretation aid	Correlations with significance level p<=0.01	Source
1st Pillar: Visual Analysis				
Stroboscopy: Glottal closure	Voice pathology (VQ & VF): • Vocal fold nodules (VF-N) • Vocal fold paralysis (VF-P) • Presbylarynx (PL) • Atrophy (A)	Presence of glottal closure insufficiency = Presence of specific voice pathology	60 to 75% (VF-N) 75% (VF-P) 61% (PL) 100% (A)	Pontes et al. (2005); Banjara et al. (2012); Sachdeva et al. (2020)
	Breathiness (VQ): • B from GRB/ABI	>Glottal closure insufficiency = > Breathiness	r = 0.74 (55%)	Uloza et al. (2013)
	Acoustics (VF): • Voice Range Profile	> Glottal closure insufficiency = < VRP contour	r = −0.76 (58%)	Uloza et al. (2013)
		> Glottal closure insufficiency = < VRP melodic range	r = −0.72 (52%)	Uloza et al. (2013)
		> Glottal closure insufficiency = < VRP dynamic range	r = −0.73 (53%)	Uloza et al. (2013)
	Voice efficiency (VQ & VF) • DSI	> Glottal closure insufficiency = < DSI	r = −0.69 (48%)	Uloza et al. (2013)

(continued)

Table 4.1 (continued)

Focus of the pathological diagnostic parameter	Correlation parameter	Ratio and interpretation aid	Correlations with significance level $p <= 0.01$	Source
	Aerodynamics (VF): • MPT	> Glottal closure insufficiency = < MPT	$r = -0.63$ (40%)	Uloza et al. (2013)
	Self-perception (VQ & VF): • VHI	> Glottal closure insufficiency = > VHI-T	$r = 0.65$ (42%)	Uloza et al. (2013)
		> Glottal closure insufficiency = > VHI-P	$r = 0.70$ (49%)	Uloza et al. (2013)
Stroboscopy: Regularity or symmetry of the phonatory pattern	Voice pathology (VQ & VF): • Vocal fold polyp (VF-P) • Reinke's edema (RE) • Ventricular phonation (VP)	Presence of irregularity/asymmetry = Presence of specific voice pathology	88% to 100% (VF-P) 43% to 86% (RE) 53% to 100% (VP)	Von Doersten et al. (1992); Banjara et al. (2012); Watanabe et al. (2016); Sachdeva et al. (2020);
	Roughness (VQ): • R from GRB	> Irregularity/SL-Symmetry = > Roughness	$r = 0.65$ (42%)	Uloza et al. (2013)

(continued)

Table 4.1 (continued)

Focus of the pathological diagnostic parameter	Correlation parameter	Ratio and interpretation aid	Correlations with significance level p<=0.01	Source
Stroboscopy: Ventricular fold activity	Perception (VQ): • Pressed voice quality • Roughness	> Ventricular fold activity = > Pressed voice quality & Roughness	100%	Maryn et al. (2003)
	Acoustics (VF): • Low head voice component • Low melodic range	> Ventricular fold activity = < lower melodic range & head voice component	In 60% of cases, an average of 22 ST of the semitone voice range, in 40% of cases not evaluable (too high ventricular fold activity)	Von Doersten et al. (1992);
2nd Pillar: Perception				
Perception: Falpation	Perception (VQ): • R from GRB • Pressed voice quality	> Elevated larynx (dynamic laryngeal hypertonus) = > Roughness	81%	Izadi and Salehi (2013)
		> reduced thyroid space (dynamic laryngeal hypertonus) = > pressed voice quality	91%	Izadi and Salehi (2013)
	Voice efficiency (VQ & VF): • DSI	> laryngeal hypertonus (static & dynamic) = < DSI	r = −0.60 (36%)	Kooijman et al. (2005)

(continued)

Table 4.1 (continued)

Focus of the patho-logical diagnostic parameter	Correlation parameter	Ratio and interpretation aid	Correlations with significance level p<=0.01	Source
	Self-perception (VQ & VF): • VHI	> static laryngeal hypertonus = > VHI-T	r = 0.50 (25%)	Bargar (2024)
	Self-perception (VQ & VF): • Vocal fatigue (VFI)	> static laryngeal hypertonus = > VFI- Part 1	r = 0.51 (26%)	Bargar (2024)
Perception: Roughness	Voice pathology (VQ & VF): • Vocal fold polyp (VF-P)	> Size of VF-P = > Roughness	r = 0.41 (before therapy) (17%)	Salmen et al. (2017)
Perception: Breathiness	Acoustics (VF): • Speaking loudness	> Breathiness = < SRP-I	r = −0.82 (67%)	Hertegard and Gauffin (1991)
3rd Pillar: Acoustics				
Acoustics: Dysphonia Severity Index	Presence of a voice pathology (VQ & VF)	< DSI = Presence of a voice pathology	88%	Barsties v. Latoszek et al. (2019)
	Self-perception (VQ & VF): • VHI	< DSI = > VHI-T	r = −0.79 (62%), 63%	Wuyts et al. (2000); Hakkesteegt et al. (2010)

(continued)

Table 4.1 (continued)

Focus of the pathological diagnostic parameter	Correlation parameter	Ratio and interpretation aid	Correlations with significance level p<=0.01	Source
Acoustics: Acoustic Voice Quality Index	Presence of a voice pathology (VQ & VF)	> AVQI = Presence of a voice pathology	79%	Barsties v. Latoszek et al. (2019)
	Self-perception (VQ & VF): • VHI	> AVQI = > VHI-T	r = 0.48 to 0.58 (23% to 34%)	Pomée et al. (2020); Englert et al. (2024)
Acoustics: Voice Range Profile	Anamnesis: • Age in years	< VRP- F0-high/ < VRP- semitone range = > Age in years	r = −0.32 to -0.53 (10% to 28%)	Berghs et al. (2013)
	Organic voice pathologies (VQ & VF)	Reduced contour = Presence of an organic voice pathology	48% to 55% reduced compared to healthy voices	Ikeda et al. (1999)
	Voice pathology (VQ & VF): • Vocal fold nodules (VF-N) • Vocal fold polyps (VF-P)	> the size of VF-N, VF-P = < VRP- semitone range (especially: < VRP- F0-high)	18% to 63% (VF-N), r = −0.30 to -0.41 (9% to 17%) (VF-P)	Shah et al. (2008) Uloza et al. (2008)

(continued)

Table 4.1 (continued)

Focus of the patho-logical diagnostic parameter	Correlation parameter	Ratio and interpretation aid	Correlations with significance level p<=0.01	Source
4th Pillar: Aerodynamics				
Aerodynamics: Maximum phonation time	Breathiness (VQ): • B from GRB & ABI	< MPT = > Breathiness	r = −0.39 to -0.75 (15% to 56%)	Fujiki and Thibeault (2021); Barsties v. Latoszek et al. (2017); Fujiki and Thibeault (2023)
	Acoustics (VF): • Voice Range Profile	< MPT = < VRP- boundaries	r = 0.42 (18%)	Ma et al. (2006)
		< MPT = < VRP-semitone range	r = 0.32 to 0.51 (10% to 26%)	Ma and Yiu (2006); Barsties v. Latoszek et al. (2017)
		< MPT = < VRP-intensityc range	r = 0.39 to 0.45 (15% to 20%)	Ma and Yiu (2006); Barsties v. Latoszek et al. (2017)
5th Pillar: Self-evaluation				
Self-evaluation: Voice Handicap Index	Presence of a voice pathology (VQ & VF)	> VHI = Presence of a voice pathology	96.4% to 100%	Behlau et al. (2016)

(continued)

Table 4.1 (continued)

Focus of the patho-logical diagnostic parameter	Correlation parameter	Ratio and interpretation aid	Correlations with significance level p<=0.01	Source
Self-evaluation: Vocal fatigue	Acoustics (VF): • Voice Range Profile	> Vocal fatigue = > Breaks/reduction in the VRP.- bounda-ries (smaller surface area)	16% to 67% expansion of the VRP-boundaries possible through targeted symptom treatment	Holmberg et al. (2007)
	Acoustics (VQ): • AVQI	>VFI cluster 1 = > AVQI	r = 0.42 (18%)	Kankare et al. (in press)
	Acoustics (VQ): • CPPS (vowel /a:/)	>VFI cluster 1 = < CPPS	r = −0.50 (25%)	Mahalingam et al. (2021)
Self-evaluation: Laryngeal discomfort (VTD)	Anamnesis: • After vocal effort at work	> VTD frequency (throat irritated) = > Vocal effort	r = 0.60 (36%)	Mendes et al. (2016)
		> VTD frequency (lump in throat) = > Vocal effort	r = 0.46 (21%)	Mendes et al. (2016)
		> VTD intensity (throat irritated) = > Vocal effort	r = 0.46 (21%)	Mendes et al. (2016)
		> VTD intensity (lump in throat) = > Vocal effort	r = 0.48 (23%)	Mendes et al. (2016)

(continued)

treatment effectiveness). When interpreting, it should be noted that the Excel voice examination protocol, due to correlations, only provides recommendations for a ranking of the top 3 voice parameters. They serve as an initial guide, and it must be finally assessed by the clinicians which critical measurement parameters are definitively collected for the top 3 assessment (see step 3). Therefore, an additional look at the entire correlation matrix in the worksheet of this Excel document should always be taken.

Based on the relationships derived from the current findings of the voice patients and on which measurement parameters most connections in the correlation matrix of Table 4.1 can be traced back to, voice treatment forms are selected according to these results. The primary choice of a suitable intervention (i.e., the start in the manner of treatment and choice of method) based on the results of the voice diagnostics is crucial to more clearly define the requirements for the treatment and to determine, beyond the diagnosis of a voice disorder, whether a voice quality or voice function problem predominantly exists.

In the third step, all results from steps 1 and 2 regarding the (high-ranking) top-3 features that represent the manifestations of an individual patient's disorder are compiled.

The selection of these top-3 features takes place on three different levels:

1. As described in step 1; if available, the determination of a primary majority of VQ or VF
   - In the case of a majority of VQ & VF, the significance of this level is omitted, as no clear focus can be placed, or there is a certain ambiguity in the weighting of the measurement parameters to shift the treatment method requirements to VQ or VF.
   - The only exception applies to very severely impaired voices, where a majority in VQ & VF without a replacement voice (e.g., ventricular phonation, voice prosthesis, etc.) is present in the diagnostic evaluation. Then, the general treatment hierarchy according to Mathiesson (2001) comes into effect, which is described as the minimal standard for this treatment strategy in Sect. 4.1.
2. As described in step 2; the measurement parameter with the most connections from the correlation matrix—derived from the columns on the "focus of the pathological diagnostic parameter" and "correlation parameter"—which is also applicable to the individual patients from the diagnostics
3. Selection of targeted measurement parameters from the context of the voice disorder, with the highest individual severity and other ICF components

These derived top-3 features are also the essential evaluation parameters by which the medical and/or therapeutic success over the start of the treatment of the individual patients is measured. Furthermore, the greatest possible effect in this phase of the treatment start (primary treatment focus) should be triggered by creating an avalanche effect.

When choosing the first intervention, it must be considered that certain organic voice disorders are primarily subject to medical interventions and thus an interdisciplinary exchange between physicians and voice therapists is essential for treatment success. These medical interventions are described in detail in Sect. 5.1.

References

Banjara H, Mungutwar V, Singh D, Gupta A, Singh S (2012) Demographic and videostroboscopic assessment of vocal pathologies. Indian J Otolaryngol Head Neck Surg. 64(2):150–157. https://doi.org/10.1007/s12070-011-0451-z

Bargar I (2024) [Die Reliabilität und Validität eines Palpationstools zur statischen laryngealen Untersuchung]. Unpublished Bachelorthesis, SRH University of Applied Sciences Heidelberg, Düsseldorf

Barsties v. Latoszek B, Maryn Y, Gerrits E, De Bodt M (2017) The Acoustic Breathiness Index (ABI): a multivariate acoustic model for breathiness. J Voice 31(4):511.e11–511.e27. https://doi.org/10.1016/j.jvoice.2016.11.017

Barsties v. Latoszek B, Ulozaitė-Stanienė N, Petrauskas T, Uloza V, Maryn Y (2019) Diagnostic accuracy of dysphonia classification of DSI and AVQI. Laryngoscope. 129(3):692–698. https://doi.org/10.1002/lary.27350

Behlau M, Madazio G, Moreti F, Oliveira G, Dos Santos Lde M, Paulinelli BR, Couto Junior Ede B (2016) Efficiency and cutoff values of self-assessment instruments on the impact of a voice problem. J Voice. 30(4):506.e9–506.e18. https://doi.org/10.1016/j.jvoice.2015.05.022

Berghs G, Creylman N, Avaux M, Decoster W, de Jong F (2013) A lifetime of professional singing: voice parameters and age in the Netherlands radio choir. Logoped Phoniatr Vocol 38(2):59–63. https://doi.org/10.3109/14015439.2012.731082

Bolton JW (2015) Varieties of clinical reasoning. J Eval Clin Pract 21(3):486–489. https://doi.org/10.1111/jep.12309

Englert M, Barsties v. Latoszek B, Behlau M (2024) Exploring the validity of acoustic measurements and other voice assessments. J Voice 38(3):567–571. https://doi.org/10.1016/j.jvoice.2021.12.014

Fujiki RB, Thibeault SL (2021) The relationship between auditory-perceptual rating scales and objective voice measures in children with voice disorders. Am J Speech Lang Pathol 30(1):228–238. https://doi.org/10.1044/2020_AJSLP-20-00188

Fujiki RB, Thibeault SL (2023) Examining relationships between GRBAS ratings and acoustic, aerodynamic and patient-reported voice measures in adults with voice disorders. J Voice 37(3):390–397. https://doi.org/10.1016/j.jvoice.2021.02.007

Gigerenzer G, Gaissmaier W (2011) Heuristic decision making. Annu Rev Psychol 62:451–482. https://doi.org/10.1146/annurev-psych-120709-145346

Hakkesteegt MM, Brocaar MP, Wieringa MH (2010) The applicability of the dysphonia severity index and the voice handicap index in evaluating effects of voice therapy and phonosurgery. J Voice 24(2):199–205. https://doi.org/10.1016/j.jvoice.2008.06.007

Hertegard S, Gauffin J (1991) Insufficient vocal fold closure as studied by inverse filtering. In: Gauffin J, Hammarberg B (Hrsg) Vocal fold physiology: acoustic, perceptual, and physiological aspects of voice mechanisms. Whurr Publishers London, pp 243–250

Higgs J, Jones MA (2000) Clinical reasoning in health professions. In: Higgs J, Jones M (Hrsg) Clinical reasoning in the health professions. 2nd edn. Butterworth Heinemann, Oxford, pp 3–14

Holmberg EB, Ihre E, Södersten M (2007) Phonetograms as a tool in the voice clinic: changes across voice therapy for patients with vocal fatigue. Logoped Phoniatr Vocol 32(3):113–127. https://doi.org/10.1080/14015430701661632

Ikeda Y, Masuda T, Manako H, Yamashita H, Yamamoto T, Komiyama S (1999) Quantitative evaluation of the voice range profile in patients with voice disorder. Eur Arch Otorhinolaryngol 256(Suppl 1):S51–S55. https://doi.org/10.1007/pl00014154

Izadi F, Salehi A (2013) Comparison between palpatory findings of the hyoid position and their acoustic, videostroboscopic, and perceptual attributes in patients with muscle tension dysphonia (with and without organic lesions). J Voice 27(1):78–83. https://doi.org/10.1016/j.jvoice.2012.06.008

Kankare E, Rantala L, Laukkanen AM (in press) Vocal Fatigue Index in Finnish-Speaking Population. *J Voice* https://doi.org/10.1016/j.jvoice.2023.02.034

Kempainen RR, Migeon MB, Wolf FM (2003) Understanding our mistakes: a primer on errors in clinical reasoning. Med Teach 25(2):177–181. https://doi.org/10.1080/0142159031000092580

Klemme B, Siegmann G (2006) [Clinical Reasoning. Therapeutische Denkprozesse lernen]. Georg Thieme, Stuttgart

Kooijman PG, de Jong FI, Oudes MJ, Huinck W, van Acht H, Graamans K (2005) Muscular tension and body posture in relation to voice handicap and voice quality in teachers with persistent voice complaints. Folia Phoniatr Logop 57(3):134–147. https://doi.org/10.1159/000084134

Ma EP, Yiu EM (2006) Multiparametric evaluation of dysphonic severity. J Voice 20(3):380–390. https://doi.org/10.1016/j.jvoice.2005.04.007

Ma EP, Yiu EM, Abbott KV (2007) Application of the ICF in voice disorders. Semin Speech Lang 28(4):343–350. https://doi.org/10.1055/s-2007-986531

Mahalingam S, Boominathan P, Arunachalam R, Venkatesh L, Srinivas S (2021) Cepstral measures to analyze vocal fatigue in individuals with hyperfunctional voice disorder. J Voice 35(6):815–821. https://doi.org/10.1016/j.jvoice.2020.02.007

Mamede S, van Gog T, van den Berge K, Rikers RM, van Saase JL, van Guldener C, Schmidt HG (2010) Effect of availability bias and reflective reasoning on diagnostic accuracy among internal medicine residents. JAMA 304(11):1198–1203. https://doi.org/10.1001/jama.2010.1276

Mamede S, van Gog T, Sampaio AM, de Faria RM, Maria JP, Schmidt HG (2014) How can students' diagnostic competence benefit most from practice with clinical cases? The effects of structured reflection on future diagnosis of the same and novel diseases. Acad Med 89(1):121–127. https://doi.org/10.1097/ACM.0000000000000076

Maryn Y, De Bodt MS, Van Cauwenberge P (2003) Ventricular dysphonia: clinical aspects and therapeutic options. Laryngoscope 113(5):859–866. https://doi.org/10.1097/00005537-200305000-00016

Mathieson L (2001) The voice and its disorders. Whurr Publishers, London

Mendes AL, Lucena BT, De Araújo AM, Melo LP, Lopes LW, Silva MF (2016) Teacher's voice: vocal tract discomfort symptoms, vocal intensity and noise in the classroom. Codas 28(2):168–175. https://doi.org/10.1590/2317-1782/20162015027

Norman GR, Monteiro SD, Sherbino J, Ilgen JS, Schmidt HG, Mamede S (2017) The causes of errors in clinical reasoning: cognitive biases, knowledge deficits, and dual process thinking. Acad Med 92(1):23–30. https://doi.org/10.1097/ACM.0000000000001421

Patel V, Arocha J, Zhang J (2005) Thinking and reasoning in medicine. In: Holyoak K, Morrison R (Hrsg.). The Cambridge handbook of thinking and reasoning. Cambridge: Cambridge University Press pp 727–750

Pontes P, Brasolotto A, Behlau M (2005) Glottic characteristics and voice complaint in the elderly. J Voice 19(1):84–94. https://doi.org/10.1016/j.jvoice.2004.09.002

Pommée T, Maryn Y, Finck C, Morsomme D (2020) The Acoustic Voice Quality Index, Version 03.01, in French and the Voice Handicap Index. *J Voice* 34(4):646.e1–646.e10. https://doi.org/10.1016/j.jvoice.2018.11.017

Rogers JC, Holm MB (1991) Occupational therapy diagnostic reasoning: a component of clinical reasoning. Am J Occup Ther 45(11):1045–1053. https://doi.org/10.5014/ajot.45.11.1045

Sachdeva K, Mittal N, Sachdeva N (2020) Role of Video Laryngostroboscopy in benign disease of larynx. Indian J Otolaryngol Head Neck Surg. 72(2):267–273. https://doi.org/10.1007/s12070-020-01827-8

Salmen T, Ermakova T, Möller A, Seipelt M, Weikert S, Rummich J, Gross M, Nawka T, Caffier PP (2017) The value of Vocal Extent Measure (VEM) assessing phonomicrosurgical outcomes in vocal fold polyps. J Voice. 31(1):114.e7–114.e15. https://doi.org/10.1016/j.jvoice.2016.03.016

Scherfer E (2006) [Forschung verstehen. Ein Grundkurs in evidenzbasierter Praxis]. Pflaum, München

Schmidt HG, Mamede S (2015) How to improve the teaching of clinical reasoning: a narrative review and a proposal. Med Educ 49(10):961–973. https://doi.org/10.1111/medu.12775

Schön DA (1983) The reflective practitioner—how professionals think in action. Basic Books, New York

Shah RK, Engel SH, Choi SS (2008) Relationship between voice quality and vocal nodule size. Otolaryngol Head Neck Surg 139(5):723–726. https://doi.org/10.1016/j.otohns.2008.08.010

ten Cate O, Durning SJ (2018) Understanding clinical reasoning from multiple perspectives: a conceptual and theoretical overview. In O. ten Cate, E. Custers, S. Durning (Hrsg) Principles and practice of case-based clinical reasoning education. Innovation and change in professional education, Bd. 15. Springer, Cham. https://doi.org/10.1007/978-3-319-64828-6_3

Uloza V, Kaseta M, Pribuisiene R, Saferis V, Jokūzis V, Gelzinis A, Bacauskiene M (2008) Quantitative microlaryngoscopic measurements of vocal fold polyps, glottal gap and their relation to vocal function. Medicina (Kaunas) 44(4):266–272

Uloza V, Vegienė A, Saferis V (2013) Correlation between the basic video laryngostroboscopic parameters and multidimensional voice measurements. J Voice 27(6):744–752. https://doi.org/10.1016/j.jvoice.2013.06.008

Von Doersten PV, Izdebski K, Ross JC, Cruz RM (1992) Ventricular dysphonia: a profile of 40 cases. Laryngoscope 102(11):1296–1301. https://doi.org/10.1288/00005537-199211000-00018

Wan X, Zeng R (2020) Clinical reasoning. In: Wan XH, Zeng R (Hrsg) Handbook of clinical diagnostics. Springer, Singapore https://doi.org/10.1007/978-981-13-7677-1_71

Watanabe T, Kaneko K, Sakaguchi K, Takahashi H (2016) Vocal-fold vibration of patients with Reinke's edema observed using high-speed digital imaging. Auris Nasus Larynx 43(6):654–657. https://doi.org/10.1016/j.anl.2016.02.007

Wuyts FL, De Bodt MS, Molenberghs G, Remacle M, Heylen L, Millet B, Van Lierde K, Raes J, Van de Heyning PH (2000) The dysphonia severity index: an objective measure of vocal quality based on a multiparameter approach. J Speech Lang Hear Res 43(3):796–809. https://doi.org/10.1044/jslhr.4303.796

Treatment of Voice Disorders According to EBM Criteria

5

The etiology of dysphonia is diverse (De Bodt et al. 2015; Martins et al. 2016) and thus determines the primary treatment approach (i.e., the start in the manner of treatment and choice of method). Treatment options include conservative voice therapy (Speyer 2008; Ruotsalainen et al. 2008; Eastwood et al. 2015; Walton et al. 2017; da Cunha Pereira et al. 2018; Barsties v. Latoszek 2020a), various medical surgical treatment approaches (Sataloff et al. 2007; Reiter and Hoffmann 2017) and/or pharmacological treatment (Schönweiler 2020).

Successful treatment of voice disorders depends on various factors. The cause of the problem (e.g., neuropathology, emotion, incorrect voice habits, structural pathology) should be determined first and foremost. Other factors that maintain the problem should also be known. The patient's motivation should be high for successful therapy. The treatment contents must be tailored to the individual patient, and the availability of appropriate treatment should be age-appropriate. The evaluation of the diagnostic analysis should significantly help determine the direction of the voice treatment to be performed. The following Sects. 5.1 to 5.3 describe detailed medical and therapeutic treatment options to provide a guideline for an EBM-based treatment focus and/or the start of the type or method of treatment for heterogeneous voice disorders.

▶ The EBM-level structure can be divided into levels and evidence based on the Oxford Centre for Evidence-Based Medicine (OCEBM) (OCEBM 2011). The OCEBM classification takes into account, among other things, the strength of the evidence of the ranking (level structure) for interventional study designs regarding their effects and harms. Regarding intervention

---

Supplementary Information The electronic version of this chapter contains supplementary material, which can be accessed via the following link https://doi.org/10.1007/978-3-662-68958-5_5. The videos can be played by clicking the DOI link in the legend of a corresponding figure, or by scanning this link with the SN More Media app.

B. Barsties v. Latoszek et al., *Diagnostic and Treatment in Voice Therapy*,
https://doi.org/10.1007/978-3-662-70162-1_5

studies, the OCEBM has the following ranking for the essential study designs (OCEBM 2011): Level 1 = (systematic) literature reviews; Level 2 = randomized controlled trials; Level 3 = non-randomized controlled trials or cohort studies with/without follow-up; Level 4 = case-control studies, case series, or historically controlled studies; Level 5 = expert opinion based on mechanistic reasoning.

The basis for the different treatment recommendations from this 5th chapter is particularly directed at research (Level 1) in the form of literature reviews, meta-analyses, and umbrella reviews. Literature reviews (review articles) synthesize information for readers, providing increased clarity and valuable insights into a topic (Sataloff et al. 2021). Most valuable are umbrella reviews, which synthesize information from previously published systematic reviews and meta-analyses into a practical paper. For a qualitative evaluation of the research situation, the systematic literature review is the most common procedure and the basis for further quantitative analyses such as a meta-analysis.

▶ A meta-analysis allows for the combination of data and the statistical summarization of the results of several clinical studies that have investigated the effectiveness of a comparable treatment approach in a similar patient group (Israel and Richter 2011).

This statistical technique, based on the results of a systematic literature review, can prove particularly useful when there are several clinical studies on a specific treatment approach with or without consistent results, or when there is a small to medium number of subjects in studies with inconclusive results. By combining the results of two or more studies, a meta-analysis can increase statistical power and provide a single numerical value for the overall effect of the treatment (Israel and Richter 2011). The result of the meta-analysis, which describes the treatment effect of an intervention, can either show a benefit or a lack of benefit of a treatment approach (e.g., through confidence intervals, effect size, or *p*-values and is thus considered a guideline for treatment recommendations in EBM). The treatment effect is the gain (or loss) observed in the experimental group compared to the control group. The positive or negative overall change can be difficult to detect in individual studies. Only in repeated comparable study designs can a treatment effect be determined, with any type of study being included in a meta-analysis. However, the approach is best suited for randomized controlled trials (RCTs). Randomized studies are often more elaborate and planning-intensive than other study types and have a lower number of potential biases compared to observational studies, which can thus weaken the treatment effect (Rosenfeld 2004).

▶ Another special form of meta-analysis is the network meta-analysis. This form allows for the comparison of multiple treatments for a specific medical or health condition in one analysis.

In a network meta-analysis, a network of both direct comparisons of interventions and indirect comparisons between studies based on a common comparator is considered (Salanti 2012). This statistical approach can be useful for meta-analyses on the effectiveness of voice therapies, as various voice treatments can be compared if the same measurement method has been applied in all studies in the same way. Furthermore, in a network meta-analysis, a ranking of interventions can be determined using a quantitative measure that represents a critical evaluation of the ranking without the need for resampling methods, for example (Rücker and Schwarzer 2015). It is an analytical method based on frequentist effect estimation and their standard errors, as well as the size and probability of inaccuracy. This statistical measure can be interpreted as a measure of the average degree of confidence, so that one treatment proves to be better than a comparable treatment.

5.1 Primary Medical Interventions Depending on the Disorder

For certain diagnoses of organic voice disorders, medical interventions are preferable for the start of treatment (primary). While conservative voice therapy is the focus for functional voice disorders, organic laryngeal pathologies are partly treated medically. The following techniques are available to physicians for this purpose: surgical (steroid injections, augmentation, biopsies, laser ablations, phonosurgery, thyroplasty, reinnervations, reconstructions, pacemaker treatments, endoscopic and open partial laryngectomies for tumors) or medicinal through the prescription of medications, and for malignant tumors also radiochemo-/immunotherapies.

The disease patterns presented in detail below are clinically relevant and are often predestined for a specific primary medical intervention with a focus on voice improvement. In addition, there is an evidence base for these interventions that can be mapped in the voice examination protocol. Less commonly used medical procedures (such as surgery for laryngeal malformations and stenoses, vocal feminization surgery for male-to-female trans*, testosterone therapy for female-to-male trans*, treatment of laryngeal trauma, hematomas, or burns) are therefore only conditionally included in this book, as the focus is on benign, organic, or functional dysphonias with phonatory deficits.

5.1.1 Acute Laryngitis

In the primary stage, the disease is an inflammation of the endolarynx caused by rhino-, adeno-, influenza, or parainfluenza viruses, provided it was not caused by phonotrauma. This results in increased vascular injection of the vocal fold mucosa and edema of the vocal folds, leading to hoarseness. Therefore, there is no causal medicinal therapy approach. The treatment is symptomatic, aimed at suppressing cough, pain relief, and possibly fever treatment, and is usually carried out through self-medication by the patient. In the case of secondary superinfections, persistent purulent rhinosinusitis, or tracheobronchitis with cough, the prescription of an antibiotic by the physicians may be useful in individual cases. An evidence-based advantage of patients treated with antibiotics regarding laryngitis symptoms could not be demonstrated in systematic literature review studies (Reveiz and Cardona 2013, 2015).

5.1.2 Vocal Fold Polyps

Vocal fold polyps are predominantly unilateral benign tissue changes on the vocal folds, which can be broad-based or pedunculated in their form. The morphological structure can also vary from gelatinous translucent to fibrous, but also hemangiomatous; the size of the findings also varies (Vasconcelos et al. 2019; Cho et al. 2011). In some regions, vocal fold polyps are among the five most common organic laryngeal diseases, with prevalence rates of up to 14% (Hah et al. 2015; Martins et al. 2016). The causes of their development are multifactorial. Smoking, reflux, shouting, or vocal overuse can play a role (Kenny et al. in press). In a network meta-analysis, phonosurgery with "cold" microsurgery or laser treatment (often CO_2 or potassium titanyl phosphate (KTP) laser) proved to be significantly more effective in treating heterogeneous features of vocal fold polyps compared to conservative voice therapy (Barsties v. Latoszek et al. 2023b). The recurrence rate after microscopic excision by "cold" microsurgery is generally considered low (11%), evaluated as gender-independent, but the rate varies across age groups (younger adults have a significantly higher recurrence rate than middle-aged or older adults) (Lee and Sulica 2020). Subsequent voice therapy rehabilitation is then considered significantly superior to phonosurgery alone if patients preoperatively exhibited a high degree of hoarseness, a significantly shortened maximum phonation time, and more pronounced values in the subscales of the VHI, the functional and emotional components (Barsties v. Latoszek et al. 2023b).

5.1.3 Laryngopharyngeal Reflux and Irritative Cough

Laryngopharyngeal reflux (LPR) is a secondary inflammatory condition caused by the backflow of acidic stomach contents into the laryngopharynx, leading to irritation of the mucosa in the upper aerodigestive tract (Koufman et al. 2002). LPR can lead to irritation of the interarytenoid region of the larynx with whitish mucosal discoloration and transverse folds in this area (posterior laryngitis). The accompanying hoarseness (measured objectively or subjectively) is explained by occurring dehiscences between epithelial cells, inflammatory infiltrates of the mucosa and epithelial thickening, reduction of the fluid content of the Reinke's space, and drying of the mucosal surface (Lechien et al. 2017).

Validated measurement methods for assessing clinical LPR findings proved challenging in a systematic literature review, as only 6 out of 16 detected measurement instruments were examined with at least one criterion of developmental measurement properties (Lechien et al. 2019). From this study, none of the 6 instruments could validly measure a complete assessment of laryngeal and extralaryngeal signs associated with LPR (Lechien et al. 2019). Therefore, at the current time, the pH-metry procedure is still used as the standard for LPR diagnosis, despite shortcomings such as high false-positive and false-negative values (Lechien et al. 2019, 2021).

In the case of LPR detection through pH-metry and after excluding a gastroesophageal underlying condition, many clinicians still recommend a trial treatment with proton pump inhibitors (PPI), although the evidence is poor. In a recent umbrella review, 7 meta-analyses and 2 systematic literature reviews were included, of which 6 out of 9 studies could not demonstrate the superiority of PPI over placebo in reducing laryngeal symptoms (Spantideas et al. 2020). As an alternative treatment based on a systematic literature review, an anti-reflux diet is recommended, while LPR patients with dominant voice problems should undergo conservative voice therapy (Huestis et al. 2020). In general, however, the effective treatment of LPR patients remains complex, even with the help of proposed treatment pathways and medical flow charts (Lechien et al. 2020, 2021).

Mechanical irritation of the larynx by extralaryngeally induced irritative cough can be managed, after excluding a treatable underlying condition, by reducing the cough reflex using gabapentin. The evidence for effectiveness and patient safety is good (Ryan 2015). In cases of neurogenic cough and post-COVID-19 cough, a new treatment option showed symptom relief through the temporary block of the superior laryngeal nerve by injection of lidocaine/triamcinolone in a placebo-controlled study (Tipton et al. 2023).

5.1.4 Reinke's Edema

Reinke's edema is a chronic, benign, vascular-related congestion and fluid overload of the Reinke's space with swelling of the vocal fold (Tavaluc and Tan-Geller 2019). Also known as polypoid corditis, polypoid laryngitis, and polypoid degeneration of the vocal fold, it is closely associated with smoking, often with vocal abuse and laryngopharyngeal reflux (Dewan et al. 2022). In the late stage of Reinke's edema, polypoid degeneration of the vocal fold occurs, where the edema decreases and is replaced by connective tissue septa, causing the polypoid appearance of the vocal folds. Due to the exposure to noxious agents, advanced findings are also associated with mucosal leukoplakia and dysplasia. The increasing polypoid degeneration leads to a lowering of pitch and a rough voice (Dewan et al. 2022). The stages of gradations for the classification of Reinke's edema are used in the literature according to Yonekawa (1988) or Tan et al. (2017).

Stages of Gradations for the Classification of Reinke's Edema

1. Yonekawa (1988)

Grade 1: An edematous swelling is observed on the upper surface of the vocal folds, while the patency of the glottis is sufficiently maintained.

Grade 2: The edematous swelling extends from the upper to the lower surface over the edges of both vocal folds, which partially touch each other.

Grade 3: The edematous swelling is more advanced, so that an opening is only visible in the posterior part of the glottis, or the swelling is so large that it hangs down into the subglottic space during inhalation.

2. Tan et al. (2017)

Grade 1: Minimal polypoid degeneration of the vocal folds up to 25% of the glottal airway;

Grade 2: Extensive polypoid lesion occupying 25% to 50% of the glottal airway;

Grade 3: Extensive polypoid lesion occupying 50% to 75% of the glottal airway;

Grade 4: Obstructive lesion, regardless of laterality, occupying more than 75% of the glottal airway.

Two systematic literature reviews reported on medical interventions (especially laser treatment) for Reinke's edema when there is a high grade of swelling of the vocal folds (e.g., *Grade 2* and *Grade 3* according to Yonekawa 1988) (Khodeir et al. 2021; Hamdan et al. in press). Both studies evaluated between 58 and 220 data points from the included studies (mostly retrospective case studies without a control group). Although significant improvements in the multidimensional voice assessment were generally observed through medical intervention, further studies with more data from subjects and randomized controlled study designs are needed before specific medical treatment procedures (e.g., certain laser treatments, cold surgery, or injection of steroids or hyaluronidase) can be recommended (Khodeir et al. 2021). While certain assessments in voice examination parameters can already be evaluated through a meta-analysis in outpatient laser treatment, fundamental recommendations are still not possible due to small data sets and low EBM levels of the included studies (Hamdan et al. in press). According to the evaluations of Hamdan et al. (in press), significant improvements are observed after outpatient laser treatment in VHI scores and certain acoustic voice quality parameters (e.g., jitter), the lesion size of the edema also achieves a significant reduction, and habitual pitch increases significantly. A clear differential indication between outpatient laser reduction with potassium titanyl phosphate (KTP) laser and the microsurgical removal of Reinke's edema with mucosal reconstruction and subsequent voice therapy must be considered.

High-grade stages of Reinke's edema should be pretreated with the laser to avoid the risk of increased airway collapse during anesthesia induction for microsurgery. Likewise, microsurgery is always advisable when dysplasia is suspected to obtain biopsies and rule out malignancy.

In Grade 1–2 of Reinke's edema, the more elaborate microsurgery should be offered to patients who do not have increased anesthesia risks. They should be willing to change their behavior regarding nicotine and voice hygiene and undergo subsequent voice therapy (Dewan et al. 2022).

5.1.5 Spasmodic Dysphonia

Segmental dystonias can prominently affect the larynx. Spasmodic dysphonias (SD) of the adductor type (the most common form at 82%) cause closure spasms with strained voice and speech flow disorder, while the abductor type (17% of cases) causes opening spasms with voice interruption (Childs et al. 2011). In addition, mixed forms also occur. SD is generally considered a rare cause of voice disorders. The estimated prevalence is 14 per 100,000, with the age group between 30 to 50 years being the most affected, women more often than men (2.5:1) (NIDCD 2010). With a latency of onset within a week, patients can indicate triggering factors (stress 42%, upper respiratory tract infections 33%, childbirth 10%, intubation during a surgical procedure 6%). In a gradual process (average 6.3 years, SD = 7.2 years), the triggering factors are unknown (Childs et al. 2011).

Symptomatic therapy is usually carried out through targeted botulinum toxin injections into the laryngeal muscles affected by the spasm, mostly EMG-guided (Kim et al. 2014). The dose used depends on the botulinum toxin preparation and the specific degree of spasm. A cohort study of a 20-year evaluation and at least 20 injections per patient showed that after the first 10 to 15 injections, the dose of botulinum toxin decreases with the duration of treatment before a stabilized dose is found (Namin et al. 2017). Despite worldwide clinical use, the evidence for botulinum toxin treatment of SD is generally only considered to be tentatively positive. A systematic literature review showed that in 13 case studies without control groups (n = 419), significant improvements in perceptual and acoustic measurement methods as well as in self-evaluation of voice-related quality of life could be demonstrated after botulinum toxin injections (van Esch et al. 2017). Further meta-analyses with similarly low EBM study designs of the included studies showed moderate to very significant improvements in multidimensional voice examination parameters through botulinum toxin injections (Whurr et al. 1998; Boutsen et al. 2002; Faham et al. 2021). The study situation regarding randomized controlled study designs is poor, so the treatment recommendation for SD with botulinum toxin can currently only be made based on clinical observation of effectiveness in case studies. The scientific proof through good case-control studies and systematic meta-analyses of the literature is still pending (Watts ct al. 2006). As a last resort, ablative surgical procedures for denervation or muscle resection of the spastic muscle parts are used in cases of significant impairment of quality of life. In Japan, a procedure for distraction of the vocal folds in the anterior commissure with titanium clips is currently being tested, which aims to interrupt the spasm by disrupting the sensory perception of vocal fold contact (Sanuki and Yumoto 2017). All newly diagnosed SD patients should be referred to a neurologist for evaluation of medication therapy options for segmental dystonia.

5.1.6 Sulcus Vocalis

The term sulcus vocalis refers to a groove that runs parallel to the free edge of the vocal fold and represents an area with reduced mucosal mobility (Soni and Dailey 2019). It is a benign anomaly of the vocal folds with varying lengths and depths. In this area, the lamina propria is reduced or absent. The result is a decreased functional capacity of vocal fold vibration (Soni and Dailey 2019).

The severity classification of a sulcus vocalis is usually based on Ford et al. (1996)

A type I sulcus is a depression of the epithelium to the upper layer of the lamina propria. Generally, this type I causes no or only minor functional impacts on phonation and is usually not considered pathological (also referred to as "physiological sulcus" or "superficial sulcus").

A type II sulcus, also called sulcus vergeture, is characterized by a loss of the upper layer of the lamina propria extending to the vocal ligament (middle and deeper layers of the lamina propria).

A type III sulcus is often referred to as a "pit" or "pocket" because it is a focal depression that extends to the vocal ligament (middle and deeper layers of the lamina propria) or deeper.

Older prevalence rates of sulcus vocalis from 1967 to 1998 showed an incidence of 0.4% to 4.9% in post-mortem analyses (Selleck et al. 2015). Later studies confirmed an increase in sulcus malformation from 19.6% to 28.5% across all types and for higher-grade types from 2.1% (type 2), 5.7% (type 3) up to 9% (Selleck et al. 2015). Whether the frequency has truly increased or the analysis has improved remains open.

Comorbid conditions (such as reflux, active rheumatologic diseases, sinus and allergic diseases) that can exacerbate the voice disorder should be considered when deciding on the therapy for sulcus vocalis (Soni and Dailey 2019). A systematic literature review examined the treatment effect of various medical interventions directly on the focal depression (e.g., laser treatments, "cold" surgery, augmentation, regenerative intervention on the lamina propria) or indirectly (e.g., injection laryngoplasty of the vocal fold or type I thyroplasty) (Medeiros et al. 2022). A large heterogeneity was found between the different included study designs (67.8% retrospective cohort studies, 16.1% prospective cohort studies, 12.9% randomized controlled trials, and 3.2% quasi-experimental studies), the different medical treatment techniques, and the multidimensional voice assessment parameters, so currently no preference for a particular procedural technique over another can be justified (Medeiros et al. 2022). Overall, considering a smaller number of exceptions from non-reproduced studies with experimental interventions, a consistent improvement in self-evaluation through various medical interventions was observed (Medeiros et al. 2022). In the other measurement methods from the multidimensional voice assessment (visual analysis, perception, acoustics, and aerodynamics), irregular significant improvements are documented, but overall, there are generally positive improvements in voice function and voice quality (Medeiros et al. 2022). To what extent conservative voice therapy can influence the treatment process preoperatively or postoperatively remains unclear and very variable (Medeiros et al. 2022).

5.1.7 Vocal Fold Scars

Vocal fold scars affect the lamina propria of the vocal fold and can be congenital or acquired. The latter occurs most frequently, such as in surgical vocal fold trauma (Allen 2010). Although sulcus vocalis and vocal fold scars share similar characteristics, vocal fold scars occur two to six times more frequently than a type 2 or type 3 sulcus vocalis (Selleck et al. 2015). According to a systematic literature review, similar to the treatment of sulcus vocalis, no specific medical procedural technique showed a preference for vocal fold scars (Medeiros et al. 2022). However, new medical treatment approaches (e.g., fibrosis-modifying drugs, stem cell therapy, and other tissue engineering approaches) could potentially offer solutions in the future. For the development of these new therapeutic approaches, knowledge of the processes of wound healing and fibrosis formation in the vocal fold wound must be improved (Allen 2021).

5.1.8 Recurrent Respiratory Papillomatosis

Recurrent respiratory (laryngeal) papillomatosis (RRP) is a rare chronic disease caused by human papillomaviruses (HPV) in at least 90% of cases, affecting the larynx and the lower respiratory tract, but less frequently the vocal cords (Coordes et al. 2023). This condition naturally occurs in children from birth (transmission in the birth canal) and in adults secondarily through sexual contact (Coordes et al. 2023). The form of treatment is exclusively medical, with prevention being the primary focus. The HPV immunization introduced for the prevention of cervical cancer in women has led to the greatest oncological progress of the past decades and, despite still unsatisfactory vaccination rates, effectively prevents other HPV-associated genital and anorectal tumor types according to a recent literature study (Henschke et al. 2022). It is often overlooked that this vaccination also provides effective prophylaxis against RRP and its malignancy risks, as well as HPV-associated oropharyngeal carcinomas. Since the introduction of HPV vaccination in Australia (the highest HPV vaccination rate worldwide), the incidence of RRP has been reduced from 0.16 to 0.02 per 100,000 children. In the USA and Europe, the reduction rates are lower due to poorer vaccination rates but are still significant. Even a single HPV immunization, as promoted in developing countries, has the potential to largely prevent this disease (Benedict and Derkay 2021).

In cases of manifest RRP, the standard treatment is microlaryngoscopic surgical removal with or without laser vaporization of the affected tissue (Derkay and Bluher 2019; Coordes et al. 2023). Due to the frequency of recurrences, surgical interventions have been combined with local injection of cidofovir (Grasso et al. 2014), systemic interferon-alpha administration (Gerein et al. 2005), and the use of HPV immunization as a therapeutic measure (Förster et al. 2008), without conclusive evidence of shortening the recurrence intervals.

Repeated surgical procedures to remove papillomas can cause permanent voice and breathing problems due to scarring, thereby impairing quality of life and increasing the severity of dysphonia. The prognosis is generally unfavorable, as recurrences are frequent. It is still unclear whether the recurrences are triggered by a new infection of neighboring cells or reactivation by infected basal cells (Derkay and Bluher 2019; Coordes et al. 2023). There is no evidence from a systematic literature study that reflux worsens the clinical course or tissue characteristics of RRP (San Giorgi et al. 2016). Significant progress in the medical treatment of RRP is currently expected. For aggressive or lung-spread RRP courses, bevacizumab is already being used systemically (Derkay et al. 2023). The efficacy and safety for pediatric patients are good, but the evidence level is currently still at level 5. Case-control studies and meta-analyses must follow. The effect of local application of bevacizumab has not yet been sufficiently proven. The greatest hope lies in the market introduction of a therapeutic vaccine (Lee et al. 2021). Studies on two preparations are currently underway in the USA, which may potentially cure the disease in the future without surgical intervention, thereby preserving the voice.

The greatest danger of RRP is the transformation into malignant laryngeal or tracheobronchial tumors. Meta-analyses have shown that infections of the larynx with HPV significantly increase the risk of developing laryngeal carcinomas (Li et al. 2013; Zhang et al. 2016).

5.1.9 Malignant Laryngeal Tumors

Malignant laryngeal tumors are heterogeneous in their prognosis and treatment. Due to the early symptom of hoarseness, they should be among the carcinomas discovered at the earliest tumor stage. In reality, however, patients often overlook this early symptom, or the tumor is located away from the vocal cords and therefore goes unnoticed. Advances in biological therapy for head and neck tumor treatment have significantly increased scientific interest in the literature (Ferlito et al. 2019).

Therefore, this book only addresses certain general factors to provide an initial overview. The incidence of squamous cell carcinomas of the larynx accounts for about 2% of all malignant tumors (Lorenz 2015). Risk factors of malignant laryngeal tumors include nicotine abuse with an average 6.98-fold (95% CI: 3.14–15.52) increased risk of disease (Gandini et al. 2008), moderate (>1 to <4 drinks per day) to heavy (≥4 drinks per day) alcohol consumption with a 1.5 to 2.5-fold increased risk of disease (Islami et al. 2010; de Menezes et al. 2013), coffee consumption with an average 1.47-fold (95% CI: 1.03–2.11) increased risk of disease (not increased with tea consumption) (Chen and Long 2014), and certain occupations (Bayer et al. 2016) such as production workers (risk factor = 1.3; 95% CI: 1.2–1.4), miners (risk factor = 1.6; 95% CI: 1.2–2.1), tailors (risk factor = 1.7; 95% CI: 1.2–2.3), blacksmiths and toolmakers (risk factor = 1.5; 95% CI: 1.2–1.7), painters (risk factor = 1.4; 95% CI: 1.1–1.9), masons and carpenters (risk factor = 1.3; 95% CI: 1.2–1.5), and certain laryngeal diseases such as chronic laryngitis and the aforementioned RRP (Reiter et al. 2015; see Sect. 5.1.8). Furthermore, significantly more men than women are affected (Steuer et al. 2017).

Compared to other carcinomas, distant metastases are less common at the time of diagnosis. The chances for cure, local tumor control, and resulting quality of life after tumor therapy depend greatly on the primary location, tumor extent, and neck lymph node status, but also on tumor biology and the general condition of the patient. In addition to surgical therapy for tumor and metastasis removal, important treatment pillars include radiation, radio-chemotherapy, and radioimmunotherapy (Lorenz 2015). For locally advanced laryngeal carcinomas, laryngeal preservation is considered if a quality of life-relevant residual function of the organ is expected after radio-chemotherapy and equal chances of cure are seen. If the tumor has already destroyed the function or infiltrated the cartilage, total laryngectomy must still be performed today (Lorenz 2015; Steuer et al. 2017). In the voice rehabilitation of laryngectomized patients, counseling on options should occur before surgery, and voice therapy should consider the patient's suitability for learning esophageal speech. With the introduction of voice shunt valves, the ability to learn good esophageal speech has unfortunately somewhat receded into the background. The advantage of a louder and more fluent replacement voice with a well-functioning voice valve is offset by the disadvantage of permanent dependence on tracheal cannulas, stoma seals, and frequent shunt valve changes. The more frequently the valve is changed, the more often leakage occurs between the fistula and the valve, and in some cases, complicated surgeries for fistula reduction or closure are necessary. Nevertheless, today, in the majority of cases, the decision to place a primary shunt valve is made during the tumor operation. A network meta-analysis confirmed that an older model of silicone voice prostheses is judged by patients to be the best choice, showing the least dislocation and granulation formation (Tawfik et al. 2021). However, patient factors such as radiation dose, nutritional status, stoma hygiene, valve location, and frequency of valve changes play a clinically much larger role than the model of the voice valve.

5.2 Surgical and Medicinal Therapy of Voice Disorders

In principle, surgical interventions, the application of substances to laryngeal structures, and the systemic administration of medications are only considered after exhausting conservative treatment alternatives. A comprehensive treatment plan must be developed for the patient, considering the timing of surgical intervention and the inclusion of supportive therapy forms. Evidence for this can be seen in the fact that for benign vocal cord lesions, a recurrence rate of 13% must be expected after surgical interventions alone. This rate significantly decreases to 7.14% when supportive therapy (e.g., conservative voice therapy) is included (Gocal et al. in press).

5.2.1 Details on Surgical Techniques

Laser Treatment

Internationally, a trend is emerging in laryngology where many treatments traditionally performed in the clinic under general anesthesia are being replaced by outpatient procedures performed on the practice chair (office-based). The reasons lie in the availability of these new options, patient preference, and the significant cost difference between outpatient and inpatient services in various countries. Lasers are finding a growing field of application in this context. Fiber-guided lasers, such as the pulsed dye laser (PDL), the diode laser (Arroyo et al. 2016), KTP laser (532 nm) (Xie et al. 2013), and the blue laser (445 nm) (Hess et al. 2018) enable use through the working channel of a flexible endoscope in mucosal anesthesia on an awake patient. While diode lasers can be used ablatively for hyperkeratoses, leukoplakias (after prior histological confirmation), papillomas, and scars, photoangiolytic lasers, such as KTP and blue laser, offer the possibility to shrink hypervascularized lesions like vascular malformations, laryngeal papillomas, contact granulomas by vessel occlusion, and exudative lesions like Reinke's edema, serous pseudocysts, or edematous polyps by fluid withdrawal. For this purpose, the laser is used in a non-contact mode until the lesion shrinks or the surface discolors "blanching." Repetition of such procedures is possible, allowing for sequential shrinking/removal of benign lesions when microlaryngoscopic excision is not possible due to exposure problems or anesthesia risks, or is rejected by the patient. A combination of laser treatment with the injection of medications for papillomas, scars, polyps, or with augmentation for contact granulomas to treat the underlying glottic closure insufficiency is possible.

Lasers are also used in microlaryngoscopic procedures under general anesthesia. The CO_2 laser has its advantages in the ablation or cutting of tissue while sparing adjacent tissue from overheating. It is used for laryngeal papillomas, synechias in the anterior commissure, laryngomalacia, and for glottic enlargement in bilateral vocal cord paralysis in benign conditions. The main application field of the CO_2 laser is in the endoscopic resection of laryngeal malignancies.

Phonosurgery

At its core, phonosurgery was understood as the microscopic correction of the vibrating edge of the vocal folds with fine microsurgical instruments under optimal magnification of the vocal folds in general anesthesia. With the advancement of technology, endoscope-supported procedures with manipulators, robotics, and 3D technology, and in the broadest sense, office-based laser procedures are now also considered part of phonosurgery (Vasan et al. 2019; Ulmschneider et al. 2020; Bohlender 2021; Arens and Gugatschka 2021). The goal of phonosurgery is the restoration or improvement of vocal function (Zeitels and Healy 2003) through, for example, the removal of benign masses while preserving adjacent structures and maintaining the mucosal cover and vibratory capacity of the vocal fold, correction of non-closable vocal fold sections (such as sulci and scars), removal of edema and excess mucosa as in Reinke's edema, or the reduction or increase of tension and volume of the vocal fold (Remacle et al. 2003). In addition to endolaryngeal microsurgery, larger procedures for the positional correction of the vocal cord, such as type I thyroplasty, arytenoid adduction, and the reconstruction of vocal cord defects or level differences of the vocal folds, as well as transgender procedures, are also part of phonosurgery. Extralaryngeal procedures, such as the non-selective reinnervation of a vocal fold paralyzed by recurrent laryngeal nerve paralysis through an ansa cervicalis nerve anastomosis, also lead to positional correction and re-toning of the vocal fold in the sense of a voice-improving intervention. In the future, neurostimulation of paralyzed vocal folds, currently being tested for bilateral paralysis, will also play a role. Due to the variety of methods, the literature on phonosurgery is dominated by heterogeneous case series. EBM-relevant literature studies exist only for transgender phonosurgery (Song and Jiang 2017), where shortening the vocal folds length in male-to-female trans* is superior, and for the treatment of vocal fold polyps (see Sect. 5.1.2).

Common Surgical Techniques for Benign Vocal Fold Lesions

At the beginning of the section, laser technology was already discussed, and at the end, the consideration of when outpatient interventions on awake patients are appropriate will be addressed. At this point, some typical so-called "cold" surgical techniques of classical phonosurgery in microlaryngoscopic technique will be briefly outlined. A common prerequisite is good exposure of the microsurgically treatable vocal fold sections. For this, a thin ventilation tube, a laryngoscope blade suitable for the individual patient, and optimal reclination of the head must be chosen to fully visualize the findings, usually located in the anterior glottis, under the microscope (Setton et al. 2019).

According to the classification of the European Laryngological Society (ELS) by Remacle et al. (2003), which rather emphasizes the heterogeneity of procedures and nomenclatures than reduces it, the following phonosurgical strategies on the vocal fold can be distinguished (see Tab. 5.1).

An important "cold" surgical procedure is the *incision* of the mucosa to reach underlying structures, such as in the suction of hematomas, edemas, the exposure of subepithelial cysts, pseudocysts, epidermoids, mesenchymal neoplasms such

Tab. 5.1 Classification of phonosurgical procedures of the ELS (Remacle et al. 2003)

Procedures	Comment
Incision	Hematomas, scar webs (congenital/acquired)
Excision (Tissue removal)	Polyps, cysts, epidermoids, scar mucosal bridges, Reinke's edema, vocal process granulomas
Dissection (microflap) (Soft tissue removal)	Scars, sulci, Reinke's edema, defects
Augmentation (Filling)	Atrophy, presbyphonia, paresis
Vaporization	Papillomas, hyperkeratoses, vascular varices
Coagulation (Treatment of bleeding)	Vascular ectasias, granulomas
Injection of pharmaceutical agents (Pharmaceutical injection)	Cortisone for bamboo nodes, granulomas, polyps, botulinum toxin for SD, hyperfunction, antivirals for papillomas
Suction	Reinke's edema, hematomas
Stenting	Scar webs
Mobilization	Cricoarytenoid joint dislocation, fixation

as lipomas, and for the purpose of cutting scar webs (congenital or acquired) and scars. Tiny sickle knives or scissors are usually used for this purpose.

The most important procedure is the *excision* of neoplasms located on the mucosal surface, such as polyps, granulomas, hyperkeratoses, leukoplakias, papillomas, mucosal excesses in Reinke's edema, and mucosal bridges, as well as subepithelial pathologies described in the incision. Tiny, angled, partially triangular grasping forceps, scissors, elevators, and double spoons are used for such procedures.

The *dissection* is another important "cold" surgical procedure, in which the epithelium is separated from subepithelial adhesions, such as in sulcus or scars, using elevators and scissors, Reinke's space compartments are connected, and the mucosa is shifted. In larger defects, such as scars and epithelial defects from previous surgeries, *micro- and miniflaps* of the mucosa are created with the aim of completely re-epithelializing the vocal fold (without excess and without tension) and restoring the vibratory capacity of the free vocal fold edge. These techniques are combined with the coagulation of vascular malformations, the augmentation or filling of local substance defects, and the injection of pharmacological substances. The mucosal wound closure is achieved by natural adhesion, tissue glue, or microsutures. Generally, various procedures are combined in phonosurgery.

Injection

The injection of pharmacologically active substances into the laryngeal muscle or vocal fold structures can be supportive for enhancing and prolonging the effects of phonosurgery, but it can also be performed as an independent procedure. Typical examples include the injection of botulinum toxin into hypertonic laryngeal muscles in spasmodic dysphonia (see Sect. 5.1.5), the local application of antiviral agents or biologics in recurrent laryngeal papillomatosis (see Sect. 5.1.8), as well as the injection of corticosteroid preparations and growth factors, which will be presented below.

To avoid systemic side effects, the intralesional corticosteroid injection for the treatment of vocal fold nodules (Ramavat et al. 2019), bamboo nodes, vocal fold polyps, and partially also Reinke's edema and scars is described in literature (Wang et al. 2015). This approach is justifiable only in cases of immunologically mediated inflammation in the vocal fold tissue, such as in sarcoidosis, lupus erythematosus, granulomatosis with polyangiitis, and bamboo nodes (Imaizumi et al. 2016) and in cases of excessive scar formation.

For vocalis atrophy or presbyphonia, all substances used so far are still in experimental phases or are not approved in Europe. The goal of the treatment is to stimulate fibroblasts, increase the matrix volume, and counteract muscle fiber atrophy. Substances with potential for future use include recombinant human *basic fibroblast growth factor* and mesenchymal stem cells from adipose tissue (Müller 2022).

Augmentation

Voice disorders due to incomplete glottal closure with the main symptom of breathiness may necessitate an intervention to approximate the vocal folds during phonation after exhausting conservative treatment options. Depending on the etiology (atrophy, lack of tension, misalignment due to paralysis or scars), the position of the vocal folds or the volume of the vocal fold in the open glottal gap must be corrected. Only external interventions on the larynx, such as type I thyroplasty with the insertion of a implant into the thyroid cartilage for medialization, arytenoid adduction, or even more invasive laryngeal framework surgeries, are considered for positional correction. For a glottal gap up to 2 mm in vocal fold paralysis (Reiter et al. 2020), presbyphonia, substance defects of the vocal folds, and atrophies, augmentation of the vocal fold, also known as injection laryngoplasty, is considered.

In cases of vocal fold paralysis, absorbable materials such as hyaluronic acid are mostly used for temporary augmentations with an effect duration of up to 3 months. The advantage of early augmentation in unilateral vocal fold paralysis is that supraglottic compensatory mechanisms and often subsequent surgeries such as thyroplasties can be reduced (Reiter et al. 2020; Müller 2022). From a clinical perspective, voice therapy can be initiated 14 days after the augmentation.

Performing these augmentations requires a learning curve to master needle guidance in the awake patient, distribution of the material in the vocal fold, and the correct volume selection. Courses and training programs are helpful (Enver et al. 2021; Shuman and Dwyer 2023). In Germany, the broad application in practice is further complicated by the fact that these procedures are currently not covered by health insurance, so inpatient procedures under anesthesia are usually preferred. For the injection of fat or permanent materials, performing the procedure under general anesthesia using microlaryngoscopy techniques is considered the gold standard from a professional perspective. Permanent augmentations are also helpful for aspiration prevention, for example, in malignant tumors with recurrent nerve paralysis such as esophageal, thyroid, or lung cancer.

Vocal fold medialization with the insertion of Gore-Tex strips, which are very popular in the USA, occupy an intermediate position between augmentation and thyroplasty, but unfortunately, they can lead to inflamatorry reactions in individual cases (Frost and Mirza 2020).

Oral Medication

The prescription of medications for the treatment of voice disorders does not occupy a large space compared to other diseases. Only in the case of proven bacterial infection and inflammatory damage to the larynx due to neighboring inflammations such as sinusitis or bronchitis is the prescription of antibiotics justified. The majority of laryngitis and pharyngitis are caused by viruses and are usually due to pathogens for which no antiviral drugs are available on the market, so the course of the disease must be awaited, the voice must be rested, and symptomatic treatment should be provided (see Sect. 5.1.1).

The administration of corticosteroid preparations is repeatedly discussed and sometimes demanded by patients who are professionally dependent on the timely restoration of their voice function.

According to the current US practice guideline on hoarseness, oral corticosteroids should never be prescribed before laryngoscopic clarification of the underlying condition of the voice disorder (Stachler et al. 2018). Due to the side effects that increase with the duration of intake (Rice et al. 2017), only short-term intake (2–3 days) of oral corticosteroids, e.g., to alleviate hoarseness for professional voice use, is justifiable after excluding contraindications. There is no conclusive evidence for the effectiveness of corticosteroids in shortening hoarseness (Dvorin and Ebell 2020).

Due to the particular risk of causing recurrent laryngeal nerve paresis through thyroid and cervical spine surgeries, the prophylactic administration of dexamethasone has been applied. However, a meta-analysis could not demonstrate risk minimization (Cheng et al. 2015). Today, the gold standard is continuous neuromonitoring of the recurrent laryngeal nerve during thyroid surgeries (Schneider et al. 2020).

To positively influence reinnervation (avoidance of synkinetic reinnervation) in iatrogenic recurrent laryngeal nerve paresis (such as from thyroid or cervical spine surgeries), nimodipine is used (Tian et al. 2022; Mattsson et al. 2018). This approach has not yet been established in clinical practice.

The administration of male sex hormones in female-to-male trans* individuals is a special form of oral medication to influence voice pitch (Cosyns et al. 2014).

5.2.2 Outpatient Intervention vs. Microlaryngoscopy

When weighing outpatient intervention on a locally anesthetized patient versus microlaryngoscopy under general anesthesia, the following aspects must be considered. First, during laryngoscopy, it must be assessed whether a longer laryngoscopy and additional intervention can be tolerated by the patient and whether the examiner has sufficient practical experience and the necessary equipment (instruments, laser, second examiner, endoscope with working channel, etc.) available at that time. Risk factors such as anticoagulant drugs, COPD with oxygen dependency, and circulatory instability must be taken into account. On the other hand, it should also be considered whether the patient has a particular general anesthesia risk and whether the larynx is likely to be well exposed during surgery (which can be difficult with a stiff cervical spine, jaw clamping, or severe sleep apnea). In such cases, flexible endoscopic intervention on the awake patient is less risky.

With minimal gag reflex in the patient, biopsies of vocal fold lesions of unclear dignity and, with sufficient experience, the removal of benign lesions on the awake patient under local anesthesia with curved forceps under magnifying laryngoscopic or flexible endoscopic view are possible. An advantage in such cases can be the immediate auditory control of the treatment effect for findings on the free edge of the vocal folds (Nawka and Hosemann 2005).

If the conditions for office based surgery are not met, microlaryngoscopy under general anesthesia should be performed (see Sect. 5.2.1 in the section on phonosurgery). In cases of suspected malignancy, this procedure can also be combined with a panendoscopy to exclude synchronous secondary carcinomas, as required by oncological guidelines (DGHNO-KHC 2019).

5.2.3 Voice Rest After Phonosurgery

Voice rest after phonosurgery is recommended because the vocal folds begin to heal immediately after the surgical procedure, and this fundamental healing process can last from 4 to 14 days (Ishikawa and Thibeault 2010). Therefore, absolute voice rest is necessary during this critical phase to prevent further trauma to the vocal folds, facilitate the healing of the mucous membranes, and limit scar formation (Kaneko and Hirano 2017). In clinical practice, it is observed that most physicians advise their voice patients to have 7 days of absolute voice rest or a combination of absolute and relative voice rest after surgery for benign lesions (Joshi and Johns 2018). However, an initial meta-analysis of randomized controlled trials ($n = 4$) showed that there are no significant differences in follow-up multidimensional voice assessment between longer ($\geq$7 days) and shorter (<7 days) voice rest (Chi et al. 2023). However, further studies are needed to determine the optimal duration and extent of postoperative voice rest.

5.2.4 Voice Disorders as a Side Effect of Medications

Pharmacological therapies can conversely cause voice disorders as a side effect. Important substances that should be queried in the medication history of a voice patient include inhaled corticosteroids in asthma therapy, substances that alter the mucous film in the throat and larynx ("drying" substances), such as anticholinergics, antihistamines, decongestants (decongestant nasal drops), contraceptives and antihypertensives (Stachler et al. 2018).

5.3 Conservative Voice Therapy

5.3.1 Concepts in Conservative Voice Therapy

In the 1930s, Van Riper described four basic principles of voice therapy (Van Riper 1939): First, a voice problem must be recognized by the patient themselves. Second, a new and appropriate voice sound should be produced. Third, the new voice behavior should be stabilized in different contexts. Fourth, the new voice behavior should be habituated in all situations. These early basic principles of voice rehabilitation have since evolved into several management concepts, which can be categorized as follows: indirect voice therapy (voice hygiene/voice care), symptomatic voice therapy, physiological voice therapy, psychogenic voice therapy, device-assisted aids in voice therapy, and eclectic voice therapy. These treatment concepts are explained in more detail in the following sections.

Vocal Hygiene (Indirect Voice Therapy)

Hygienic voice therapy, voice care, or indirect voice therapy focuses on exploring the causes of voice disorders in conversation with the patient (Stemple et al. 2014). Some examples of behaviors that constitute poor vocal hygiene are shouting, loud speaking, frequent coughing, throat clearing, insufficient fluid intake, smoking, alcohol abuse, etc. When poor vocal hygiene behaviors are identified, vocal symptoms can improve even without direct voice techniques or exercises for the subsystems of the voice (i.e., respiration, phonation, and resonance) (Stemple et al. 2014). This type of therapy aims to incorporate healthy vocal behaviors into the patient's habitual speech patterns. Good vocal hygiene also ensures the health of the vocal fold surface through adequate internal hydration and reduction of airborne pollutants. Evidence on vocal hygiene has been researched for individual vocal hygiene training, group vocal hygiene training, and specific goals in vocal hygiene (e.g., fluid intake, quiet coughing, and voice rest) (Thomas and Stemple 2007). However, vocal hygiene as a standalone therapy is less successful in treating heterogeneous voice disorders compared to direct voice therapy (Barsties v. Latoszek et al. 2020, 2023a, b). Various network meta-analyses have shown that vocal hygiene, compared to various voice therapies, did not exhibit a statistically significant therapeutic effect in treating adults with dysphonia. It ranks among the top-3 in low-ranking evaluations using VHI (mean difference = −7.00; 95% confidence interval = −15.35 to 1.34) (Barsties v. Latoszek et al. 2020) and maximum phonation time (mean difference = 1.36; 95% confidence interval = −4.81 to 7.54) (Barsties v. Latoszek et al. 2023a, b).

However, vocal hygiene seems to be of greater importance in the treatment of juvenile vocal fold nodules, as comparable results in various multidimensional measurement parameters of direct and indirect voice therapy have been demonstrated (Hartnick et al. 2018).

Additionally, the combination of indirect and direct voice therapy or the integration of vocal hygiene into comprehensive eclectic voice therapy programs seems to be an effective method to comprehensively treat a voice disorder (Ruotsalainen et al. 2008; Stemple et al. 2014).

Symptomatic Voice Therapy

Symptomatic voice therapy focuses on changing the symptoms of a voice disorder or the unfavorable voice components identified during voice diagnostics (Stemple et al. 2014), such as habitual inefficient pitch or intensity, breathy phonation, glottal fry, etc. (Boone et al. 2010). Symptomatic voice therapy is based on the assumption that most voice disorders are caused by functional misuse of voice components (e.g., respiration, phonation, resonance) or by hyperfunctional dysphonia (Stemple et al. 2014). In this therapy, the voice therapist uses facilitating techniques (i.e., direct voice therapy techniques) to help the patient find and use their best voice production. It is a continuous trial-and-error process to find the voice that sounds appropriate or normal and that the patient can produce with relatively low effort. Some supportive techniques (e.g., humming) have been evaluated separately and showed good short-term results in the therapy of non-structural (Ogawa et al. 2013, 2014) and structural voice disorders (Yiu and Ho 2002; Vlot et al. 2017). However, the evidence for the effectiveness of this approach is still insufficient for the following reasons: First, case studies were often reported (Brodnitz and Fröschels 1954; McFarlane 1988; Fisher and Logemann 1970); second, no specific method for improving the voice was identified (Aghadoost et al. 2020); third, in some studies, voice-improving techniques were tested only on vocally healthy subjects (Boone and McFarlane 1993; Meerschman et al. 2016a, b, 2017). In summary, all these techniques have been used clinically for many years, but the effectiveness of this form of therapy as an initial treatment for heterogeneous voice disorders according to EBM criteria appears to be insufficient for most of the single techniques to be used as a stand-alone therapy.

Physiological Voice Therapy

Physiological voice therapy includes voice exercises that directly change or modify the physiology of the voice mechanism. Normal voice production depends on the balance and coordination between airflow (i.e., the supply by the respiratory system), laryngeal muscles, endurance, and supraglottic resonance structures of the pharynx, oral cavity, and nasal cavity (Stemple et al. 2014). The change in voice production can be the result of disturbances in physiological balance.

These disturbances can affect the respiratory system (e.g., volume, performance, pressure, and flow), the phonation system (e.g., vocal fold tone, mass, stiffness, flexibility, and glottal closure), and the resonance system (e.g., coupling of the supraglottic resonators with each other and the subglottic resonator as well as tone placement). The cause can be mechanical, neurological, or psychological. In this type of voice therapy concept, causality is secondary, as the voice exercises directly change the inappropriate physiological activity. Most physiological voice therapy programs that take a holistic approach attempt to balance the three subsystems of voice production simultaneously: for example, the Vocal Function Exercises (Angadi et al. 2019), approaches of resonance voice therapy (Yiu et al. 2017), and the accent method (Thyme-Frøkjær and Frøkjær-Jensen 2014). These physiological concepts of voice therapy are currently fundamentally better supported in research than other forms of voice therapy (Stemple et al. 2014; Barsties v. Latoszek 2020a).

Psychogenic Voice Therapy

Psychogenic voice therapy is based on the assumption of underlying emotional or psychosocial behavioral causes or psychogenic trigger situations of voice problems (Stemple et al. 2014). Additionally, patients with psychogenic voice disorders may also have a conversion disorder, where the patient is convinced that the cause of the voice disorder is organic, although there is no basis for this assumption. There is an unconscious inner conflict of the patient, which is maintained by the factor of stress (unconscious emotions are usually suppressed anger) (van Harten and Schutte 1992).

On the one hand, psychogenic voice therapy focuses on identifying and changing the emotional and psychosocial disorders associated with the occurrence and persistence of voice disorders (Aronson 1980; Colton and Casper 1996). The interventions include conversational and counseling techniques to address the psychogenic causes or identify triggers that can lead to an improvement in voice problems. A therapist must be able to recognize when the emotional or psychosocial problem requires more intensive evaluation and therapy by other disciplines (e.g., psychotherapists).

On the other hand, in cases of psychogenic aphonia, the symptom can also be treated directly by starting from natural and unconscious vocalization fragments (such as coughing or throat clearing), which usually lead to phonation. Subsequently, the duration of this vocalization is extended, requiring a longer exhalation, preferably through abdominal breathing. Hierarchically, the voice is built up at the sound level, syllable level, word level, text level, and spontaneous speech level (van Harten and Schutte 1992; Aronson 1980).

The evidence for the therapy of psychogenic voice disorder is low (Miller et al. 2014; Gray et al. 2024). A systematic literature review on this topic showed that there is a high heterogeneity of interventions and measurement instruments used. The study quality of the included studies ($n = 23$) was overall low to critical, as many cohort and case studies lacked control groups, blinding, and robust measurements (Gray et al. 2024).

However, patients diagnosed with a psychogenic voice disorder can be successfully treated with various voice exercises from other voice therapy approaches. While direct voice therapy alone does not effectively treat all voice patients or prevent a recurrence of dysphonia, this suggests that a more holistic approach, including psychotherapy, may be necessary (Tezcaner et al. 2019).

Device-Assisted Aids in Voice Therapy

In modern voice therapy, the use of devices or other aids is very popular. They can be used to treat various voice symptoms (e.g., voice amplifiers) or to support or promote the voice (e.g., Water Resistance Therapy, transcutaneous electrical nerve stimulation, or external local vibration).

Speaking loudly against noise, improper vocalization, or shouting occur more frequently in certain professions (such as teachers) and can cause voice problems (Ziegler et al. 2010). An adequately high voice intensity can be limited in diseases such as vocal fold paralysis. Instrumental voice amplification is a form of indirect voice therapy when the phonation volume is insufficient for daily speaking or in certain professional situations. Evidence for voice improvements through voice amplifiers has currently been investigated in teachers with dysphonia (Roy et al. 2002, 2003; Bovo et al. 2013; Teixeira and Behlau 2015; Masson and de Araújo 2018). This professional group has a higher risk of developing voice disorders than others (Roy et al. 2004; Thibeault et al. 2004). In almost all studies, voice amplification over 4 to 12 weeks led to significant improvements (Roy et al. 2002, 2003; Bovo et al. 2013; Teixeira and Behlau 2015). Some studies also reported improvements in perceptual voice quality assessment (Roy et al. 2002, 2003; Bovo et al. 2013) and in acoustic analyses (Roy et al. 2002), but no improvements in stroboscopy (Teixeira and Behlau 2015). In summary, voice amplifiers improve voice function in teachers with dysphonia when used continuously.

Water Resistance Therapy (WRT) is a form of Semi-Occluded Vocal Tract Exercises (SOVTE). In this, a tube is used to produce sound, with one end submerged in water. SOVTE are attributed with the following effects: a) generation of high acoustic impedance (Story et al. 2000; Titze and Laukkanen 2007), b) promotion of vocal efficiency, based on the ratio of oral acoustic output power to aerodynamic subglottic input power (Titze and Laukkanen 2007), c) achieving high vocal economy (Titze and Laukkanen 2007), expressed by the ratio of maximized vocal output to minimized intraglottal impact stress (Titze 2002, 2006), d) an altered configuration of the vocal tract, such as a lower vertical laryngeal position, a stronger narrowing of the aryepiglottic folds, and a wider pharynx (Guzman et al. 2013). High vocal economy is associated with minimal respiratory effort and muscle strain of the larynx, as well as effortless voice production and a healthy voice (Laukkanen et al. 2009). In WRT, it is additionally assumed that the fluctuations of supraglottic pressure associated with bubbling modulate the vibrations of the vocal folds and relax the walls of the vocal tract, which could be interpreted as a massage effect (Enflo et al. 2013; Radolf et al. 2014; Granqvist et al. 2015; Wistbacka et al. 2016). Furthermore, it is assumed that WRT promotes blood circulation, which could be associated with a massage and healing effect (Enflo et al. 2013). WRT led to more pronounced changes in various laryngoscopic variables compared to most other SOVT exercises (Guzman et al. 2013). These results were confirmed in an MRI study (Yamasaki et al. 2017). Here, the experimental group—women with vocal fold nodules—showed a greater distance between the epiglottis and the posterior pharyngeal wall after WRT than the control group. Additionally, a larger area of the laryngeal vestibule was observed, while the inclination of the vocal folds decreased due to a lower elevation of the anterior commissure of the larynx.

In view of the numerous studies on the underlying physiology of WRT, there is some evidence of its clinical therapeutic efficacy (Batista et al. 2024). Mainly, functional dysphonia has been investigated in individual studies. The results showed significant improvements in auditory-perceptual assessment (Simberg et al. 2006; Paes et al. 2013; Guzman et al. 2017), self-evaluation (Simberg et al. 2006; Paes et al. 2013; Guzman et al. 2017), and aerodynamic parameters (Guzman et al. 2017) after WRT. This therapy form will be revisited later, as data from meta-analyses are already available to further assess the effect of this voice therapy (see Sect. 5.3.2).

Transcutaneous electrical nerve stimulation (TENS) is a non-invasive procedure used to alleviate pain symptoms in various clinical situations. Additionally, it is used to promote muscle relaxation, improve local vascularization, and reduce muscle hyperactivity (Sluka and Walsh 2003; Santos et al. 2016; Gibson et al. 2019). Typically, two types of TENS settings are applied in clinical practice: low frequency ($\leq$10 Hz) and high frequency ($\geq$50 Hz). Low-frequency TENS induces muscle contractions, while high-frequency TENS inhibits discomfort. However, both mechanisms produce similar effects in analgesia (Sluka and Walsh 2003; Gibson et al. 2019). In the voice treatment of dysphonia patients, TENS is used to reduce the muscle tone of the cervical and perilaryngeal muscles, which can lead to an improvement in voice quality (Alves Silverio et al. 2015; Mansuri et al. 2020). The effectiveness of this technology is based on a reduction in pain and an improvement in voice quality when used in combination with voice exercises (Mansuri et al. 2020). A systematic review of the effectiveness of TENS in voice treatment confirmed positive results in 7 out of 8 included studies (Stangherlin et al. 2021). Low-frequency TENS of 200 μs and 10 Hz was used for 20 minutes with variable stimulus intensity depending on the sensitivity of the users. As a result, pain in several areas (e.g., neck, shoulders, back, masseter muscle, larynx) decreased, the auditory-perceptual assessment of several voice quality parameters (e.g., strain, breathiness, roughness, instability, asthenia), and various types of discomfort in the larynx (e.g., burning, lump in the throat, and effort when speaking) decreased after TENS treatment (Stangherlin et al. 2021).

External local vibration is also a non-invasive procedure for successful pain treatment (Lundeberg et al. 1984, 1987; Lundeberg 1984). Additionally, it promotes movement, motor activity, and motor learning after a stroke (Tavernese et al. 2013). Finally, external local vibration can also reduce muscle tension and spasticity in neurological disorders (Murillo et al. 2014; Caliandro et al. 2012; Casale et al. 2014). Mechanical oscillating vibration devices can either promote or inhibit muscle activity when applied externally to a muscle or tendons (Bishop 1974, 1975). High-frequency vibrations (e.g., 100 Hz) are known to induce a tonic response such as muscle contraction (Bishop 1974, 1975; Clark 2003), while low-frequency vibrations (e.g., 20–50 Hz) inhibit muscle activity and facilitate the release of hypertonic muscle tension (Bishop 1974, 1975; Homma 1973). Local vibration activates three physiological effects, which are believed to have additional benefits in the treatment of voice disorders. First, vibration on the skin surface stimulates deeper mechanoreceptors (Hansson and Lundeberg 1993), which, according to the gate control theory of pain (non-painful input closes the "nerve gates" to painful input, preventing the pain sensation from being transmitted to the central nervous system), allows for high selectivity of the involved sensors (Melzack and Wall 1965) to treat symptoms such as odynophonia.

Second, local vibration triggers a muscle contraction via the stretch reflex (Ritzmann et al. 2010). It is believed that this increases physical performance, especially through type II muscle fibers (Rittweger et al. 2000). Type II fibers have a high concentration in the vocalis muscle and the cricothyroid muscle (Hoh 2005), which regulate glottal closure and vocal fold tension.

In voice therapy, for example, the Novafon device (Novafon GmbH, Weinstadt) has been successfully evaluated. It is a sound wave appliance for local vibration therapy. Its mechanical vibrations penetrate six centimeters deep into the tissue (Fuchs et al. 1984). On the one hand, local vibration with the Novafon device was investigated in the treatment of vocal fatigue (Yiu et al. 2021). The cause of vocal fatigue is, among other things, excessive tension of the perilaryngeal muscles (Solomon 2008), which impairs laryngeal alignment, for example, during the production of high-pitched tones. Furthermore, the viscosity of the vocal fold tissue can increase, and the mucosal wave propagation can be impaired in individuals with vocal fatigue, making the phonation of soft and high pitches difficult (Milbrath and Solomon 2003). The performance of vocal functions improved in subjects with vocal fatigue after vibration therapy, suggesting that vibrations reduce excessive muscle tension and increase blood flow and metabolism in the fatigued muscles (Yiu et al. 2021). Reduced blood flow to the larynx could be a possible underlying physiological mechanism contributing to vocal fatigue (Welham and Maclagan 2003). If blood flow to the muscles is increased, lactic acid could be broken down (Clark et al. 1998), which can lead to improved recovery from muscle fatigue.

On the other hand, further studies have found that the combination of voice exercises and the Novafon sound wave appliance (Novafon Local Vibration Voice Therapy Program [NLVVT]) reduces the severity of a voice disorder (Barsties v. Latoszek 2020a, b). Furthermore, it was shown that the voice quality improved significantly more in combination with the Novafon sound wave appliance and voice exercises than with voice exercises alone (Barsties v. Latoszek 2020b). In a single case, symptoms of a superior nerve paresis also improved through NLVVT (Barsties v. Latoszek and Watts 2021).

The NLVVT is described in more detail in Sect. 5.3.2, as data from meta-analyses are already available here to further assess the effect of this voice therapy.

Eclectic Voice Therapy

Eclectic voice therapy is a combination of all the concepts described above. The clinical decision on which type and form of voice therapy to use depends on the therapist, who employs a selection of voice therapy techniques that seem suitable for successful treatment of the individual patient. Although the diagnoses of voice patients can be classified into certain treatment groups, the personalities, vocal needs, emotional and/or compensatory responses, and causes of the patients' voice problems are different. Therefore, various therapy approaches are required to treat patients with the same voice pathology. The applicability of a wide range of voice therapy techniques is, in most cases, dependent on the individualization, skills, and experience of the therapist.

In general, eclectic voice therapy approaches are undefined in studies because, on the one hand, no standardization takes place or has taken place (e.g., van Gogh et al. 2006; Stier 2011) and, on the other hand, only essential features, exercises, or specific methods are specifically mentioned (e.g., Schindler et al. 2008; Zhuge et al. 2016). A precise hierarchical structure with frequency, duration, and procedure is rare, as previously described, the choice and adaptation of voice treatment forms are freely tailored to the individual patient. An eclectic concept form examined in meta-analyses is the Comprehensive Vocal Rehabilitation Program from Brazil. This is a therapy model based on the consolidation and experiences of the Brazilian Larynx Institute of the 1970s, the Ambulatories of Larynx and Voice of Universidade Federal de São Paulo, and the Center for the Study of Voice of the 1990s (Behlau et al. 2013). This approach was mainly developed for functional voice disorders and is a holistic voice therapy concept. Further details on this voice therapy concept are explained in Sect. 5.3.2.

5.3.2 Voice Therapy Programs Based on Systematic Literature Studies: EBP

Programs or methods for voice treatment with a clear hierarchy, which use direct voice therapies or voice exercises in the treatment, mostly follow the concept of physiological voice therapy. This conclusion was reached by a literature study, in which significant improvements in stroboscopy, voice quality, voice function, and self-perception were shown in 9 out of 17 voice therapy methods (Barsties v. Latoszek 2020a). The duration of these voice therapy methods ranged from one day to ten weeks. The most frequently investigated voice therapy method with 13 studies was the Vocal Function Exercises (VFE). This method can be used for heterogeneous voice disorders and contains only four exercises (see later section on VFE). Other evaluated physiological voice therapy methods were the Accent Method, the Stretch-and-Flow Phonation (SFP), and two approaches to resonance therapy (Lessac-Madsen Resonant Voice Therapy and Stemple's Resonance Therapy) (Barsties v. Latoszek 2020a).

A more specialized form of voice therapy is the manual approach, which improves the physiology of voice production and individual symptoms or laryngeal discomfort such as the globus sensation. If one were to classify the manual approach in voice therapy among the previously mentioned treatment concepts, it would most likely be counted as symptomatic voice therapy (Barsties v. Latoszek et al. 2024). The most evaluated manual voice therapy approach is the Manual Circumlaryngeal Therapy according to Roy (2008) for the treatment of primary and secondary hyperfunctional voice disorders (Barsties v. Latoszek et al. 2024) and puberphonia (Barsties v. Latoszek 2021).

In reviewing further systematic literature studies for the evaluation of voice therapies in voice disorders, the following 39 studies up to September 2023 could be identified in the English-language bibliographic database Pubmed (Medline) of the *National Library of Medicine* (sorted chronologically):

> Speyer (2008), *Ruotsalainen et al.* (2008), Ziegler et al. (2010), Van Houtte et al. (2011), Eastwood et al. (2015), Walton et al. (2017), Yiu et al. (2017), Desjardins et al. (2017), da Cunha Pereira et al. (2018), Mansuri et al. (2018), ***Ribeiro et al.*** (2018),***Angadi et al.*** (2019), Alves et al. (2019), Desjardins and Bonilha (2020), ***Barsties v. Latoszek et al.*** (2020),*Alegria et al.* (2020a), Alegria et al. (2020b), ***Yuan et al.*** (2020),*Alegria et al.* (2021), Feinstein and Abbott (2021), *Kim* (2021), *Nolan et al.* (2019),***Pu et al.*** (2021), Stangherlin et al. (2021), Adriaansen et al. (2022), Al-Kadi et al. (2022), Almeida et al. (2022), Vermeulen et al. (2022), ***Barsties v. Latoszek et al.*** (2023a), *Barsties v. Latoszek et al.* (2023b), ***Barsties v. Latoszek and Hetjens*** (2023), Lester-Smith et al. (2023), *Schwarz et al.* (2023), Bhatt et al. (2023), White et al. (2023), Gray et al. (2024), *Pozzali et al.* (2024),***Barsties v. Latoszek et al.*** (2024), Batista et al. (2024).

Only 16 out of 39 systematic literature reviews also included a meta-analysis (italicized), of which only 8 of the 16 studies (bold and italicized) were applied and analyzed on specific voice therapy methods.

These 8 meta analyses of specific voice therapy methods yielded demonstrable results for various voice disorders and their indications

1. Ribeiro et al. (2018) analyzed in their meta-analysis the approach of laryngeal manual therapy according to Mathieson et al. (2009) from two RCT studies out of 2128 studies (excluding duplicates), in which the perceptual degree of hoarseness and the intensity of voice and laryngeal paraesthesia were evaluated. The treatment effect of laryngeal manual therapy from this meta-analysis showed no significant differences compared to the control groups of TENS or voice training (such as tongue or lip trills, humming, overarticulation, and chewing).
2. Angadi et al. (2019) identified three voice diagnostic parameters from a total of 21 included studies for the evaluation of VFE, most of which were case-control studies in their meta-analysis. Firstly, the results from the meta-analysis confirmed a significant improvement in VHI through VFE treatment. An effect size, summarized from four studies, showed a mean VHI-T difference of about -10 points after VFE treatment. However, at

least 13 points between pre- and post-treatment are required to confirm a clinically significant improvement (as described in Sect. 2.5). Secondly, another questionnaire on voice-related quality of life, which has a comparable focus to the VHI, was analyzed. This questionnaire also confirmed a significant treatment effect through VFE. Finally, the maximum phonation time was examined. A significant mean increase of 6.5 seconds after VFE voice therapy was measured.

However, the evidence level of this meta-analysis is somewhat lower, as only a few RCT studies were included and important quantitative information such as heterogeneity, publication bias, overall effect, and confidence intervals are missing.

3. Barsties v. Latoszek et al. (2020) examined in one of the first network meta-analyses on voice therapies a ranking of 8 voice therapy methods from 13 RCT studies considering the measurement parameter VHI-T. A total of n = 389 in the intervention groups and n = 51 from a control group of dysphonic patients, who either received no voice therapy or a sham therapy, were identified. The results showed that the voice therapy Stretch and Flow Phonation (mean difference = −28.37 points), resonance therapy (mean difference = -21.84 points), the Comprehensive Voice Rehabilitation Program (mean difference = −22.01 points), and Vocal Function Exercises (mean difference = −13.00 points) effectively improved the VHI-T value, with Stretch and Flow Phonation ranking first and exceeding the clinical significance of the necessary difference including the 95% confidence interval between pre- and post-treatment of 13 points in VHI-T as the only method in this study. Other voice therapy approaches such as respiratory muscle training, water resistance therapy, lip trills, voice hygiene, and SOVTE with the straw and its distal end in the air did not lead to significant or clinically relevant treatment effects in the VHI result. Thus, this first presented network meta-analysis was able to filter the number of effective interventions from a larger pool of voice therapy approaches for individuals with predominantly functional voice disorders, which were based on the self-assessment of a perceived vocal handicap, and conduct an initial efficacy proof with a ranking.
4. Yuan et al. (2020) explored the effectiveness of the Lee Silverman Voice Treatment (LSVT) in patients with Parkinson's disease suffering from dysarthrophonia, which includes vocal parameters as key symptoms in communication, such as loudness and self-evaluation. Only RCT studies were considered, which included another voice therapy concept (e.g., respiratory therapy) or no therapy as control groups to LSVT. A total of 8 out of 505 studies (excluding duplicates) were used for the meta-analysis. After 1 month of LSVT, significant improvements in intensity from an average of 3.31 dB to 8.87 dB were observed in all voice production variants (sustained phonation to conversational speech). This effect is

still present after 6 to 7 months. No significant difference in the improvement of volume between online therapy or in-person therapy was found. Compared to breathing therapy, LSVT proved to be more effective in improving loudness in all voice production variants (3.19 dB to 13.39 dB) after 1 month of therapy. The effect of LSVT therapy seems to be more successful over another 6 to 24 months compared to respiratory therapy, but this effect was only demonstrated in one study. In addition to the improvement in volume, the VHI values also significantly improved after 1 to 3 months through LSVT compared to no therapy (VHI-T: mean difference = −15.91 points [95% confidence interval = −20.22 points to −11.59 points]).

5. Pu et al. (2021) also investigated the effectiveness of LSVT in Parkinson's disease. Only RCT studies were considered, in which the control group consisted of patients with other voice therapy or no therapy. In this study, as in Yuan et al. (2020), a significant improvement in loudness through LSVT compared to no therapy or breathing therapy was observed (*immediately after treatment:* mean difference = 7.36 dB [95% confidence interval = 6.60 dB to 8.12 dB]; *after 1 to 6 months:* mean difference = 5.19 dB [95% confidence interval = 3.23 dB to 7.15 dB]; *after 6 to 12 months:* mean difference = 3.88 dB [95% confidence interval = 2.60 dB to 5.16 dB]). The VHI-T evaluations also yielded comparable results to Yuan et al. (2020), which also showed a significantly stronger improvement after LSVT compared to the control groups. Additionally, this study evaluated the semitone range aspect of the speaking voice range and other questionnaires on functional communication (such as intelligibility) in Parkinson's disease. It appears that the speaking melody during reading significantly expands after LSVT compared to control groups, but not significantly during conversational speech. Other communication aspects from the self-evaluation questionnaires as well as the VHI also achieved significantly better values after LSVT compared to the control groups.
6. Barsties v. Latoszek et al. (2023a) investigated in a second network meta-analysis the ranking of 8 voice therapy methods from 12 RCT studies considering the measurement parameter MPT. A total of n = 285 in the intervention groups and n = 62 from a control group of dysphonic patients, who either received no voice therapy or a sham therapy, were identified. Only Vocal Function Exercises (mean difference = 6.16 sec [95% confidence interval = 1.18 sec to 11.13 sec]) achieved an effective improvement and clinical significance of the necessary difference including the 95% confidence interval between pre- and post-treatment. This result in the mean difference also corresponds to the research result of Angadi et al. (2019). Other approaches to voice therapy such as respiratory therapy, accent method, finger kazoo, Liuzijue Qigong, resonance therapy, stretch and flow phonation, and voice hygiene did not lead

to significant or clinically relevant treatment effects in the MPT result. It thus seems that an improvement in MPT can only be achieved if it is specifically practiced and integrated into the therapy. In the VFE approach, MPT is an essential component, where patients control their phonation (in exercises No. 1 and No. 4 and home exercises) by sustaining a sound (usually lip buzzing on the modified vowel /o/) as long as possible. The VFE therapy thus has a positive impact on MPT measurements by increasing the strength of the inspiratory muscles and improving muscular coordination, strength, and endurance during exhalation compared to other voice therapy methods.

7. Barsties v. Latoszek and Hetjens (2023) investigated in this network meta-analysis the treatment effect of two different therapy approaches with device-assisted aids in voice therapy on voice-related quality of life with the four different areas of the VHI (see Sect. 2.5). For this purpose, 5 out of 65 studies (without duplicates) were selected, which examined the therapy effect in Water Resistance Therapy ($n = 42$) and Novafon Local Vibration Voice Therapy ($n = 22$). Both therapies showed highly significant improvements in all subareas of the VHI ($p < 0.01$), but in direct comparison, NLVVT achieved significantly stronger results in three areas than WRT ($p < 0.01$). Only in the physical subaspect of the VHI (VHI-P) there was no significant difference ($p = 0.28$). Additionally, NLVVT as well as Stretch and Flow Phonation achieved the clinical significance of a necessary difference including the 95% confidence interval between pre- and post-treatment of over 13 points in the VHI-T (mean difference = −23.893 points [95% confidence interval = −29.387 points to −18.398 points]).
   Although in a first network meta-analysis by Barsties v. Latoszek et al. (2020) the improvement of the VHI-T through Water Resistance Therapy was determined to be minor compared to other therapy variants, this new study, considering newer study results on the VHI-T (mean difference = −17.385 points [95% confidence interval= −24.121 points to −10.649 points]), was able to demonstrate highly significant improvements in all aspects of the VHI (p-values< 0.01).
8. Barsties v. Latoszek et al. (2024) investigated the effect of Manual Circumlaryngeal Therapy in patients with functional dysphonia. The acoustics were checked regarding voice quality and SRP-F0 during sustained phonation. For this purpose, six out of an initial 30 studies (excluding duplicates) from the systematic literature search were included, with a patient range of $n = 65$ to 119 for the individual measurement parameters, with predominantly women being examined. Basically, a large treatment effect for the improvement of acoustic voice quality parameters could be achieved with this manual therapy method ($d > 0.8$). However, this effect could only be significantly demonstrated for two out of three

measurement parameters (shimmer and harmonics-to-noise ratio) ($p < 0.05$) when natural variability fluctuations in the voice during single and multiple voice recordings (test-retest studies), as investigated by Pierce et al. (2021), are taken into account. A change in the SRP-F0 is not to be expected in functional dysphonia through Manual Circumlaryngeal Therapy.

The voice therapy methods and approaches that have been classified as effective from the meta-analyses described above are compactly presented in the following sections in terms of form, content, structure, objectives, indication, duration and frequency, and difficulties/risks/contraindications. They serve as a basis for the therapist to inform themselves about the individual interventions with a high level of evidence in voice therapy. With this basic knowledge from the following overview for practical application, an initial aid for therapists is to be provided.

Vocal Function Exercises
Description
The Vocal Function Exercises are a physiological voice therapy program that trains the laryngeal muscles through conditioning training at the sound level using lip buzzing, lip trills, or tongue trills (Stemple et al. 2014). This program includes only 4 basic exercises related to pitch changes (glides) and maximum sound prolongation (max. phonation time).

These exercises consider 3 main components for phonation: respiration, phonation, and resonance. A high coordination of these mechanisms is promoted, leading to maximum vocal performance with minimal effort.

A demonstration video from Prof. Dr. Joseph Stemple's DVD on VFE can be found, for example, at https://www.pluralpublishing.com/publications/vocal-function-exercises.

Additionally, all VFE exercises including instructions are prepared as audio recordings by the first author of the book and made available for streaming, offering a self-explanatory application for female and male patients and/or therapists (see section: Structure/Instruction).

Objectives

- Minimize strain/tension in the laryngeal area
- Strengthening and coordination of the laryngeal muscles
- Improvement of the efficiency between airflow, vocal fold movement, and supraglottic preparation for phonation can be enabled

Indication

- Heterogeneous voice disorders
- Pathological objective voice quality
- Reduced quality of life
- Increased VHI
- Shortened max. phonation time

Structure/Instruction

General introduction to VFE (see Fig. 5.1)

1. Exercise 1: Warm-Up (see Figs. 5.2 and 5.3)

Introduction to the vocal technique of lip buzzing (Lip Buzz) (see Fig. 5.4)

2. Exercise 2: Stretching (see Fig. 5.5)
3. Exercise 3: Contraction (see Fig. 5.6)

Introduction to the last and most important exercise of VFE (see Fig. 5.7)

4. Exercise 4: Power Exercise

Tone C (see Figs. 5.8 and 5.9)
Tone D (see Figs. 5.10 and 5.11)
Tone E (see Figs. 5.12 and 5.13)
Tone F (see Figs. 5.14 and 5.15)
Tone G (see Figs. 5.16 and 5.17)

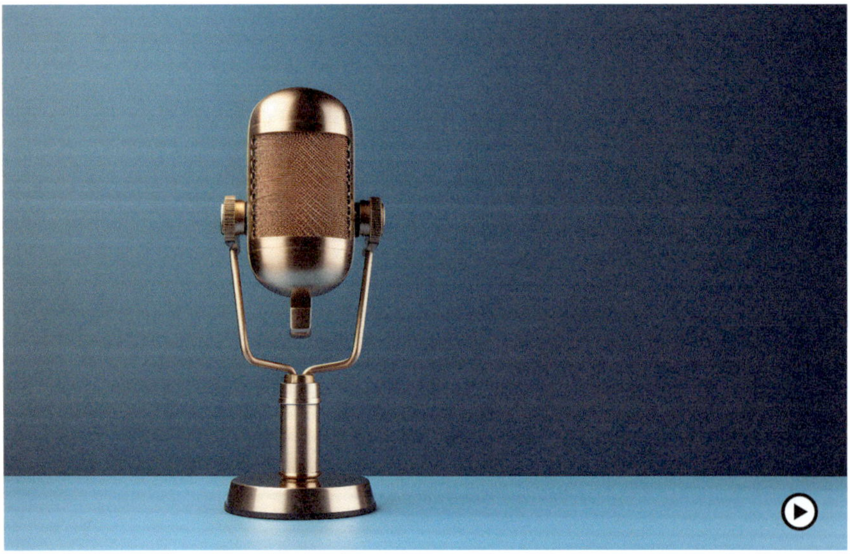

Fig. 5.1 General introduction to VFE (▶ https://doi.org/10.1007/000-dx9)

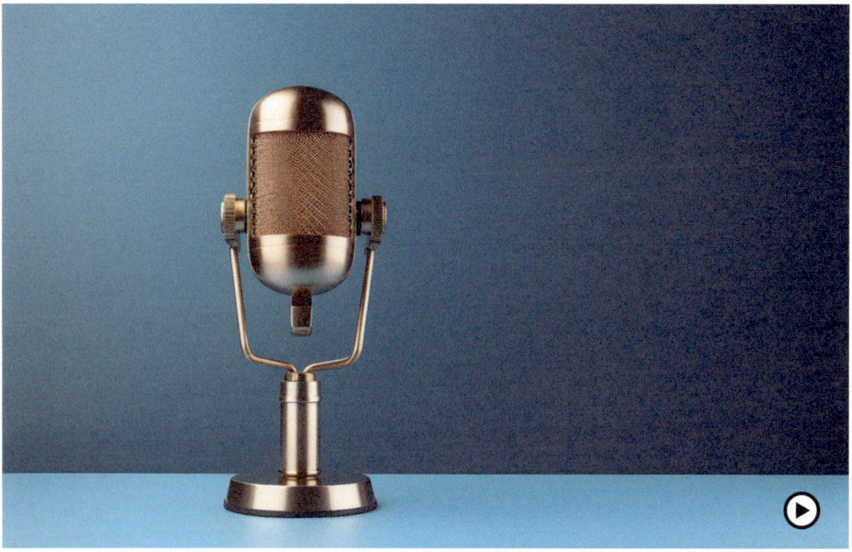

Fig. 5.2 VFE – Exercise 1: Warm-Up for Women (▸ https://doi.org/10.1007/000-dwv)

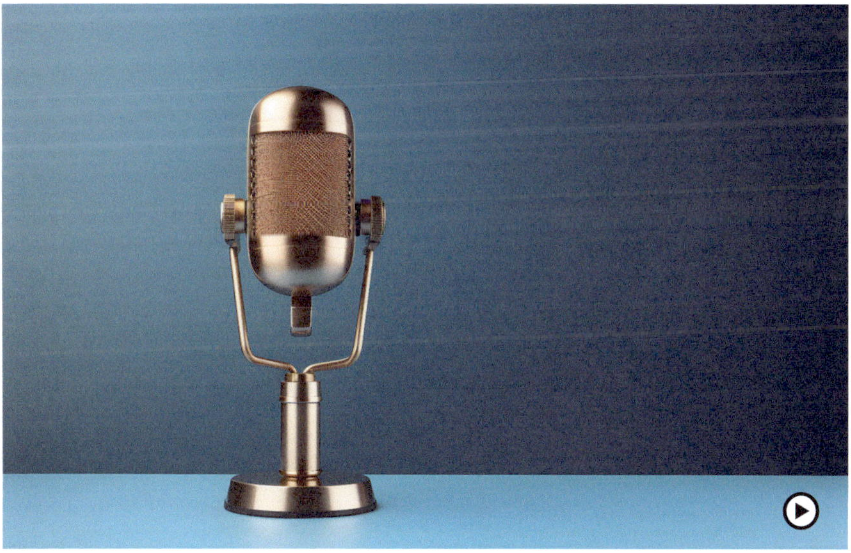

Fig. 5.3 VFE – Exercise 1: Warm-Up for Men (▸ https://doi.org/10.1007/000-dww)

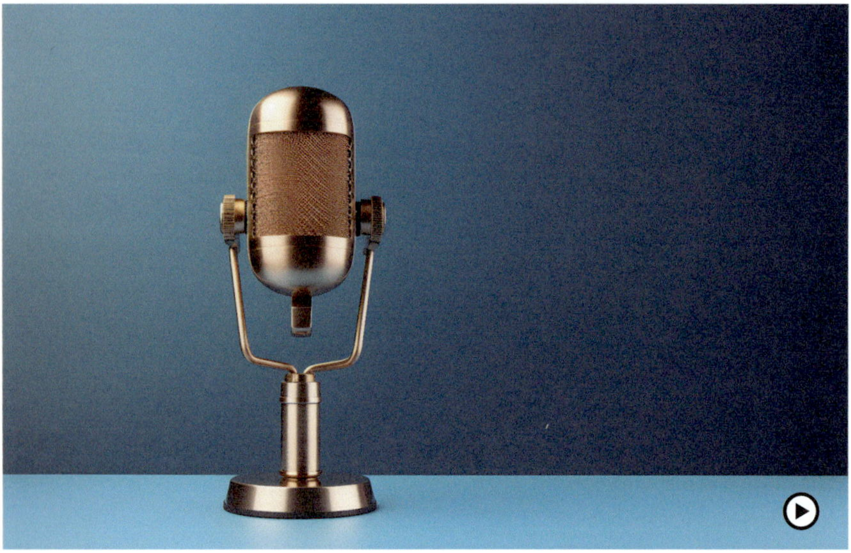

Fig. 5.4 Introduction to the vocal technique of lip buzzing (Lip Buzz) (▸ https://doi.org/10.1007/000-dwx)

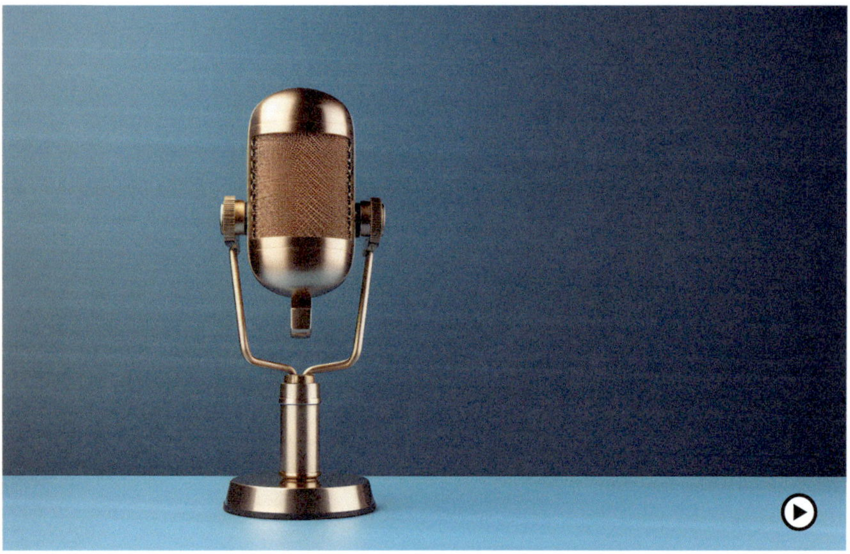

Fig. 5.5 VFE – Exercise 2: Stretching (▸ https://doi.org/10.1007/000-dwy)

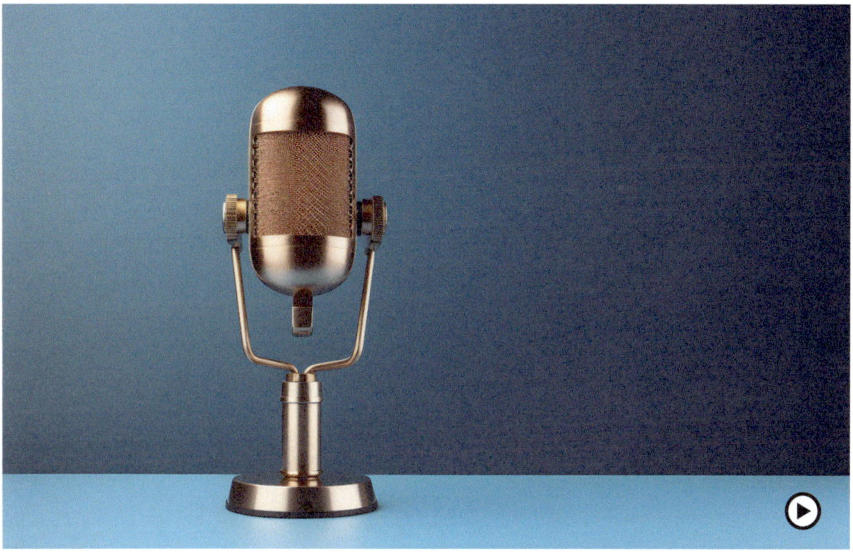

Fig. 5.6 VFE – Exercise 3: Contraction (▸ https://doi.org/10.1007/000-dwz)

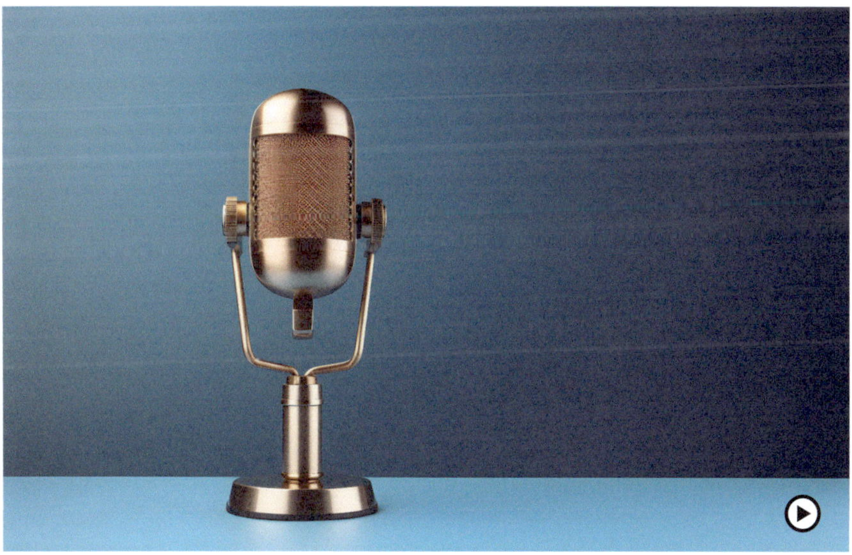

Fig. 5.7 Introduction to the last and most important exercise of VFE (Power Exercise) (▸ https://doi.org/10.1007/000-dx0)

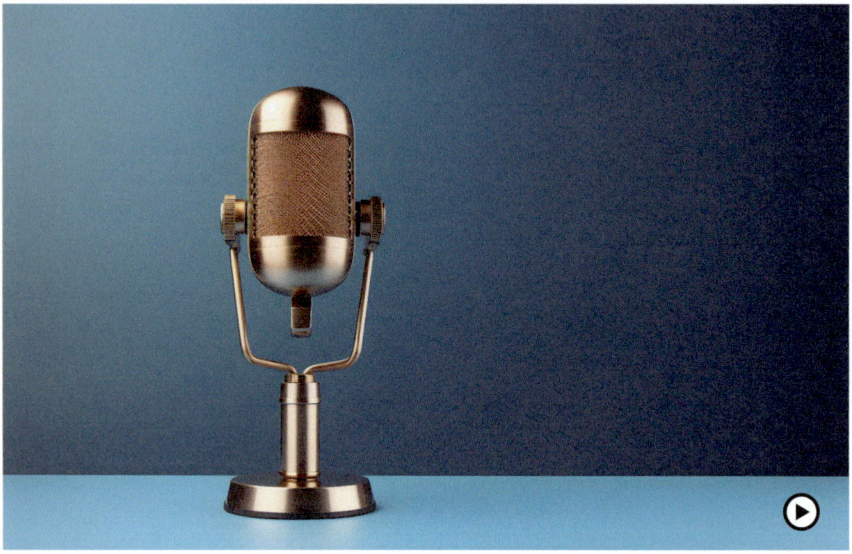

Fig. 5.8 VFE – Exercise 4: Tone C for women (▸ https://doi.org/10.1007/000-dx1)

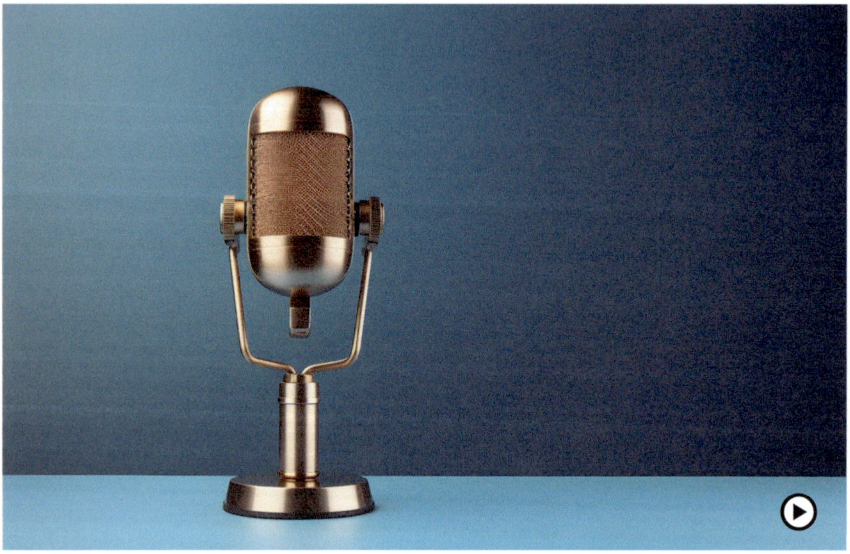

Fig. 5.9 VFE – Exercise 4: Tone C for men (▸ https://doi.org/10.1007/000-dx2)

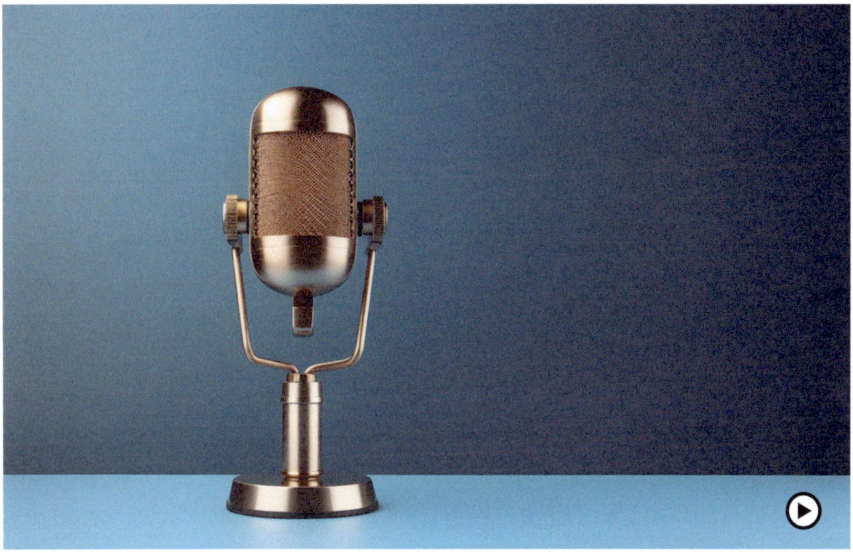

Fig. 5.10 VFE – Exercise 4: Tone D for women (▸ https://doi.org/10.1007/000-dx3)

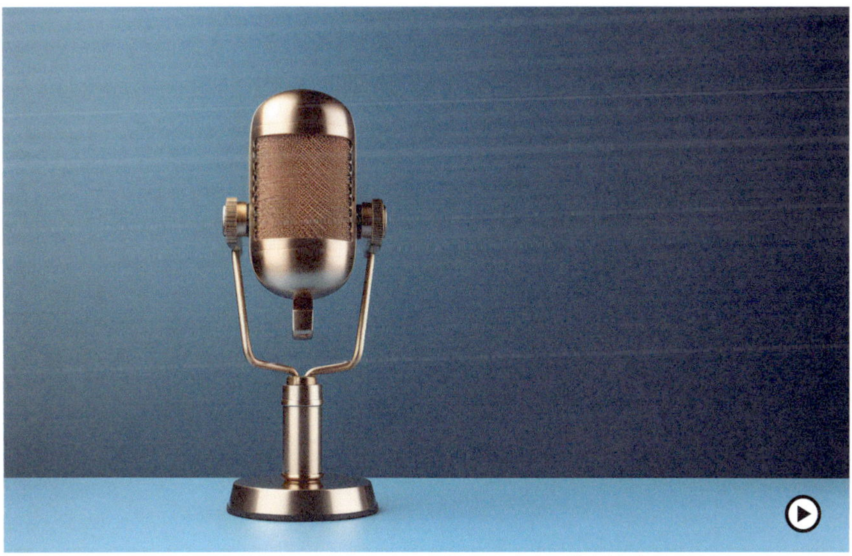

Fig. 5.11 VFE – Exercise 4: Tone D for men (▸ https://doi.org/10.1007/000-dx4)

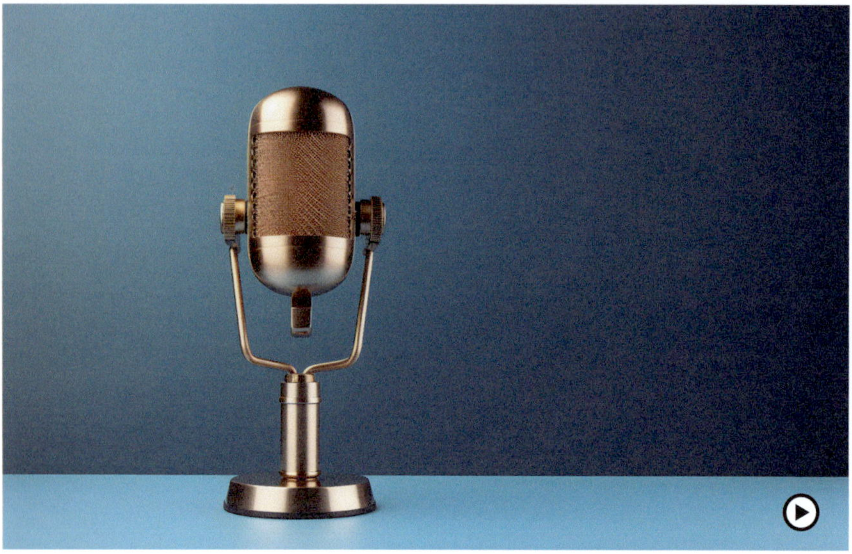

Fig. 5.12 VFE – Exercise 4: Tone E for women (▸ https://doi.org/10.1007/000-dx5)

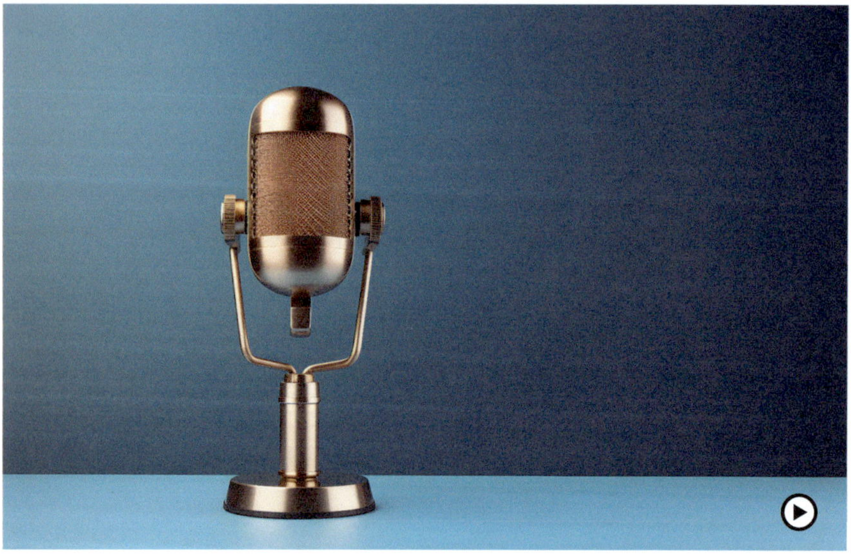

Fig. 5.13 VFE – Exercise 4: Tone E for men (▸ https://doi.org/10.1007/000-dx6)

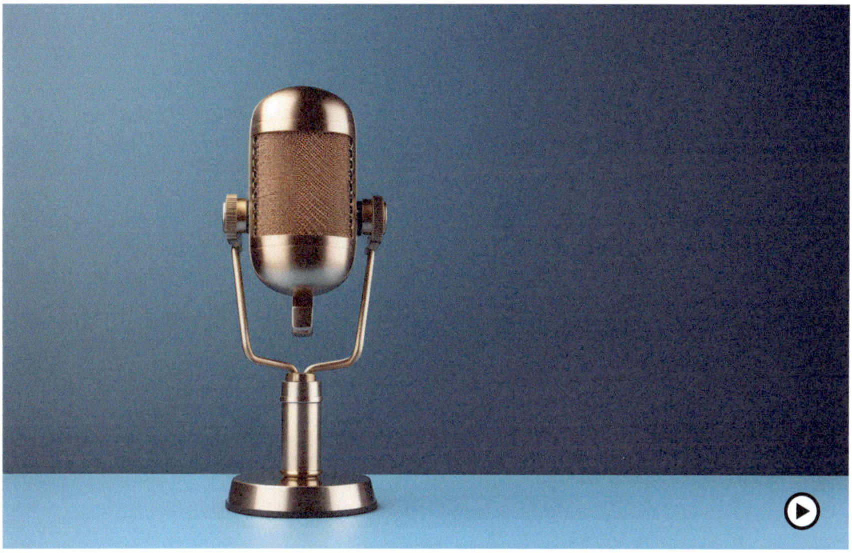

Fig. 5.14 VFE – Exercise 4: Tone F for women (▸ https://doi.org/10.1007/000-dx7)

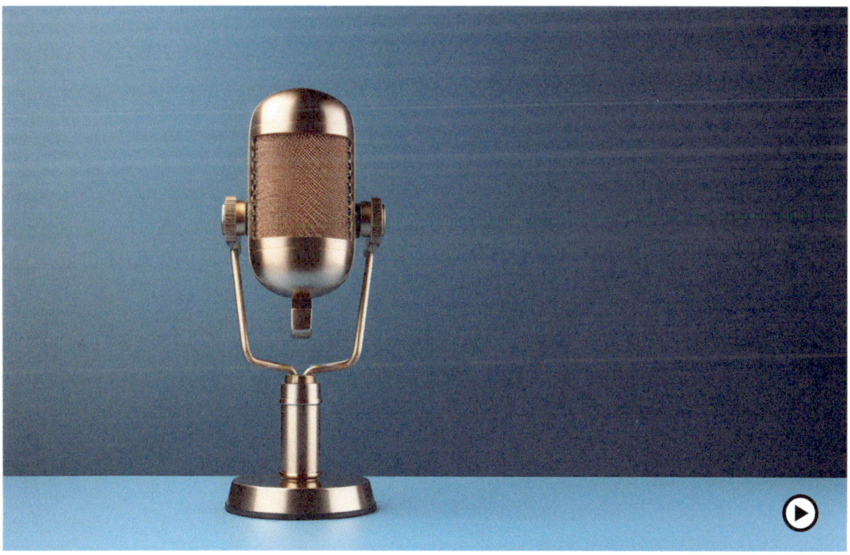

Fig. 5.15 VFE – Exercise 4: Tone F for men (▸ https://doi.org/10.1007/000-dx8)

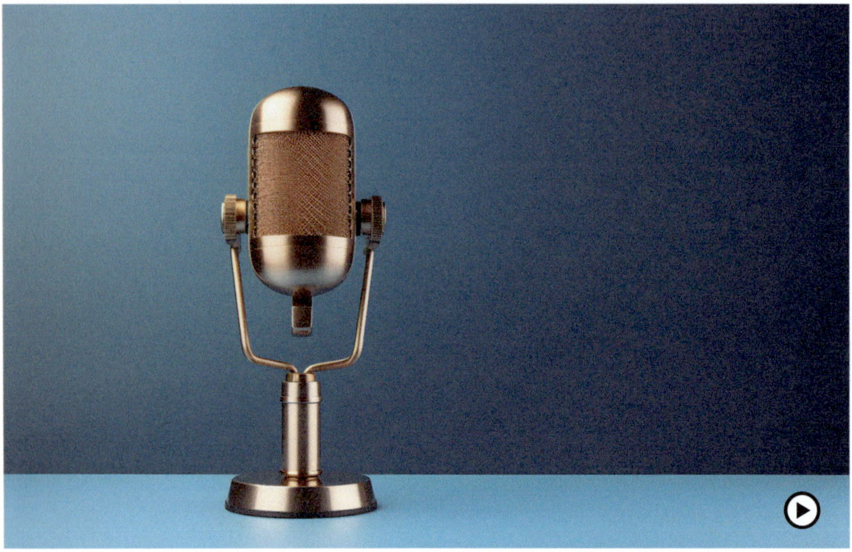

Fig. 5.16 VFE – Exercise 4: Tone G for women (▸ https://doi.org/10.1007/000-dwt)

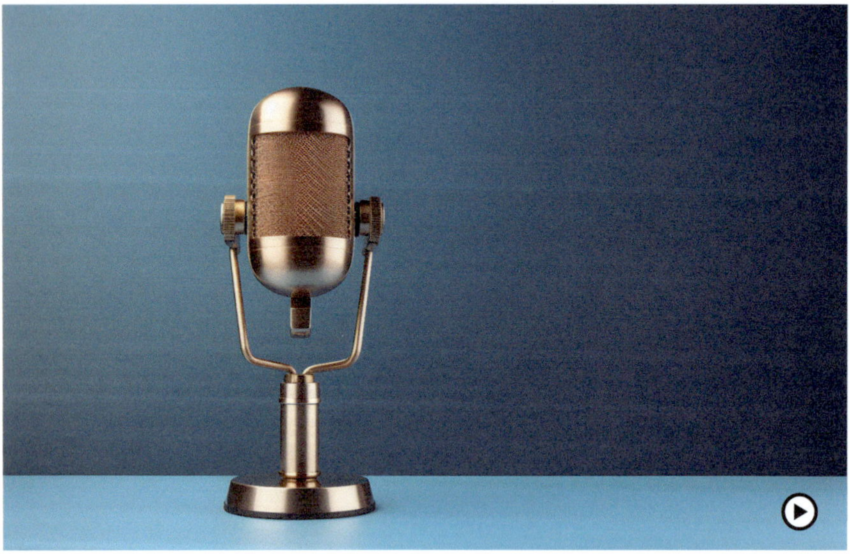

Fig. 5.17 VFE – Exercise 4: Tone G for men (▸ https://doi.org/10.1007/000-dxa)

The sound in exercises 2 to 4 is demonstrated only by lip buzzing, which is preferred by the developer and judged to be the most effective and efficient technique compared to other variants (Bane et al. 2019a).

Duration and Frequency

- Twice daily (Bane et al. 2019b)

Difficulties/ Risk/ Contraindications

As long as the sound is performed correctly, no risk is to be expected during the execution.

Meta-analyses on Effectiveness

- Angadi et al. (2019), Barsties v. Latoszek et al. (2020, 2023a, b)

Stretch- and Flow-Phonation

Description

Stretch- and Flow-Phonation was first described by Stone and Casteel in the early 1980s as a method for treating functional dysphonias (Watts et al. 2019).

As the name of the therapy suggests, the key concept of the treatment is an intentional focus on airflow to train the kinesthetic awareness of phonation physiology and the connection between the vocal subsystems. Proper physiological control of airflow is crucial for efficient voice production. The transglottal airflow is influenced by the activity of the laryngeal muscles. Imbalances in the activation of these muscles are etiological for functional voice disorders.

Stretch and Flow Phonation directly targets the control of airflow to reduce the excessive activation of the laryngeal muscles and to balance the laryngeal functions through breathing and resonance during phonation.

Objective

- The control of airflow and vocal fold contact
- Increasing complexity from voiceless to exaggerated airflow to normal articulation and vowel production
- Perception of a light, effortless airflow while speaking

Indication

- (Hyper)Functional dysphonia
- Increased VHI

Structure/Instruction

1. Cut a sheet from the kitchen roll or a cosmetic tissue into a strip, which serves as airflow control and is held about 10 cm in front of the mouth using the index and middle fingers
2. Airflow control: Voiceless /u/ (as heard in "tree rustling") loosely tone so that the tissue moves in the airflow
3. Airflow control with light phonation (as in yawning): Vowel /u/
4. High extension/stretching and airflow control (voiceless) at the corresponding levels: automatic speech, tongue twisters, reading text
5. High extension/stretching and airflow control (voiced, soft) at the corresponding levels: automatic speech, tongue twisters, reading text
6. Light extension/stretching with still high airflow control (voiced, engaged/medium loud) at the corresponding levels: automatic speech, tongue twisters, reading text
7. Light to no extension/stretching with lower airflow control (voiced, target voice) at the corresponding levels: automatic speech, tongue twisters, reading text

Duration and Frequency

- Treatment duration 6 weeks
- Once per week
- Patients are instructed and encouraged to practice daily at home during the treatment period and to keep a homework protocol to monitor practice.

Difficulties/Risks/Contraindications
As long as no hypertension occurs during phonation, no risk is expected during the procedure.

Meta-analyses on Effectiveness

- Barsties v. Latoszek et al. (2020)

Resonance Therapy Concepts
Description
Resonance therapy concepts train the patient to produce a sonorous and clear voice that can be perceived sensorily in the face and in the bone structures of the face. It is a technique that allows the patient to perceive vocal vibrations (in the area: lips/tongue/nose) and enables better voice projection.

All resonance therapy concepts are based on the same principle, namely to use the nasal and oral resonance spaces to improve voice quality and voice function. Targeted programs such as the Lessac-Madsen Resonant Voice Therapy (Verdolini-Abbott 2008), Pahn's Nasalization Method (Pahn and Pahn 1998), or

Stemple's Resonance Voice (Stemple et al. 2014) are the most well-known published resonance therapy programs.

Resonance therapies are also often the subject of eclectic voice therapy concepts as well as device-assisted aids, such as in the Novafon Local Vibration Voice Therapy or the Comprehensive Voice Rehabilitation Program.

Objective

- The goal of this form of therapy is to achieve a clear and strong voice, based on economical tension with as low tonus impact on the vocal folds as possible.
- Resonance therapy concepts aim to enable a more efficient glottal closure and reduce perilaryngeal tensions, so that the voice gains more carrying power and penetration.

Indication

- Heterogeneous voice disorders
- Increased VHI

Structure/Instruction

The basis of resonance in voice therapy is founded on the consonants /m/, /n/, and /ŋ/ to increase vibratory resonance and create a high effect on phonation. Sometimes, the therapy begins with the humming sound "m-hmm" to make the resonance principle easily perceptible for patients, which can then be further built upon in therapy. In this therapy, the sensory perception of vibration and voice sound is more emphasized than the analysis of physiology.

Lessac-Madsen Resonant Voice Therapy:

The Lessac-Madsen Resonant Voice Therapy is a specific form of resonance therapy, named in honor of two mentors/voice teachers (Prof. Dr. Arthur Lessac and Dr. Mark Madsen) of the developer of the voice therapy program, Prof. Dr. Katherine Verdolini-Abbott. Two primary goals of this therapy for patients are formulated:

1. A strong and clear voice that can be heard over a greater distance and up close, and also overcomes ambient noise.
2. Either to prevent future disorders of the vocal folds or to reverse voice disorders where they exist.

The therapy consists of 8 therapy units, offered once or twice a week for 30 to 45 minutes. Here is a rough overview:

TU	VH (30–45 min)	Stretching (5–10 min)	RV Core (5–10 min)	RV Singing (5–10 min)	RV VC (5–10 min)	RS Mini (5 min)	RS MdV (5–10 min)	CL (5–20 min)	OT (15–20 min)
I	✓	(✓)	(✓)						
II		✓	✓	✓	✓			CL1	
II		✓	✓	✓	✓	✓		CL2	
IV		✓	✓		✓	(✓)	✓	CL1 + 2	
V		✓	✓		✓	(✓)	✓	CL3	
VI		✓	✓			(✓)	✓	CL4	
VII		✓	✓				✓	CL5	
VIII		✓	✓					CL6	✓

Abbreviations/Explanations: TU = Therapy unit, VH = Voice hygiene (hydration therapy consisting of monitoring water intake throughout the day and steam inhalation and reflux management); RV = Resonance voice; VC = Vocal Communicator; MdV = Messa di Voce; CL = Conversation level (CL1 = normal conversation; CL2 = quiet conversation on the phone; CL3 = loud voice over a greater distance, relevant to the patients; CL4 = speaking in ambient noise, relevant to the patients; CL5 = speaking in an emotional context, relevant to the patients; CL6 = conversation with "challenge"); OT = own text

Nasalization Method

The term "nasalization"/"nasalizing"/"nasality" refers to a different placement of resonance in vowels and nasal consonants, where the airflow can escape through the mouth and nasal cavity simultaneously during phonation. In this form of therapy, resonance is trained as an exercise voice (pre-exercises up to level 3) until the target voice (level 4) is developed.

- *Pre-exercises:*
  Posture correction, relaxation exercises for neck and throat muscles, relaxation of the larynx, pharynx, and mouth area
- *Level 1:*
  Nasalizing on the indifferent sound (base tone), voice play including pitch variations
- *Level 2:*
  Chewing and jaw shaking exercises (sound and syllable level)
- *Level 3:*
  Chewing articulation at word, sentence, text, and spontaneous speech levels
- *Level 4:*
  Denasalizing in 5 steps (at word, sentence, text, and conversational levels):
  a) Complete nasalization with minimal articulation movement (only high jaw mobility)
  b) Enhanced mouth resonance used as nasal resonance with minimal articulation movement and only high jaw mobility

c) Mainly mouth resonance as nasal resonance with normal articulation movement (while jaw mobility is still high)
d) Intonation and normal voice, speech production (target voice)

Stemple's Resonance Voice:
This is a 7-step program based on the work of Lessac-Madsen Resonant Voice Therapy but further developed by Stemple (2000).

- *Basic Training Gesture:*
  After comfortable inhalation and in an eutonous standing or sitting position, patients should repeat a vocal sigh from high to low pitch on: /molm/
- *Step 1 (voiced):*
  For all exercises, the pitch should be slightly higher than the habitual speaking voice. This can also be specified on a piano or a piano app.
  a) Repetition of /molm – molm – molm/ in tempo variations (slow-fast-slow), perception of vibrations, reduce vocal effort
  b) Repetition of /molm – molm – molm/ in tempo variations (slow-fast-slow) and loudness (soft-loud-soft)
  c) Apply the vocalization /molm – molm – molm/ to the intonation (natural loudness and pitch variations) of existing sentences, but only speak on /molm/
  d) Chanting at the sentence level with a high proportion of /m/ and /n/ sounds
  e) The same sentences from d) without singing; during practice, ensure that a connection is made from abdominal breathing to the face
- *Step 2 (voiced vs. voiceless contrast):*
  The vocalization is now /mamapapa/ instead of /molm – molm – molm/, going through the same 5 subpoints as in Step 1
- *Step 3 (sentence level)*
  a) Chanting on 5–7 syllables in a sentence at habitual speaking voice
  b) Reflecting on the same sentences as in a) with a strongly forward-directed voice projection
  c) Repetition of b), but now in a more natural manner of forward-directed voice production
- *Step 4 (reading texts):*
  a) Read text with marked points where individual comfortable inhalation occurs
  b) Voice production of sentences as in Step 3 b) and c)
  c) Repetition of a) without marked inhalation points
- *Step 5 (controlled conversation):*
  Practice conversation with a forward-directed manner of speaking. Voice anomalies such as glottal stops, creaking, etc. are not allowed and must be avoided.
- *Step 6 (environmental changes):*
  Repetition of Step 5, but now with simulated environmental noises or sounds that patients experience in everyday life. These can be played back, for example, through headphones.

- *Step 7 (emotional changes):*
  Repetition of Step 5, but the conversation is conducted on different emotional levels, such as topics for laughing, loud speaking, anger, outrage, etc. These topics can be tailored to the patient's personality, interests, work experience, or passions.

Duration and Frequency

- Based on the example of Lessac-Madsen Resonant Voice Therapy, one treatment per week for a total of 8 weeks is suggested, along with daily home practice.
- In Stemple's Resonance Voice, it is suggested to practice twice daily for 5–10 minutes each: Basic Training Gesture and the current hierarchy level (i.e., Step 1 to 7).
- Resonance exercises are generally integrated into holistic or eclectic voice therapy programs. The duration and frequency are specified differently in each case.

Difficulties/ Risk/ Contraindications
If the exercises are performed correctly, no risk is to be expected.

Meta-analyses on Effectiveness

- Barsties v. Latoszek et al. (2020)

Novafon Local Vibration Voice Therapy
Description
The Novafon Local Vibration Voice Therapy (NLVVT) program combines 100 Hz local vibration with the Novafon sound wave appliance and voice exercises over a five-week treatment period (Barsties v. Latoszek 2020c). The intensity of the vibration is individually adjusted to the highest vibration pressure that is comfortable for the user. The Novafon is placed on the thyroid cartilage side plate. During phonation, an additional buzzing noise can be heard, which is caused by the local vibration of the Novafon. This buzzing sound is the control for the user to ensure that the vocal folds are being stimulated by the local vibration. The NLVVT program includes evidence-based voice exercises such as humming, chewing, tongue trills, lip trills, a combination of tongue trills, hand-over-mouth approach, and resonance. These voice exercises vary each week and are language-independent, as they are practiced at the sound, syllable, and pseudoword level.

NLVVT is offered in Germany as a certified workshop by the company Novafon and other partners from training institutes (https://novafon.com/de/fortbildungen).

Objective

- Treatment of physical laryngeal fitness
- The local vibration triggers muscle contractions of type-2 muscle fibers, due to stretch reflexes
- Improvement of vocal functions

Indication

- Heterogeneous voice disorders
- Increased VHI

Structure/Instruction according to Barsties v. Latoszek(2020c)
Week 1

- Passive use of the Novafon in the neck area
- Novafon + voice exercises in habitual pitch (such as humming, lip trills, tongue trills, and tongue trills + hand-over-mouth approach)

Week 2

- Modification in pitch of the voice exercises + Novafon
- Modification in loudness of the voice exercises + Novafon

Week 3

- Resonance therapy in habitual pitch + Novafon
- Variation of resonance voice exercises in tempo (slow vs. fast)

Week 4

- Modification of pitch in resonance therapy + Novafon
- Modification of loudness in resonance therapy + Novafon

Week 5

- Simultaneous modification of pitch + loudness in resonance therapy + Novafon
- Longer syllable chains (pseudowords)

Duration and Frequency according to Barsties v. Latoszek(2020c)

- Therapy frequency: Once per week
- Home practice: Twice daily for 10 minutes each

Difficulties/Risks/Contraindications

- Observe contraindications for sound wave therapy (e.g. https://novafon.com/en/contraindications)
- Do not exceed the treatment duration with the sound wave device, as this may cause unwanted side effects in the patient or the sound wave device to overheat

Meta-analyses on Effectiveness

- Barsties v. Latoszek and Hetjens (2023)

Water Resistance Therapy
Description

Water Resistance Therapy consists of various phonatory exercises that are performed through a tube made of glass or plastic. The distal end of the tube is immersed in water (Tyrmi et al. 2017). Other synonyms that work on the same principle include Resonance Voice Tube, Lax Vox®, or Doctor Vox®. Besides material differences, the diameter, the length of the tube, and the water depth play a crucial role. In particular, the diameter and the water depth are two critical variables that affect the glottal resistance (da Silva et al. 2019; Tyrmi and Laukkanen 2017).

A positive side effect of using Water Resistance Therapy is a massaging effect on the vocal folds and the tissue of the vocal tract due to the water bubbles that form during phonation (Ramalkhan et al. 2014). The enhancement of the massage effect of Water Resistance Therapy could be due to the formation of larger bubbles when tubes with a larger diameter are used, which would result in stronger oral pressure oscillations (higher amplitude and lower frequency of air oscillations in the vocal tract) (Radolf et al. 2014; Tyrmi et al. 2017).

The procedure of this voice therapy is not uniformly formulated and is used differently in hierarchy and program structure for different patient groups (e.g., Mailänder et al. 2017; Meerschman et al. 2019; Wu and Chan 2020; Guzman et al. 2023).

More practical information on this voice therapy are offered by various institutes, including the *Doctor Vox®Ltd.,* (https://www.doctorvox.com/).

Objectives

- Due to the supraglottic pressure changes, a more comfortable and higher quality voice production is expected.
- The change in water depth and possibly other diameters of the tube are to be used significantly to control the glottal closure/resistance as well as the massage effect.

Indication

- (Hyper-)Functional Dysphonia
- Increased VHI

Structure/Instruction according to Mailänder et al. (2017)

1. ***Perception of body posture***
   Achieving a correct body posture (recommended in an eutonous sitting position)
2. ***Preparing for phonation by bubbling***
   Patients should tone with the tube between their closed lips, with the distal end of the tube in a bottle of water. The water depth depends on the therapeutic goal. Inhale through the nose and exhale through the mouth.
3. ***Phonation***
   Water bubbling with phonation: /hhhooo/; varying the pitch while bubbling; bubbling familiar melodies/songs
4. ***Advanced level in phonation***
   Gliding tones; changing the resistance by changing the position of the tube (up to max. 4–6 cm)
5. ***Preparation for transfer to everyday life***
   Continuation of phonation without immersing the tube in water
6. ***Transfer to everyday life***
   Continued phonation without the tube

Duration and Frequency
The exercises should be performed several times a day for a few minutes. Once the exercises are learned, patients should also perform them independently. There is no clear data on the overall duration of the therapy. As part of warm-up and conditioning exercises, they are regularly repeated.

Difficulties/Risks/Contraindications
As long as the exercises are performed without excessive force or hypertension due to an excessive airflow, no risk is expected.

Meta-analyses on Effectiveness

- Barsties v. Latoszek and Hetjens (2023)

Manual Circumlaryngeal Therapy
Description:
This voice therapy consists of various manual techniques to bring the larynx into a lowered position with the therapist's hands. It aims primarily to achieve a reduction in the tone of the (peri)laryngeal muscles, which affects the voice production. Manual Circumlaryngeal Therapy was first described by Aronson (1980) and then

further developed by Roy et al. (1997). In particular, three techniques are to be highlighted from this therapy ("Push-back," "Pull-down," and "Circumlaryngeal massage") and are described in more detail in *Structure/Instruction*.

In Germany, for example, the first author offers workshops at various training institutes on this manual therapy approach to learn these techniques theoretically and practically.

Objective

- Reduction of muscular tension associated with vocal hyperfunction
- Relaxation of high muscular tension around the larynx, which is intended to improve voice production

Indication

- (Hyper-)Functional dysphonia/aphonia
- Pathological objective voice quality
- Pathological DSI value
- Increased VRP-1-min

Structure/Instruction

Patients are thoroughly instructed before the start of treatment and informed about the goal and course of the exercises. They need to know that these applications will have a noticeable impact on the laryngeal area and can be interrupted at any time. The intense high-pressure sensation from the manual techniques will subside immediately, but a possible desired voice effect, along with the alleviation of various laryngeal discomfort (e.g., pain, burning, globus sensation, etc.), can be lasting. Which techniques are most suitable for the patient is determined by examination through palpation. Palpation is the diagnostic basis for the application of manual techniques (see Sect. 2.2.2).

Hyoid Push-Back

During sustained phonation of /a:/, /e:/, /o:/, or /m:/, the hyoid bone is pushed back. The finger or thumb is positioned above the laryngeal prominence and then a posterior movement is performed to further enlarge the thyrohyoid space. The finger strength required for this can be relatively high, as the resistance of the laryngeal muscle activity can also be very high.

Thyroid Pull-down

This technique consists of a combination of compression and caudal-circumlaryngeal movement. The index fingers and thumbs are positioned at the superior cornu in front of the thyroid cartilage. The movement is first performed without phonation and later with phonation. As with the Hyoid Push-back, the phonation sounds described above are to be used. During phonation, this procedure is repeated several times to enable a quick and permanent repositioning of the laryngeal structures during phonation to minimize laryngeal muscle tone.

Circumlaryngeal massage

This technique involves circular movements (with thumb and index finger) over the edges of the hyoid bone and is further extended to the thyrohyoid space and over the posterior edges of the thyroid. It is crucial to recognize voice changes in a timely manner. The work should proceed gradually from superficial to deep pressure. Location and pressure should vary according to the patient's tolerance. Patients should be allowed to vocalize simultaneously and increase the complexity of the vocal demand (from sounds to sequential speaking to words and sentences).

Duration and Frequency

This depends on the patient. Some patients achieve significant results after just a few minutes, while others require several therapy sessions and even corresponding self-application, considering cognitive and motor sensitivity in performing certain manual techniques. Shorter sessions are preferred and serve as a starting phase for further voice therapy.

Difficulties/Risks/Contraindications

- The extent to which patients respond to Manual Circumlaryngeal Therapy cannot be precisely predicted.
- Caution is advised when applying pressure in general (the more experience, the more confident the practitioners become in handling the techniques) and the manipulative repositioning movements in children and patients with increased pain sensitivity and fibromyalgia.
- Contraindications for the application of manual techniques include, for example, fractures in the head-neck, shoulder area, radiochemotherapy in the head-neck area, and osteoporosis.

Meta-analyses on Effectiveness

- Kim (2021), Barsties v. Latoszek et al. (2024)

Lee Silverman Voice Treatment

Description

The Lee Silverman Voice Treatment (LSVT©) is a very specific and intensive treatment program that particularly focuses on the criterion of "loud speaking" in patients with dysarthria with reduced voice loudness and incomplete glottal closure (e.g., oval gap). The therapy developed from this was named after one of the first patients who suffered from Parkinson's disease and wanted to improve her speech intelligibility (Ramig et al. 1994). LSVT© has been developed in the USA and internationally, there are various options for obtaining certification. In Germany, for example a certification is possible since the year 2000, and workshops are offered with more than 1,300 trained therapists. Further information can also be found at LSVT-Global (https://www.lsvtglobal.com/).

Objectives

- Improve voice loudness
- Improve glottal closure
- Increase speech intelligibility through more power and intensity

Indication

- Parkinson's disease
- Increased VHI
- Lower SRP-I

Structure/Instruction

- The treatment begins with holding vowels at high volume (10–12 repetitions), then progresses to word, sentence level, and conversational speaking.
- Hierarchical speech and volume drill structure:
  1. Week: single words or phrases
  2. Week: sentences
  3. Week: reading texts
  4. Week: spontaneous speech
     1st to 3rd week: in each therapy session, 30 words/phrases/sentences are spoken, each repeated 3× (a total of 80–120 repetitions)
- Maximum frequency range of high and low tones using vowels (repeat 10× and hold the maxima of the tones for 2–3 seconds)
- Patients are continuously reminded to speak loudly (under the motto: "Think loud")
- To maintain intensity, biofeedback is used (e.g., a dB meter).
- The new loud voice should be quickly implemented in everyday life with functional phrases, greetings, thanking, phone calls, etc.

Duration and Frequency

- The therapy is based on a dose of 16 units of 60 minutes each on 4 consecutive days for a total of 4 weeks.
- Additionally, patients must practice daily at home and should continue to do so after completing the 16 therapy units.

Difficulties/Risks/Contraindications

- Possible vocal overstrain
- Difficulties in maintaining (not becoming too quiet) and higher loudness levels (not shouting too loudly)
- Risk of relapse due to lack of/too long breaks in therapeutic support
- Inappropriate or too high habitual pitch during/after practice

Meta-analyses on Effectiveness

- Yuan et al. (2020), Pu et al. (2021)

Comprehensive Voice Rehabilitation Program
Description
The Brazilian concept of the Comprehensive Voice Rehabilitation Program includes an eclectic voice therapy approach with a six-week application (Behlau et al. 2013). Main aspects of the program are indirect voice therapy units, psychodynamic analyses, and voice training. The treatment includes the identification, awareness, and modification of negative voice habits, the development of techniques for the interaction between body and voice, vocal adjustment, and resonance balancing.

Objective

- To understand behavioral changes in a comprehensive manner, that voice disorders are multifactorial and thus various perspectives of treatment forms are considered
- Structure and design correspond to a segmented learning method to follow the therapeutic process

Indication

- (Hyper-)Functional Dysphonia
- Increased VHI

Structure/Instruction according to (Behlau et al.2013)
Week 1: Working with the voice source

- Orientation: Finding norms of vocal well-being and identifying controllable situations; designing a chart to record the occurrence of the most altered aspects;
- Psychodynamics: Analyzing the impact of the altered voice; quick training in the perception of voice deviations and reviewing the impact of voice problems within the areas of the VHI

Week 2: Working with source/filter

- Evaluation of the effect and results of the exercises performed at home
- Orientation on the use of the voice
- Movement exercises in the waist and stretching of the arms, shoulders, and cervical spine for 5 min
- Tongue or lip trills or prolongation of modulated fricative sounds for 1 min or 10×
- Nasal resonance of /m/ or /n/ sounds held for 1 min

- Repetitions of the techniques: 20×
- Sounded blow technique for 1 min or 10×
- Chewing method with nasal sounds for 2 min or 20×

Week 3: Working with source/filter, breath-voice coupling, and articulation

- Evaluation of the effects and results of the exercises performed at home
- Orientation on the use of the voice
- Movement exercises in the waist and stretching of the arms, shoulders, and cervical spine for 5 min
- Tongue, lip trills or prolongation of fricative sounds without modulation along with movements of the cervical spine for 1 min or 10×
- Tongue, lip trills or prolongation of modulated fricative sounds for 1 min or 10×
- Nasal glides for 1 min or 10×
- Sounded blow technique with rounded vowels for 2 min or 2 sequences with 7 vowels;
- Nasal resonance technique for 1 min or 10×
- Soft and sonorous fricative sounds with vowels for 2 min or 2 sequences with 7 vowels

Week 4: Working with source/filter, breath-voice coupling, and articulation

- Evaluation of the effect and results of the exercises performed at home
- Orientation on the use of the voice
- Movement exercises in the waist and stretching of the arms, shoulders, and cervical spine for 5 min
- Tongue, lip trills or prolongation of fricative sounds with ascending and descending glides for 1 min or 10×
- Sounded blow technique with rounded lips for 2 min or 20×
- Soft and sonorous fricative sounds with vowels for 2 min or 2 sequences with 7 vowels and repeat this twice
- Nasal resonance technique of /m/ or /n/ sounds in phonatory units for 2 min or 20×
- General nasal resonance technique in phonatory units with vowels for 2 min or a seven-vowel sequence repeated twice

Week 5: Working with Source/Filter, Breath-Voice Coupling, and Articulation

- Evaluation of the effects and results of the exercises performed at home
- Orientation on the use of the voice
- Movement exercises in the waist and stretching of the arms, shoulders, and cervical spine for 5 min
- Tongue vibration technique alternated with lip trill or extension of fricative sounds with ascending and descending glides for 1 min or 10×

- Sounded blow technique with rounded lips and short vowels for 2 min or 2 sequences with 7 vowels
- Masticated nasal sound technique with vowels for 1 min or 10×
- Sonorous fricative sounds with vowels for 1 min or 1 sequence with 7 vowels
- Nasal resonance technique on vowels for 2 min: Twice repetition of the exercise with 7 vowels
- Resonance technique of nasal sound sequences followed by consonant groups for 3 min (pataka, peteké, petekê, pitiki, potokó, potokô, putuku…)

Week 6: Working with Source/Filter, Breath-Voice Coupling, and Articulation

- Evaluation of the effects and results of the exercises performed at home
- Orientation on the use of the voice
- Movement exercises in the waist and stretching of the arms, shoulders, and cervical spine for 5 min
- Tongue vibration technique alternated with lip trill or extension of fricative sounds with ascending and descending glides for 1 min or 10×
- Sounded blow technique with rounded lips and short vowels for 2 min
- Masticated nasal sound technique with vowels for 1 min or one sequence with 7 vowels
- Sonorous fricative sounds with vowels for 1 min or 1 sequence with 7 vowels
- Resonance technique with nasal sounds on vowels for 2 min or 2 sequences with 7 vowels
- Resonance technique of nasal and sonorous sound sequences followed by consonant groups for 3 min

Duration and frequency according to Behlau et al. (2013)
Daily home practice
Week 1

- Lip, tongue trills or extension of (modulated) fricative sounds each for 1 min or 10 repetitions

Week 2

- Start: Tongue, lip trills or extension of modulated fricative sounds for 1 min or 10×
- Chewing phonation for 1 min or 10×
- Sounded blow technique for 1 min or 10×
- End: Tongue, lip trills or extension of modulated fricative sounds for 1 min or 10×

Week 3

- Tongue, lip trills or extension of fricative sounds without modulation together with movements of the cervical spine for 1 min or 10×

- Glides with the nasal /m/ sound for 1 min or 10×
- Sounded blow technique with rounded vowels for 1 min or a seven-vowel sequence
- Soft and sonorous fricative sounds with vowels for 2 min or 2 sequences with 7 vowels

Week 4

- Tongue, lip trills or extension of fricative sounds with ascending and descending glides for 1 min or 10×
- Sounded blow technique with rounded lips for 1 min or 10×
- Sonorous fricative sounds with vowels for 1 min or 1 sequence with 7 vowels
- Nasal resonance technique in phonatory units together with vowels for 2 min or 2 seven-vowel sequences

Week 5

- Tongue trill alternating with lip trill or prolongation of fricative sounds with ascending and descending glides for 1 min or 10×
- Aspirated phonation with rounded lips and short vowels for 2 min or 2 seven-vowel sequences
- Resonance technique of nasal sound sequences, followed by consonant groups, for 2 min

Week 6

- Tongue trill alternating with lip trill or fricative sounds with ascending and descending glides for 1 min
- Slow blow technique with rounded lips and short vowels for 1 min or 1 sequence of 7 vowels
- Resonance technique of nasal sound sequences followed by consonant groups for 2 min

Difficulties/ Risk/ Contraindications
As long as the exercises and the procedure are carried out correctly, no risk is to be expected.

Meta-analyses on Effectiveness

- Barsties v. Latoszek et al. (2020)

References

Adriaansen A, Meerschman I, Van Lierde K, D'haeseleer E (2022) Effects of voice therapy in children with vocal fold nodules: a systematic review. Int J Lang Commun Disord 57(6):1160–1193. https://doi.org/10.1111/1460-6984.12754

Allen J (2010) Cause of vocal fold scar. Curr Opin Otolaryngol Head Neck Surg 18(6):475–480. https://doi.org/10.1097/MOO.0b013e32833fecd1

Allen J (2021) Current approaches to management of vocal fold scar. Curr Opin Otolaryngol Head Neck Surg 29(6):465–472. https://doi.org/10.1097/MOO.0000000000000769

Al-Kadi M, Alfawaz MA, Alotaibi FZ (2022) Impact of voice therapy on pediatric patients with dysphonia and vocal nodules: a systematic review. Cureus 14(4):e24433. https://doi.org/10.7759/cureus.24433

Almeida ANS, Cunha DAD, Ferreira SLS, Guimarães BTL, Balata PMM, Silva HJD (2022) Effect of electrical stimulation on the treatment of dysphonia: a systematic review. J Voice 36(5):650–660. https://doi.org/10.1016/j.jvoice.2020.08.002

Alegria R, Freitas SV, Manso MC (2020a) Is there an improvement on acoustic voice parameters in patients with bilateral vocal fold nodules after voice therapy? A meta-analysis. Eur Arch Otorhinolaryngol 277(8):2163–2172. https://doi.org/10.1007/s00405-020-05956-2

Alegria R, Vaz Freitas S, Manso MC (2020b) Effectiveness of voice therapy in patients with vocal fold nodules: a systematic search and narrative review. Eur Arch Otorhinolaryngol 277(11):2951–2966. https://doi.org/10.1007/s00405-020-06059-8

Alegria R, Vaz Freitas S, Manso MC (2021) Efficacy of speech language therapy intervention in unilateral vocal fold paralysis – a systematic review and a meta-analysis of visual-perceptual outcome measures. Logoped Phoniatr Vocol 46(2):86–98. https://doi.org/10.1080/14015439.2020.1762730

Alves Silverio KC, Brasolotto AG, Thaís Donalonso Siqueira L, Carneiro CG, Fukushiro AP, Roberto de Jesus Guirro R (2015) Effect of application of transcutaneous electrical nerve stimulation and laryngeal manual therapy in dysphonic women: clinical trial. J Voice 29(2):200–208. https://doi.org/10.1016/j.jvoice.2014.06.003

Alves M, Krüger E, Pillay B, van Lierde K, van der Linde J (2019) The effect of hydration on voice quality in adults: a systematic review. J Voice 33(1):125.e13–125.e28. https://doi.org/10.1016/j.jvoice.2017.10.001

Aghadoost S, Jalaie S, Khatoonabadi AR, Dabirmoghaddam P, Khoddami SM (2020) A study of vocal facilitating techniques compared to Manual Circumlaryngeal Therapy in teachers with muscle tension dysphonia. J Voice 34(6):963.e11–963.e21. https://doi.org/10.1016/j.jvoice.2019.06.002

Angadi V, Croake D, Stemple J (2019) Effects of vocal function exercises: a systematic review. J Voice 33(1):124.e13–124.e34. https://doi.org/10.1016/j.jvoice.2017.08.031

Arens C, Gugatschka M (2021) [New developments in phonosurgery and laryngology]. HNO 69(9):693–694. https://doi.org/10.1007/s00106-021-01080-7

Arroyo HH, Neri L, Fussuma CY, Imamura R (2016) Diode laser for laryngeal surgery: a systematic review. Int Arch Otorhinolaryngol. 20(2):172–179. https://doi.org/10.1055/s-0036-1579741

Aronson A (1980) Clinical voice disorders: an interdisciplinary approach. Brian C. Decker, New York

Bane M, Brown M, Angadi V, Croake DJ, Andreatta RD, Stemple JC (2019a) Vocal function exercises for normal voice: with and without semi-occlusion. Int J Speech Lang Pathol 21(2):175–181. https://doi.org/10.1080/17549507.2017.1416176

Bane M, Angadi V, Dressler E, Andreatta R, Stemple J (2019b) Vocal function exercises for normal voice: the effects of varying dosage. Int J Speech Lang Pathol 21(1):37–45. https://doi.org/10.1080/17549507.2017.1373858

Barsties v. Latoszek B (2020a) [Evidenced-based voice therapy programs for the treatment of dysphonia: A systematic literature review]. Sprache-Stimme-Gehör 44(1):16–22. https://doi.org/10.1055/a-0949-6520
Barsties v. Latoszek B (2020b) Treatment effectiveness of Novafon local vibration voice therapy for dysphonia treatment. J Voice. 34(1):160.e7–160.e14. https://doi.org/10.1016/j.jvoice.2018.05.009
Barsties v. Latoszek B (2020c) Preliminary study of Novafon local vibration voice therapy for dysphonia treatment. Logoped Phoniatr Vocol 45(1):1–9. https://doi.org/10.1080/14015439.2018.1453541
Barsties v. Latoszek B (2021) [Larynxmanipulationstechniken bei Mutationsfalsettdysphonien]. Sprache-Stimme-Gehör 45(4):166–168. https://doi.org/10.1055/a-1542-6678
Barsties v. Latoszek B, Hetjens S (2023) Effektivität der Novafon Local Vibration Voice Therapy & Water Resistance Therapy: eine Meta-Analyse. Laryngorhinootologie 102(9):662–668. https://doi.org/10.1055/a-1976-9766
Barsties v. Latoszek B, Watts CR (2021) A case of nervus laryngeus superior paresis treated with Novafon local vibration voice therapy. J Voice 35(3):406–410. https://doi.org/10.1016/j.jvoice.2019.10.013
Barsties v. Latoszek B, Watts CR, Neumann K (2020) The effectiveness of voice therapy on voice-related handicap: a network meta-analysis. Clin Otolaryngol 45(5):796–804. https://doi.org/10.1111/coa.13596
Barsties v. Latoszek B, Watts CR, Schwan K, Hetjens S (2023a) The maximum phonation time as marker for voice treatment efficacy: a network meta-analysis. Clin Otolaryngol 48(2):130–138. https://doi.org/10.1111/coa.14019
Barsties v. Latoszek B, Watts CR, Hetjens S, Neumann K (2023b) The efficacy of different voice treatments for vocal fold polyps: a systematic review and meta-analysis. J Clin Med 12(10):3451. https://doi.org/10.3390/jcm12103451
Barsties v. Latoszek B, Watts CR, Hetjens S (2024) The efficacy of the Manual Circumlaryngeal Therapy for Muscle Tension Dysphonia: a systematic review and meta-analysis. Laryngoscope 134(1):18–26. https://doi.org/10.1002/lary.30850
Batista DJ, da Silva RC, Ostolin TLVDP, Behlau M, Ribeiro VV (2024) Mapping of the execution of resonance tubes phonation immersed in water exercise in adults: a scoping review. J Voice 38(6):1521.e15-1521.e37. https://doi.org/10.1016/j.jvoice.2022.06.010
Bayer O, Cámara R, Zeissig SR, Ressing M, Dietz A, Locati LD, Ramroth H, Singer S (2016) Occupation and cancer of the larynx: a systematic review and meta-analysis. Eur Arch Otorhinolaryngol 273(1):9–20. https://doi.org/10.1007/s00405-014-3321-y
Behlau M, Pontes P, Vieira VP, Yamasaki R, Madazio G (2013) Presentation of the comprehensive vocal rehabilitation program for the treatment of behavioral dysphonia. Codas 25(5):492–496. https://doi.org/10.1590/S2317-17822013000500015
Benedict JJ, Derkay CS (2021) Recurrent respiratory papillomatosis: a 2020 perspective. Laryngoscope Investig Otolaryngol 6(2):340–345. https://doi.org/10.1002/lio2.545
Bhatt NK, Garber D, Baertsch H, Beard L, Giliberto JP, Meyer TK, Merati AL, Sauder C (2023) Treatments for age-related vocal atrophy: a systematic review. Laryngoscope 133(11):2846–2855. https://doi.org/10.1002/lary.30653
Bishop B (1974) Vibratory stimulation: part 1. Neurophysiology of motor responses evoked by vibratory stimulation. Phys Ther 54(12):1273–1282
Bishop B (1975) Vibratory stimulation: part III. Possible applications of vibration in treatment of motor dysfunctions. Phys Ther 55(2):139–143
Bohlender JE (2021) [Office-based phonosurgery]. HNO 69(9):719–725. https://doi.org/10.1007/s00106-021-01081-6
Boone DR, McFarlane SC (1993) A critical view of the yawn-sigh as a voice therapy technique. J Voice 7(1):75–80. https://doi.org/10.1016/s0892-1997(05)80114-6
Boone DR, Mc Farlane SC, Von Berg SL, Zraick RI (2010) The voice and voice therapy, 8. Aufl. Pearson, Boston

Boutsen F, Cannito MP, Taylor M, Bender B (2002) Botox treatment in adductor spasmodic dysphonia: a meta-analysis. J Speech Lang Hear Res 45(3):469–481. https://doi.org/10.1044/1092-4388(2002/037)

Bovo R, Trevisi P, Emanuelli E, Martini A (2013) Voice amplification for primary school teachers with voice disorders: a randomized clinical trial. Int J Occup Med Environ Health 26(3):363–372. https://doi.org/10.2478/s13382-013-0115-1

Brodnitz FS, Fröschels E (1954) Treatment of nodules of vocal cords by chewing method. AMA Arch Otolaryngol 59(5):560–565. https://doi.org/10.1001/archotol.1954.00710050572006

Caliandro P, Celletti C, Padua L, Minciotti I, Russo G, Granata G, La Torre G, Granieri E, Camerota F (2012) Focal muscle vibration in the treatment of upper limb spasticity: a pilot randomized controlled trial in patients with chronic stroke. Arch Phys Med Rehabil 93(9):1656–1661. https://doi.org/10.1016/j.apmr.2012.04.002

Casale R, Damiani C, Maestri R, Fundarò C, Chimento P, Foti C (2014) Localized 100 Hz vibration improves function and reduces upper limb spasticity: a double-blind controlled study. Eur J Phys Rehabil Med 50(5):495–504

Chen J, Long S (2014) Tea and coffee consumption and risk of laryngeal cancer: a systematic review meta-analysis. PLoS One 9(12):e112006. https://doi.org/10.1371/journal.pone.0112006

Cheng SP, Liu TP, Yang PS, Lee KS, Liu CL (2015) Effect of perioperative dexamethasone on subjective voice quality after thyroidectomy: a meta-analysis and systematic review. Langenbecks Arch Surg 400(8):929–936. https://doi.org/10.1007/s00423-015-1354-3

Chi HW, Cho HC, Yang AY, Chen YC, Chen JW (2023) Effects of different voice rest on vocal function after microlaryngeal surgery: a systematic review and meta-analysis. Laryngoscope 133(1):154–161. https://doi.org/10.1002/lary.30082

Childs L, Rickert S, Murry T, Blitzer A, Sulica L (2011) Patient perceptions of factors leading to spasmodic dysphonia: a combined clinical experience of 350 patients. Laryngoscope 121(10):2195–2198. https://doi.org/10.1002/lary.22168

Cho KJ, Nam IC, Hwang YS, Shim MR, Park JO, Cho JH, Joo YH, Kim MS, Sun DI (2011) Analysis of factors influencing voice quality and therapeutic approaches in vocal polyp patients. Eur Arch Otorhinolaryngol 268(9):1321–1327. https://doi.org/10.1007/s00405-011-1618-7

Clark HM (2003) Neuromuscular treatments for speech and swallowing: a tutorial. Am J Speech Lang Pathol 12(4):400–415. https://doi.org/10.1044/1058-0360(2003/086)

Clark MG, Rattigan S, Newman JM, Eldershaw TP (1998) Vascular control of nutrient delivery by flow redistribution within muscle: implications for exercise and post-exercise muscle metabolism. Int J Sports Med 19(6):391–400. https://doi.org/10.1055/s-2007-971935

Colton R, Casper J (1996) Understanding voice problems: a physiological perspective for diagnosis and treatment. Williams & Wilkins, Baltimore

Coordes A, Grund D, Mainka A, Olze H, Hanitsch L, von Bernuth H, Dommerich S (2023) [Recurrent laryngeal papillomatosis]. HNO 71(2):77–82. https://doi.org/10.1007/s00106-022-01250-1

Cosyns M, Van Borsel J, Wierckx K, Dedecker D, Van de Peer F, Daelman T, Laenen S, T'Sjoen G (2014) Voice in female-to-male transsexual persons after long-term androgen therapy. Laryngoscope 124(6):1409–1414. https://doi.org/10.1002/lary.24480

da Cunha PG, de Oliveira LI, Dalbosco Gadenz C, Cassol M (2018) Effects of voice therapy on muscle tension dysphonia: a systematic literature review. J Voice 32(5):546–552. https://doi.org/10.1016/j.jvoice.2017.06.015

De Bodt M, Van den Steen L, Mertens F, Raes J, Van Bel L, Heylen L, Pattyn J, Gordts F, van de Heyning P (2015) Characteristics of a dysphonic population referred for voice assessment and/or voice therapy. Folia Phoniatr Logop 67(4):178–186. https://doi.org/10.1159/000369339

Derkay CS, Bluher AE (2019)Update on recurrent respiratory papillomatosis. Otolaryngol Clin N Am 52(4):669–679. https://doi.org/10.1016/j.otc.2019.03.011

Derkay CS, Wikner EE, Pransky S, Best SR, Zur K, Sidell DR, Klein A, Rosen C, Dikkers FG, Johnson R (2023) Systemic use of bevacizumab for recurrent respiratory papillomatosis: who, what, where, when, and why? Laryngoscope 133(1):2–3. https://doi.org/10.1002/lary.30180

Desjardins M, Bonilha HS (2020) The impact of respiratory exercises on voice outcomes: a systematic review of the literature. J Voice 34(4):648.e1–648.e39. https://doi.org/10.1016/j.jvoice.2019.01.011

Desjardins M, Halstead L, Cooke M, Bonilha HS (2017) A systematic review of voice therapy: what „effectiveness" really implies. J Voice 31(3):392.e13–392.e32. https://doi.org/10.1016/j.jvoice.2016.10.002

Dewan K, Chhetri DK, Hoffman H (2022) Reinke's edema management and voice outcomes. Laryngoscope Investig Otolaryngol 7(4):1042–1050. https://doi.org/10.1002/lio2.840

DGHNO-KHC (2019) S3-Leitlinie Diagnostik, Therapie und Nachsorge des Larynxkarzinoms – Langfassung, 1.1 Aufl. https://register.awmf.org/assets/guidelines/017-076OLl_S3_Larynxkarzinom_2019-11.pdf. Accessed 1 Nov 2023

Dvorin EL, Ebell MH (2020) Short-term systemic corticosteroids: appropriate use in primary care. Am Fam Physician 101(2):89–94

Eastwood C, Madill C, Mccabe P (2015) The behavioural treatment of muscle tension voice disorders: a systematic review. Int J Speech Lang Pathol 17(3):287–303. https://doi.org/10.3109/17549507.2015.1024169

Enflo L, Sundberg J, Romedahl C, McAllister A (2013) Effects on vocal fold collision and phonation threshold pressure of resonance tube phonation with tube end in water. J Speech Lang Hear Res 56(5):1530–1538. https://doi.org/10.1044/1092-4388(2013/12-0040)

Enver N, Ramaswamy A, Sulica L, Pitman MJ (2021) Office-based procedure training in laryngology fellowship programs. Laryngoscope 131(9):2054–2058. https://doi.org/10.1002/lary.29170

van Esch BF, Wegner I, Stegeman I, Grolman W (2017) Effect of botulinum toxin and surgery among spasmodic dysphonia patients. Otolaryngol Head Neck Surg 156(2):238–254. https://doi.org/10.1177/0194599816675320

Faham M, Ahmadi A, Silverman E, Harouni GG, Dabirmoghaddam P (2021) Quality of life after botulinum toxin injection in patients with adductor spasmodic dysphonia; a systematic review and meta-analysis. J Voice 35(2):271–283. https://doi.org/10.1016/j.jvoice.2019.07.025

Feinstein H, Abbott KV (2021) Behavioral treatment for benign vocal fold lesions in children: a systematic review. Am J Speech Lang Pathol 30(2):772–788. https://doi.org/10.1044/2020_AJSLP-20-00304

Ferlito A, Devaney KO, Hunt JL, Hellquist H (2019) Some considerations on the WHO histological classification of laryngeal neoplasms. Adv Ther 36(7):1511–1517. https://doi.org/10.1007/s12325-019-00978-7

Fisher HB, Logemann JA (1970) Objective evaluation of therapy for vocal nodules: a case report. J Speech Hear Disord 35(3):277–285. https://doi.org/10.1044/jshd.3503.277

Ford CN, Inagi K, Khidr A, Bless DM, Gilchrist KW (1996) Sulcus vocalis: a rational analytical approach to diagnosis and management. Ann Otol Rhinol Laryngol 105(3):189–200. https://doi.org/10.1177/000348949610500304

Förster G, Boltze C, Seidel J, Pawlita M, Müller A (2008) [Juvenile laryngeal papillomatosis--immunisation with the polyvalent vaccine gardasil]. Laryngorhinootologie 87(11):796–799. https://doi.org/10.1055/s-2008-1077527

Frost A, Mirza N (2020) Gore-Tex implant extrusion following revision medialization thyroplasty: case report and review of the literature. World J Otorhinolaryngol Head Neck Surg 8(3):213–216. https://doi.org/10.1016/j.wjorl.2020.08.001

Fuchs HV, König N, Shaw S, Völkel D (1984) Report Fraunhofer Institute for building physics. Fraunhofer Institute

Gandini S, Botteri E, Iodice S, Boniol M, Lowenfels AB, Maisonneuve P, Boyle P (2008) Tobacco smoking and cancer: a meta-analysis. Int J Cancer 122(1):155–164. https://doi.org/10.1002/ijc.23033

Gerein V, Rastorguev E, Gerein J, Jecker P, Pfister H (2005) Use of interferon-alpha in recurrent respiratory papillomatosis: 20-year follow-up. Ann Otol Rhinol Laryngol 114(6):463–471. https://doi.org/10.1177/000348940511400608

Gibson W, Wand BM, Meads C, Catley MJ, O'Connell NE (2019) Transcutaneous electrical nerve stimulation (TENS) for chronic pain – an overview of Cochrane Reviews. Cochrane Database Syst Rev 2(2):CD011890. https://doi.org/10.1002/14651858.CD011890.pub2

Gocal WA, Tong JY, Maxwell PJ, Sataloff RT (in press) Systematic review of recurrence rates of benign vocal fold lesions following surgery. J Voice. https://doi.org/10.1016/j.jvoice.2022.10.015

van Gogh CD, Verdonck-de Leeuw IM, Boon-Kamma BA, Rinkel RN, de Bruin MD, Langendijk JA, Kuik DJ, Mahieu HF (2006) The efficacy of voice therapy in patients after treatment for early glottic carcinoma. Cancer 106(1):95–105. https://doi.org/10.1002/cncr.21578

Granqvist S, Simberg S, Hertegård S, Holmqvist S, Larsson H, Lindestad PÅ, Södersten M, Hammarberg B (2015) Resonance tube phonation in water: high-speed imaging, electroglottographic and oral pressure observations of vocal fold vibrations–a pilot study. Logoped Phoniatr Vocol 40(3):113–121. https://doi.org/10.3109/14015439.2014.913682

Grasso M, Remacle M, Bachy V, Van Der Vorst S, Lawson G (2014) Use of cidofovir in HPV patients with recurrent respiratory papillomatosis. Eur Arch Otorhinolaryngol 271(11):2983–2990. https://doi.org/10.1007/s00405-014-3055-x

Gray H, Coman L, Walton C, Thorning S, Cardell E, Weir KA (2024) A comparison of voice and psychotherapeutic treatments for adults with functional voice disorders: a systematic review. J Voice 38(2):542.e9–542.e27. https://doi.org/10.1016/j.jvoice.2021.09.018

Guzman M, Castro C, Testart A, Muñoz D, Gerhard J (2013) Laryngeal and pharyngeal activity during semioccluded vocal tract postures in subjects diagnosed with hyperfunctional dysphonia. J Voice 27(6):709–716. https://doi.org/10.1016/j.jvoice.2013.05.007

Guzman M, Jara R, Olavarria C, Caceres P, Escuti G, Medina F, Medina L, Madrid S, Muñoz D, Laukkanen AM (2017) Efficacy of water resistance therapy in subjects diagnosed with behavioral dysphonia: a randomized controlled trial. J Voice 31(3):385.e1-385.e10. https://doi.org/10.1016/j.jvoice.2016.09.005

Guzman M, Denizoglu I, Fridman D, Loncon C, Rivas C, García R, Morán C, Quezada C, Rodriguez L (2023) Physiologic voice rehabilitation based on water resistance therapy with connected speech in subjects with vocal fatigue. J Voice 37(2):300.e1–300.e10. https://doi.org/10.1016/j.jvoice.2020.12.022

Hah JH, Sim S, An SY, Sung MW, Choi HG (2015) Evaluation of the prevalence of and factors associated with laryngeal diseases among the general population. Laryngoscope 125(11):2536–2542. https://doi.org/10.1002/lary.25424

Hamdan AL, Abi Zeid Daou C, Ghanem A, Ar Feghali P, Hosri J, Sataloff RT (in press) Office-based laser therapy in Reinke's Edema: a systematic review and meta-analysis. J Voice. https://doi.org/10.1016/j.jvoice.2022.12.003

Hansson P, Lundeberg T (1993) Transcutanous electrical nerve stimulation, vibration, and acupuncture as pain-relieving measures. In: Wall PD, Melzack R (Hrsg) Textbook of pain, 5. Aufl. Churchill-Livingstone, New York, S 1341–1351

van Harten PN, Schutte HK (1992) [Psychogenic aphonia; an effective and rapidly treatable conversion]. Ned Tijds Geneesk 136(16):790–793

Hartnick C, Ballif C, De Guzman V, Sataloff R, Campisi P, Kerschner J, Shembel A, Reda D, Shi H, Sheryka Zacny E, Bunting G (2018) Indirect vs direct voice therapy for children with vocal nodules: a randomized clinical trial. JAMA Otolaryngol Head Neck Surg 144(2):156–163. https://doi.org/10.1001/jamaoto.2017.2618

Henschke N, Bergman H, Villanueva G, Loke YK, Golder SP, Crosbie EJ, Kyrgiou M, Dwan K, Morrison J (2022) Effects of human papillomavirus (HPV) vaccination programmes on community rates of HPV-related disease and harms from vaccination. Cochrane Database Syst Rev 5:CD015363. https://doi.org/10.1002/14651858.CD015363

Hess MM, Fleischer S, Ernstberger M (2018) New 445 nm blue laser for laryngeal surgery combines photoangiolytic and cutting properties. Eur Arch Otorhinolaryngol 275(6):1557–1567. https://doi.org/10.1007/s00405-018-4974-8

Hoh JF (2005) Laryngeal muscle fibre types. Acta Physiol Scand 183(2):133–149. https://doi.org/10.1111/j.1365-201X.2004.01402.x

Homma S (1973) A survey of Japanese research on muscle vibration. In: Desmedt JE (Hrsg) Human reflexes, pathophysiology of motor systems, methodology of human reflexes. Karger Publishers, S 463–468

Huestis MJ, Keefe KR, Kahn CI, Tracy LF, Levi JR (2020) Alternatives to acid suppression treatment for laryngopharyngeal reflux. Ann Otol Rhinol Laryngol 129(10):1030–1039. https://doi.org/10.1177/0003489420922870

Imaizumi M, Tada Y, Okano W, Tani A, Omori K (2016) Effectiveness of steroid injections for bamboo nodules: a case report. Ear Nose Throat J 95(4–5):E21–E23

Islami F, Tramacere I, Rota M, Bagnardi V, Fedirko V, Scotti L, Garavello W, Jenab M, Corrao G, Straif K, Negri E, Boffetta P, La Vecchia C (2010) Alcohol drinking and laryngeal cancer: overall and dose-risk relation: a systematic review and meta-analysis. Oral Oncol 46(11):802–810. https://doi.org/10.1016/j.oraloncology.2010.07.015

Ishikawa K, Thibeault S (2010) Voice rest versus exercise: a review of the literature. J Voice 24(4):379–387. https://doi.org/10.1016/j.jvoice.2008.10.011

Israel H, Richter RR (2011) A guide to understanding meta-analysis. J Orthop Sports Phys Ther 41(7):496–504. https://doi.org/10.2519/jospt.2011.3333

Joshi A, Johns MM 3rd (2018) Current practices for voice rest recommendations after phonomicrosurgery. Laryngoscope 128(5):1170–1175. https://doi.org/10.1002/lary.26979

Kaneko M, Hirano S (2017) Voice rest after laryngeal surgery: what's the evidence? Curr Opin Otolaryngol Head Neck Surg 25(6):459–463. https://doi.org/10.1097/MOO.0000000000000407

Kenny HL, Friedman L, Blake Simpson C, McGarey PO (in press) Vocal fold polyps: a scoping review. J Voice. https://doi.org/10.1016/j.jvoice.2023.06.007

Kim J (2021) Effects of laryngeal massage on muscle tension dysphonia: a systematic review and meta-analysis. J Korean Soc Laryngol Phoniatr Logop. Korean Soc Laryngol Phoniatr Logop 32(2):64–74. https://doi.org/10.22469/jkslp.2021.32.2.64

Kim JW, Park JH, Park KN, Lee SW (2014) Treatment efficacy of electromyography versus fiberscopy-guided botulinum toxin injection in adductor spasmodic dysphonia patients: a prospective comparative study. ScientificWorldJournal 2014:327928. https://doi.org/10.1155/2014/327928

Khodeir MS, Hassan SM, El Shoubary AM, Saad MNA (2021) Surgical and nonsurgical lines of treatment of Reinke's Edema: a systematic literature review. J Voice 35(3):502.e1–502.e11. https://doi.org/10.1016/j.jvoice.2019.10.016

Koufman JA, Aviv JE, Casiano RR, Shaw GY (2002) Laryngopharyngeal reflux: position statement of the committee on speech, voice, and swallowing disorders of the American Academy of Otolaryngology-Head and Neck Surgery. Otolaryngol Head Neck Surg 127(1):32–35. https://doi.org/10.1067/mhn.2002.125760

Laukkanen AM, Maki E, Leppanen K (2009) Electroglottogram-based estimation of vocal economy: „quasi-output-cost ratio". Folia Phoniatr Logop 61(6):316–322. https://doi.org/10.1159/000252847

Lechien JR, Saussez S, Harmegnies B, Finck C, Burns JA (2017) Laryngopharyngeal reflux and voice disorders: a multifactorial model of etiology and pathophysiology. J Voice 31(6):733–752. https://doi.org/10.1016/j.jvoice.2017.03.015

Lechien JR, Schindler A, De Marrez LG, Hamdan AL, Karkos PD, Harmegnies B, Barillari MR, Finck C, Saussez S (2019) Instruments evaluating the clinical findings of laryngopharyngeal reflux: a systematic review. Laryngoscope 129(3):720–736. https://doi.org/10.1002/lary.27537

Lechien JR, Bock JM, Carroll TL, Akst LM (2020) Is empirical treatment a reasonable strategy for laryngopharyngeal reflux? A contemporary review. Clin Otolaryngol 45(4):450–458. https://doi.org/10.1111/coa.13518

Lechien JR, Mouawad F, Bobin F, Bartaire E, Crevier-Buchman L, Saussez S (2021) Review of management of laryngopharyngeal reflux disease. Eur Ann Otorhinolaryngol Head Neck Dis 138(4):257–267. https://doi.org/10.1016/j.anorl.2020.11.002

Lee M, Sulica L (2020) Recurrence of benign phonotraumatic vocal fold lesions after microlaryngoscopy. Laryngoscope 130(8):1989–1995. https://doi.org/10.1002/lary.28349

Lee MY, Metenou S, Brough DE, Sabzevari H, Bai K, Jochems C, Schlom J, Allen CT (2021) Preclinical study of a novel therapeutic vaccine for recurrent respiratory papillomatosis. NPJ Vaccines 6(1):86. https://doi.org/10.1038/s41541-021-00348-x

Lester-Smith RA, Miller CH, Cherney LR (2023) Behavioral therapy for tremor or dystonia affecting voice in speakers with hyperkinetic dysarthria: a systematic review. J Voice 37(4):561–573. https://doi.org/10.1016/j.jvoice.2021.03.026

Li X, Gao L, Li H et al (2013) Human papillomavirus infection and laryngeal cancer risk: a systematic review and meta-analysis. J Infect Dis 207(3):479–488. https://doi.org/10.1093/infdis/jis698

Lorenz KJ (2015) [Voice rehabilitation after total laryngectomy: A chronological review of medical history]. HNO 63(10):663–680. https://doi.org/10.1007/s00106-015-0043-4

Lundeberg T (1984) Long-term results of vibratory stimulation as a pain relieving measure for chronic pain. Pain 20(1):13–23. https://doi.org/10.1016/0304-3959(84)90807-8

Lundeberg T, Nordemar R, Ottoson D (1984) Pain alleviation by vibratory stimulation. Pain 20(1):25–44. https://doi.org/10.1016/0304-3959(84)90808-X

Lundeberg T, Abrahamsson P, Bondesson L, Haker E (1987) Vibratory stimulation compared to placebo in alleviation of pain. Scand J Rehabil Med 19(4):153–158

Mailänder E, Mühre L, Barsties B (2017) Lax Vox as a voice training program for teachers: a pilot study. J Voice 31(2):262.e13–262.e22. https://doi.org/10.1016/j.jvoice.2016.04.011

Mansuri B, Tohidast SA, Soltaninejad N, Kamali M, Ghelichi L, Azimi H (2018) Nonmedical treatments of vocal fold nodules: a systematic review. J Voice 32(5):609–620. https://doi.org/10.1016/j.jvoice.2017.08.023

Mansuri B, Torabinejhad F, Jamshidi AA, Dabirmoghaddam P, Vasaghi-Gharamaleki B, Ghelichi L (2020) Transcutaneous electrical nerve stimulation combined with voice therapy in women with muscle tension dysphonia. J Voice 34(3):490.e11–490.e21. https://doi.org/10.1016/j.jvoice.2018.11.003

Martins RH, do Amaral HA, Tavares EL, Martins MG, Gonçalves TM, Dias NH (2016) Voice disorders: etiology and diagnosis. J Voice 30(6):761.e1–761.e9. https://doi.org/10.1016/j.jvoice.2015.09.017

Masson MLV, de Araújo TM (2018) Protective strategies against dysphonia in teachers: preliminary results comparing voice amplification and 0.9% NaCl nebulization. J Voice 32(2):257.e1–257.e10. https://doi.org/10.1016/j.jvoice.2017.04.013

Mathieson L, Hirani SP, Epstein R, Baken RJ, Wood G, Rubin JS (2009) Laryngeal manual therapy: a preliminary study to examine its treatment effects in the management of muscle tension dysphonia. J Voice 23(3):353–366. https://doi.org/10.1016/j.jvoice.2007.10.002

Mattsson P, Frostell A, Björck G et al (2018) Recovery of voice after reconstruction of the recurrent laryngeal nerve and adjuvant Nimodipine. World J Surg 42(3):632–638. https://doi.org/10.1007/s00268-017-4235-9

McFarlane SC (1988) Treatment of benign laryngeal disorders with traditional methods and techniques of voice therapy. Ear Nose Throat J 67(6):425–435

Meerschman I, D'haeseleer E, De Cock E, Neyens H, Claeys S, Van Lierde K (2016a) Effectiveness of chewing technique on the phonation of female speech-language pathology students: a pilot study. J Voice 30(5):574–578. https://doi.org/10.1016/j.jvoice.2015.06.016

Meerschman I, Bettens K, Dejagere S, Tetaert L, D'haeseleer E, Claeys S, Van Lierde K (2016b) Effect of two isolated vocal-facilitating techniques chant talk and pitch inflections on the phonation of female speech-language pathology students: a pilot study. J Voice 30(6):771.e17–771.e25. https://doi.org/10.1016/j.jvoice.2015.11.007

Meerschman I, D'haeseleer E, Catry T, Ruigrok B, Claeys S, Van Lierde K (2017) Effect of two isolated vocal facilitating techniques glottal fry and yawn-sigh on the phonation of female speech-language pathology students: a pilot study. J Commun Disord 66:40–50. https://doi.org/10.1016/j.jcomdis.2017.03.004

Meerschman I, Van Lierde K, Ketels J, Coppieters C, Claeys S, D'haeseleer E (2019) Effect of three semi-occluded vocal tract therapy programmes on the phonation of patients with dysphonia: lip trill, water-resistance therapy and straw phonation. Int J Lang Commun Disord 54(1):50–61. https://doi.org/10.1111/1460-6984.12431

Medeiros N, Castro MEM, van Lith-Bijl JT, Desuter GRR (2022) A systematic review on surgical treatments for sulcus vocalis and vocal fold scar. Laryngoscope 132(4):822–830. https://doi.org/10.1002/lary.29665

Melzack R, Wall PD (1965) Pain mechanisms: a new theory. Science 150(3699):971–979. https://doi.org/10.1126/science.150.3699.971

de Menezes RF, Bergmann A, Thuler LC (2013) Alcohol consumption and risk of cancer: a systematic literature review. Asian Pac J Cancer Prev 14(9):4965–4972. https://doi.org/10.7314/apjcp.2013.14.9.4965

Milbrath RL, Solomon NP (2003) Do vocal warm-up exercises alleviate vocal fatigue? J Speech Lang Hear Res 46(2):422–436. https://doi.org/10.1044/1092-4388(2003/035)

Miller T, Deary V, Patterson J (2014) Improving access to psychological therapies in voice disorders: a cognitive behavioural therapy model. Curr Opin Otolaryngol Head Neck Surg 22(3):201–205. https://doi.org/10.1097/MOO.0000000000000056

Müller A (2022) [Active and passive bioimplants for vocal fold paralysis]. Laryngorhinootologie 101(S 01):S144–S159. https://doi.org/10.1055/a-1708-2881

Murillo N, Valls-Sole J, Vidal J, Opisso E, Medina J, Kumru H (2014) Focal vibration in neurorehabilitation. Eur J Phys Rehabil Med 50(2):231–242

Namin AW, Christopher KM, Eisenbeis JF (2017) Botulinum toxin dosing trends in spasmodic dysphonia over a 20-year period. J Voice 31(1):107–110. https://doi.org/10.1016/j.jvoice.2016.01.006

Nawka T, Hosemann W (2005) Surgical procedures for voice restoration. GMS Curr Top Otorhinolaryngol Head Neck Surg 4:Doc14

NIDCD Fact Sheet (2010) Spasmodic dysphonia. National Institutes of Health, Bethesda

Nolan IT, Morrison SD, Arowojolu O, Crowe CS, Massie JP, Adler RK, Chaiet SR, Francis DO (2019) The role of voice therapy and phonosurgery in transgender vocal feminization. J Craniofac Surg 30(5):1368–1375. https://doi.org/10.1097/SCS.0000000000005132

OCEBM Levels of Evidence Working Group (2011) The Oxford 2011 levels of evidence. Oxford centre for evidence-based medicine. http://www.cebm.net/index.aspx?o=5653. Accessed 1 Nov 2023

Ogawa M, Hosokawa K, Yoshida M, Yoshii T, Shiromoto O, Inohara H (2013) Immediate effectiveness of humming on the supraglottic compression in subjects with muscle tension dysphonia. Folia Phoniatr Logop 65(3):123–128. https://doi.org/10.1159/000353539

Ogawa M, Hosokawa K, Yoshida M, Iwahashi T, Hashimoto M, Inohara H (2014) Immediate effects of humming on computed electroglottographic parameters in patients with muscle tension dysphonia. J Voice 28(6):733–741. https://doi.org/10.1016/j.jvoice.2014.02.004

Paes SM, Zambon F, Yamasaki R, Simberg S, Behlau M (2013) Immediate effects of the Finnish resonance tube method on behavioral dysphonia. J Voice 27(6):717–722. https://doi.org/10.1016/j.jvoice.2013.04.007

Pahn J, Pahn E (1998) Education and treatment of the speaking and singing voice according to the Nasality Method. Log Phon Vocol 23(1):30–32. https://doi.org/10.1080/140154398434013

Pierce JL, Tanner K, Merrill RM, Shnowske L, Roy N (2021) A field-based approach to establish normative acoustic data for healthy female voices. J Speech Lang Hear Res 64(3):691–706. https://doi.org/10.1044/2020_JSLHR-20-00490

Pozzali I, Pizzorni N, Ruggeri A, Schindler A, Dal Farra F (2024) Effectiveness of semi-occluded vocal tract exercises (SOVTEs) in patients with dysphonia: a systematic review and meta-analysis. J Voice 38(1):245.e17–245.e35. https://doi.org/10.1016/j.jvoice.2021.06.009

Pu T, Huang M, Kong X, Wang M, Chen X, Feng X, Wei C, Weng X, Xu F (2021) Lee Silverman Voice Treatment to improve speech in Parkinson's disease: a systemic review and meta-analysis. Parkinsons Dis 2021:3366870. https://doi.org/10.1155/2021/3366870

Radolf V, Laukkanen AM, Horáček J, Liu D (2014) Air-pressure, vocal fold vibration and acoustic characteristics of phonation during vocal exercising. Part 1: measurement in vivo. Eng Mech 21(3):53–59

Ramalkhan JT, Oosterbaan-Beks MJA, Goes de Graaff BE, Arendse JW, Mudde RF (2014) [Voice bubbling therapy]. Logopedie en Foniatrie 86(10):22–26

Ramavat AS, Tiwana H, Banumathy N, Bakshi J, Panda N, Goel A (2019) Efficacy of intralesional steroid injection in small benign vocal fold lesions. J Voice 33(5):767–772. https://doi.org/10.1016/j.jvoice.2018.04.008

Ramig LO, Bonitati C, Lemke J, Horii Y (1994) Voice treatment for patients with Parkinson disease: development of an approach and preliminary efficacy data. J Med Speech-Lang Path 2:191–209

Reiter R, Hoffmann TK, Pickhard A, Brosch S (2015) Hoarseness-causes and treatments. Dtsch Arztebl Int 112(19):329–337. https://doi.org/10.3238/arztebl.2015.0329

Reiter R, Hoffmann T (2017) [Phonomicrosurgery - a retrospective analysis of 400 cases] . Laryngorhinootologie 96(9):597–606. https://doi.org/10.1055/s-0043-110859

Reiter R, Pickhard A, Heyduck A, Brosch S, Hoffmann TK (2020) [Update on vocal fold augmentation] . HNO 68(6):461–472. https://doi.org/10.1007/s00106-020-00863-8

Remacle M, Friedrich G, Dikkers FG, de Jong F (2003) Phonosurgery of the vocal folds: a classification proposal. Eur Arch Otorhinolaryngol 260(1):1–6. https://doi.org/10.1007/s00405-002-0507-5

Reveiz L, Cardona AF (2013) Antibiotics for acute laryngitis in adults. Cochrane Database Syst Rev 3:CD004783. https://doi.org/10.1002/14651858.CD004783.pub4

Reveiz L, Cardona AF (2015) Antibiotics for acute laryngitis in adults. Cochrane Database Syst Rev 2015(5):CD004783. https://doi.org/10.1002/14651858.CD004783.pub5

Ribeiro VV, Pedrosa V, Silverio KCA, Behlau M (2018) Laryngeal manual therapies for behavioral dysphonia: a systematic review and meta-analysis. J Voice 32(5):553–563. https://doi.org/10.1016/j.jvoice.2017.06.019

Rice JB, White AG, Scarpati LM, Wan G, Nelson WW (2017) Long-term systemic corticosteroid exposure: a systematic literature review. Clin Ther 39(11):2216–2229. https://doi.org/10.1016/j.clinthera.2017.09.011

Rittweger J, Beller G, Felsenberg D (2000) Acute physiological effects of exhaustive whole-body vibration exercise in man. Clin Physiol 20(2):134–142. https://doi.org/10.1046/j.1365-2281.2000.00238.x

Ritzmann R, Kramer A, Gruber M, Gollhofer A, Taube W (2010) EMG activity during whole body vibration: motion artifacts or stretch reflexes. Eur J Appl Physiol 110(1):143–151. https://doi.org/10.1007/s00421-010-1483-x

Rosenfeld RM (2004) Meta-analysis. ORL J Otorhinolaryngol Relat Spec 66(4):186–195. https://doi.org/10.1159/000079876

Roy N (2008) Assessment and treatment of musculoskeletal tension in hyperfunctional voice disorders. Int J Speech Lang Pathol 10(4):195–209. https://doi.org/10.1080/17549500701885577

Roy N, Bless DM, Heisey D, Ford CN (1997) Manual circumlaryngeal therapy for functional dysphonia: an evaluation of short- and long-term treatment outcomes. J Voice 11(3):321–331. https://doi.org/10.1016/s0892-1997(97)80011-2

Roy N, Weinrich B, Gray SD et al (2002) Voice amplification versus vocal hygiene instruction for teachers with voice disorders: a treatment outcomes study. J Speech Lang Hear Res 45(4):625–638. https://doi.org/10.1044/1092-4388(2002/050)

Roy N, Weinrich B, Gray SD, Tanner K, Stemple JC, Sapienza CM (2003) Three treatments for teachers with voice disorders: a randomized clinical trial. J Speech Lang Hear Res 46(3):670–688. https://doi.org/10.1044/1092-4388(2003/053)

Roy N, Merrill RM, Thibeault S, Parsa RA, Gray SD, Smith EM (2004) Prevalence of voice disorders in teachers and the general population. J Speech Lang Hear Res 47(2):281–293. https://doi.org/10.1044/1092-4388(2004/023)

Rücker G, Schwarzer G (2015) Ranking treatments in frequentist network meta-analysis works without resampling methods. BMC Med Res Methodol 15:58. https://doi.org/10.1186/s12874-015-0060-8

Ruotsalainen J, Sellman J, Lehto L, Verbeek J (2008) Systematic review of the treatment of functional dysphonia and prevention of voice disorders. Otolaryngol Head Neck Surg 138(5):557–565. https://doi.org/10.1016/j.otohns.2008.01.014

Ryan NM (2015) A review on the efficacy and safety of gabapentin in the treatment of chronic cough. Expert Opin Pharmacother 16(1):135–145. https://doi.org/10.1517/14656566.2015.981524

Salanti G (2012) Indirect and mixed-treatment comparison, network, or multiple-treatments meta-analysis: many names, many benefits, many concerns for the next generation evidence synthesis tool. Res Synth Methods 3(2):80–97. https://doi.org/10.1002/jrsm.1037

San Giorgi MR, Helder HM, Lindeman RJ, de Bock GH, Dikkers FG (2016) The association between gastroesophageal reflux disease and recurrent respiratory papillomatosis: a systematic review. Laryngoscope 126(10):2330–2339. https://doi.org/10.1002/lary.25898

Santos JK, Silvério KC, Diniz Oliveira NF, Gama AC (2016) Evaluation of electrostimulation effect in women with vocal nodules. J Voice 30(6):769.e1–769.e7. https://doi.org/10.1016/j.jvoice.2015.10.023

Sanuki T, Yumoto E (2017) Long-term evaluation of type 2 thyroplasty with titanium bridges for Adductor Spasmodic Dysphonia. Otolaryngol Head Neck Surg 157(1):80–84. https://doi.org/10.1177/0194599817705612

Sataloff RT, Hawkshaw MJ, Divi V, Heman-Ackah YD (2007) Voice surgery. Otolaryngol Clin N Am 40(5):1151–ix. https://doi.org/10.1016/j.otc.2007.05.015

Sataloff RT, Bush ML, Chandra R, Chepeha D, Rotenberg B, Fisher EW, Goldenberg D, Hanna EY, Kerschner JE, Kraus DH, Krouse JH, Li D, Link M, Lustig LR, Selesnick SH, Sindwani R, Smith RJ, Tysome J, Weber PC, Bradley WD (2021) Systematic and other reviews: criteria and complexities. J Voice 35(4):509–511. https://doi.org/10.1016/j.jvoice.2021.04.027

Schindler A, Bottero A, Capaccio P, Ginocchio D, Adorni F, Ottaviani F (2008) Vocal improvement after voice therapy in unilateral vocal fold paralysis. J Voice 22(1):113–118. https://doi.org/10.1016/j.jvoice.2006.08.004

Schneider R, Machens A, Lorenz K, Dralle H (2020) Intraoperative nerve monitoring in thyroid surgery-shifting current paradigms. Gland Surg 9(Suppl 2):S120–S128. https://doi.org/10.21037/gs.2019.11.04

Schönweiler R (2020) [An update of medication in voice treatment and side effects on voice relating to medication]. Sprache-Stimme-Gehör 44(1):23–28. https://doi.org/10.1055/a-0949-7081

Schwarz K, Cielo CA, Spritzer PM, Villas-Boas AP, Costa AB, Fontanari AMV, Costa Gomes B, da Silva DC, Schneider MA, Lobato MIR (2023) A speech therapy for transgender women: an updated systematic review and meta-analysis. Syst Rev 12(1):128. https://doi.org/10.1186/s13643-023-02267-5

Selleck AM, Moore JE, Rutt AL, Hu A, Sataloff RT (2015) Sulcus vocalis (Type III): prevalence and strobovideolaryngoscopy characteristics. J Voice 29(4):507–511. https://doi.org/10.1016/j.jvoice.2014.09.015

Setton ARF, D'avila JS, Gurgel RQ, Tsuji DH, D'avila DV, Góis CRT, Meurer ATO, Gurgel HP (2019) Variant of the technique for laryngeal microsurgery in cases of difficult laryngoscopy. Int Arch Otorhinolaryngol 23(1):18–24. https://doi.org/10.1055/s-0038-1660825

Simberg S, Sala E, Tuomainen J, Sellman J, Rönnemaa AM (2006) The effectiveness of group therapy for students with mild voice disorders: a controlled clinical trial. J Voice 20(1):97–109. https://doi.org/10.1016/j.jvoice.2005.01.002

Shuman EA, Dwyer CD (2023) Training for awake, office-based laryngeal procedures-the Laryngology fellow's perspective. Laryngoscope. https://doi.org/10.1002/lary.31033.10.1002/lary.31033

da Silva AR, Ghirardi AC, Reiser MR, Paul S (2019) An exact analytical model for the relationship between flow resistance and geometric properties of tubes used in semi-occluded vocal tract exercises. J Voice 33(5):585–590. https://doi.org/10.1016/j.jvoice.2018.03.016

Sluka KA, Walsh D (2003) Transcutaneous electrical nerve stimulation: basic science mechanisms and clinical effectiveness. J Pain 4(3):109–121. https://doi.org/10.1054/jpai.2003.434

Solomon NP (2008) Vocal fatigue and its relation to vocal hyperfunction. Int J Speech Lang Pathol 10(4):254–266. https://doi.org/10.1080/14417040701730990

Soni RS, Dailey SH (2019) Sulcus vocalis. Otolaryngol Clin N Am 52(4):735–743. https://doi.org/10.1016/j.otc.2019.03.016

Song TE, Jiang N (2017) Transgender phonosurgery: a systematic review and meta-analysis. Otolaryngol Head Neck Surg 156(5):803–808. https://doi.org/10.1177/0194599817697050

Spantideas N, Drosou E, Bougea A, AlAbdulwahed R (2020) Proton pump inhibitors for the treatment of laryngopharyngeal reflux. A systematic review. J Voice 34(6):918–929. https://doi.org/10.1016/j.jvoice.2019.05.005

Speyer R (2008) Effects of voice therapy: a systematic review. J Voice 22(5):565–580. https://doi.org/10.1016/j.jvoice.2006.10.005

Stachler RJ, Francis DO, Schwartz SR, Damask CC, Digoy GP, Krouse HJ, McCoy SJ, Ouellette DR, Patel RR, Reavis CCW, Smith LJ, Smith M, Strode SW, Woo P, Nnacheta LC (2018) Clinical practice guideline: hoarseness (dysphonia) (update) executive summary. Otolaryngol Head Neck Surg 158(3):409–426. https://doi.org/10.1177/0194599817751031

Stangherlin DAC, Lemos IO, Bello JZ, Cassol M (2021) Transcutaneous electrical nerve stimulation in dysphonic patients: a systematic review. J Voice 35(6):876–885. https://doi.org/10.1016/j.jvoice.2020.03.003

Stemple JC (2000) Voice therapy: clinical studies, 2. Aufl. Singular Publishing, San Diego

Stemple JC, Roy N, Klaben BK (2014) Clinical voice pathology: theory and management, 5. Aufl. Plural Publishing, San Diego

Steuer CE, El-Deiry M, Parks JR, Higgins KA, Saba NF (2017) An update on larynx cancer. CA Cancer J Clin 67(1):31–50. https://doi.org/10.3322/caac.21386

Stier KH (2011) [Treatment of dysphonia patients with the Accent Method in comparison with the non-method-oriented and direct treatment]. Sprache Stimme Gehör 35:e68–e76. https://doi.org/10.1055/s-0031-1275730

Story BH, Laukkanen AM, Titze IR (2000) Acoustic impedance of an artificially lengthened and constricted vocal tract. J Voice 14(4):455–469. https://doi.org/10.1016/s0892-1997(00)80003-x

Tan M, Bryson PC, Pitts C, Woo P, Benninger MS (2017) Clinical grading of Reinke's edema. Laryngoscope 127(10):2310–2313. https://doi.org/10.1002/lary.26647

Tavaluc R, Tan-Geller M (2019) Reinke's edema. Otolaryngol Clin N Am 52(4):627–635. https://doi.org/10.1016/j.otc.2019.03.006

Tavernese E, Paoloni M, Mangone M, Mandic V, Sale P, Franceschini M, Santilli V (2013) Segmental muscle vibration improves reaching movement in patients with chronic stroke. A randomized controlled trial. NeuroRehabilitation 32(3):591–599. https://doi.org/10.3233/NRE-130881

Tawfik GM, Makram OM, Zayan AH, Ghozy S, Eid PS, Mahmoud MH, Abdelaal A, Abdelghany SM, Sayed AM, Sang TK, Kassem M, Ho QLM, Eltanany HH, Ali AF, Hassan OG, Elsherbiny KE, Shafik AG, Hirayama K, Huy NT (2021) Voice rehabilitation by voice prostheses after total laryngectomy: a systematic review and network meta-analysis for 11,918 patients. J Speech Lang Hear Res 64(7):2668–2681. https://doi.org/10.1044/2021_JSLHR-20-00597

Teixeira LC, Behlau M (2015) Comparison between vocal function exercises and voice amplification. J Voice 29(6):718–726. https://doi.org/10.1016/j.jvoice.2014.12.012

Tezcaner ZÇ, Gökmen MF, Yıldırım S, Dursun G (2019) Clinical features of psychogenic voice disorder and the efficiency of voice therapy and psychological evaluation. J Voice 33(2):250–254. https://doi.org/10.1016/j.jvoice.2017.09.022

Thibeault SL, Merrill RM, Roy N, Gray SD, Smith EM (2004) Occupational risk factors associated with voice disorders among teachers. Ann Epidemiol 14(10):786–792. https://doi.org/10.1016/j.annepidem.2004.03.004

Thomas L, Stemple J (2007) Voice therapy: does science support the art. Comm Dis Rev 1(1):51–79

Thyme-Frøkjær K, Frøkjær-Jensen B (2014) Die Akzentmethode: theorie und Praxis, 4.Aufl. Schulz-Kirchner Verlag, Idstein

Tian H, Pan J, Chen L, Wu Y (2022) A narrative review of current therapies in unilateral recurrent laryngeal nerve injury caused by thyroid surgery. Gland Surg 11(1):270–278. https://doi.org/10.21037/gs-21-708

Tipton CB, Walters R, Gudipudi R, Smyre D, Nguyen S, O'Rourke AK (2023) The efficacy of superior laryngeal nerve block for neurogenic cough: a placebo-controlled trial. Laryngoscope 133(11):3068–3074. https://doi.org/10.1002/lary.30739

Titze IR (2002) Regulating glottal airflow in phonation: application of the maximum power transfer theorem to a low dimensional phonation model. J Acoust Soc Am 111(1 Pt 1):367–376. https://doi.org/10.1121/1.1417526

Titze IR (2006) Voice training and therapy with a semi-occluded vocal tract: rationale and scientific underpinnings. J Speech Lang Hear Res 49(2):448–459. https://doi.org/10.1044/1092-4388(2006/035)

Titze IR, Laukkanen AM (2007) Can vocal economy in phonation be increased with an artificially lengthened vocal tract? A computer modeling study. Logoped Phoniatr Vocol 32(4):147–156. https://doi.org/10.1080/14015430701439765

Tyrmi J, Laukkanen AM (2017) How stressful is „deep bubbling"? J Voice 31(2):262.e1–262.e6. https://doi.org/10.1016/j.jvoice.2016.04.013

Tyrmi J, Radolf V, Horáček J, Laukkanen AM (2017) Resonance tube or LAX vox? J Voice 31(4):430–437. https://doi.org/10.1016/j.jvoice.2016.10.024

Ulmschneider C, Baker J, Vize I, Jiang J (2020) Phonosurgery: a review of current methodologies. World J Otorhinolaryngol Head Neck Surg 7(4):344–353. https://doi.org/10.1016/j.wjorl.2020.09.001

Van Houtte E, Van Lierde K, Claeys S (2011) Pathophysiology and treatment of muscle tension dysphonia: a review of the current knowledge. J Voice 25(2):202–207. https://doi.org/10.1016/j.jvoice.2009.10.009

Van Riper C (1939) Speech correction principles and methods. Prentice-Hall, Englewood Cliffs

Vasan N, Sharum M, Rodney JP (2019) Potential of robotic systems in phonosurgery. Robot Surg 6:3–8. https://doi.org/10.2147/RSRR.S177698

Vasconcelos D, Gomes AOC, Araújo CMT (2019) Vocal fold polyps: literature review. Int Arch Otorhinolaryngol 23(1):116–124. https://doi.org/10.1055/s-0038-1675391

Verdolini-Abbott K (2008) Lessac-Madsen resonant voice therapy: clinician manual. Plural Publishing, San Diego

Vermeulen R, du Toit M, van Lierde K, van der Linde J (2022) The effect of vocal hygiene education programs on voice quality in professional voice users: a systematic review. J Speech Lang Hear Res 65(12):4700–4713. https://doi.org/10.1044/2022_JSLHR-22-00097

Vlot C, Ogawa M, Hosokawa K, Iwahashi T, Kato C, Inohara H (2017) Investigation of the immediate effects of humming on vocal fold vibration irregularity using electroglottography and high-speed laryngoscopy in patients with organic voice disorders. J Voice 31(1):48–56. https://doi.org/10.1016/j.jvoice.2016.03.010

Wang CT, Lai MS, Hsiao TY (2015) Comprehensive outcome researches of intralesional steroid injection on benign vocal fold lesions. J Voice 29(5):578–587. https://doi.org/10.1016/j.jvoice.2014.11.002

Watts C, Nye C, Whurr R (2006) Botulinum toxin for treating spasmodic dysphonia (laryngeal dystonia): a systematic Cochrane review. Clin Rehabil 20(2):112–122. https://doi.org/10.1191/0269215506cr931oa

Watts CR, Hamilton A, Toles L, Childs L, Mau T (2019) Intervention outcomes of two treatments for muscle tension dysphonia: a randomized controlled trial. J Speech Lang Hear Res 62(2):272–282. https://doi.org/10.1044/2018_JSLHR-S-18-0118

Walton C, Conway E, Blackshaw H, Carding P (2017) Unilateral vocal fold paralysis: a systematic review of speech-language pathology management. J Voice 31(4):509.e7–509.e22. https://doi.org/10.1016/j.jvoice.2016.11.002

Welham NV, Maclagan MA (2003) Vocal fatigue: current knowledge and future directions. J Voice 17(1):21–30. https://doi.org/10.1016/s0892-1997(03)00033-x

White AC, Awad R, Carding P (2023) Pre and post-operative voice therapy intervention for benign vocal fold lesions: a systematic review. J Voice 37(6):857–874. https://doi.org/10.1016/j.jvoice.2021.06.005

Wistbacka G, Sundberg J, Simberg S (2016) Vertical laryngeal position and oral pressure variations during resonance tube phonation in water and in air. A pilot study. Logoped Phoniatr Vocol 41(3):117–123. https://doi.org/10.3109/14015439.2015.1028101

Whurr R, Nye C, Lorch M (1998) Meta-analysis of botulinum toxin treatment of spasmodic dysphonia: a review of 22 studies. Int J Lang Commun Disord 33(Suppl):327–329. https://doi.org/10.3109/13682829809179445

Wu CH, Chan RW (2020) Effects of a 6-week straw phonation in water exercise program on the aging voice. J Speech Lang Hear Res 63(4):1018–1032. https://doi.org/10.1044/2020_JSLHR-19-00124

Xie X, Young J, Kost K, McGregor M (2013) KTP 532 nm laser for laryngeal lesions. a systematic review. J Voice 27(2):245–249. https://doi.org/10.1016/j.jvoice.2012.11.006

Yamasaki R, Murano EZ, Gebrim E, Hachiya A, Montagnoli A, Behlau M, Tsuji D (2017) Vocal tract adjustments of dysphonic and non-dysphonic women pre- and post-flexible resonance tube in water exercise: a quantitative MRI study. J Voice 31(4):442–454. https://doi.org/10.1016/j.jvoice.2016.10.015

Yiu EML, Ho EYY (2002) Short-term effect of humming on vocal quality. Asia Pac J Speech Lang Hear 7(3):123–137

Yiu EM, Lo MC, Barrett EA (2017) A systematic review of resonant voice therapy. Int J Speech Lang Pathol 19(1):17–29. https://doi.org/10.1080/17549507.2016.1226953

Yiu EML, Liu CCY, Chan CYP, Barrett E, Lu D (2021) Vibrational therapies for vocal fatigue. J Voice 35(1):29–39. https://doi.org/10.1016/j.jvoice.2019.07.009

Yonekawa H (1988) A clinical study of Reinke's edema. Auris Nasus Larynx 15(1):57–78. https://doi.org/10.1016/s0385-8146(88)80010-5

Yuan F, Guo X, Wei X et al (2020) Lee Silverman Voice Treatment for dysarthria in patients with Parkinson's disease: a systematic review and meta-analysis. Eur J Neurol 27(10):1957–1970. https://doi.org/10.1111/ene.14399

Zeitels SM, Healy GB (2003) Laryngology and phonosurgery. N Engl J Med 349(9):882–892. https://doi.org/10.1056/NEJMra035148

Ziegler A, Gillespie AI, Abbott KV (2010) Behavioral treatment of voice disorders in teachers. Folia Phoniatr Logop 62(1–2):9–23. https://doi.org/10.1159/000239059

Zhang C, Deng Z, Chen Y, Suzuki M, Xie M (2016) Is there a higher prevalence of human papillomavirus infection in Chinese laryngeal cancer patients? A systematic review and meta-analysis. Eur Arch Otorhinolaryngol 273(2):295–303. https://doi.org/10.1007/s00405-014-3345-3

Zhuge P, You H, Wang H, Zhang Y, Du H (2016) An analysis of the effects of voice therapy on patients with early vocal fold polyps. J Voice 30(6):698–704. https://doi.org/10.1016/j.jvoice.2015.08.013

Case Studies

6

The following seven cases illustrate the Scientific Clinical Reasoning (see Sect. 4.1) from the proposed voice diagnostics (see Sect. 3.1) and the resulting top-3 voice parameters (see Sect. 4.2), which emerge as primary critical parameters for treatment and its evaluation for effectiveness and thus, in addition to the medical indication, are crucial for the start of treatment. The treatment options proposed for the cases are based on the contents of Chap. 5.

For better understanding and transparency of the individual results of each case, 7 different voice diagnostic files are provided for each case, which are listed in detail after the brief description of each case.

This material is available for download at the link https://doi.org/10.1007/978-3-662-68958-5_6.

For each case, there are also video and audio recordings (see Figs. 6.1, 6.2, 6.3, 6.4, 6.5, 6.6, 6.7, 6.8, 6.9, 6.10, 6.11, 6.12, 6.13, 6.14, 6.15, 6.16, 6.17, 6.18, 6.19, 6.20, 6.21, 6.22, 6.23, 6.24, 6.25, 6.26, 6.27 and 6.28).

- 6.1 Voice examination protocol-Case-1.xlsm—the already completed voice examination protocol according to Table 3.1 and the correlation matrix according to Table 4.1
- 6.2 Voice quality profile-Case-1.png—voice quality evaluation in the field of acoustics with the software VOXplot
- 6.3 Voice range profiles-Case-1.png—voice function evaluation of SRP and VRP with the software Vox Phonetography
- 6.4 VHI-VFI-VTD forms-Case-1.pdf—the three completed questionnaires in the field of self-evaluation

---

Supplementary Information The electronic version of this chapter contains supplementary material, which can be accessed via the following link https://doi.org/10.1007/978-3-662-70162-1_6. The videos can be played by clicking the DOI link in the legend of a corresponding figure, or by scanning this link with the SN More Media app.

B. Barsties v. Latoszek et al., *Diagnostic and Treatment in Voice Therapy*, https://doi.org/10.1007/978-3-662-70162-1_6

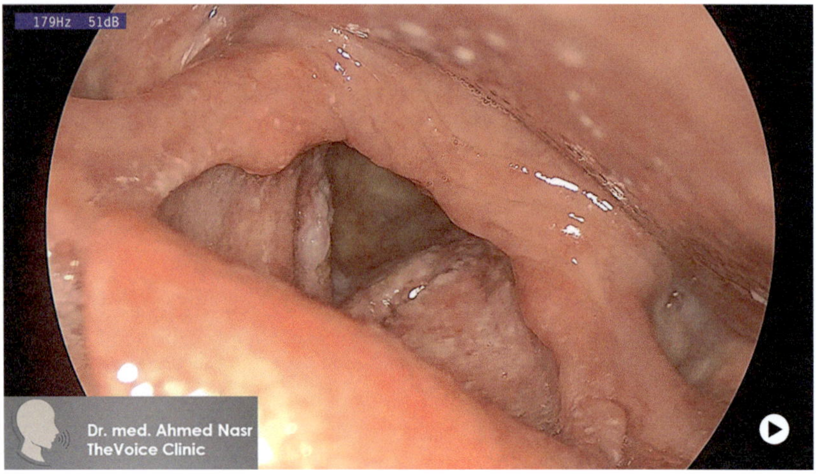

Fig. 6.1 Stroboscopic video recording for visual analysis—Case-1 (▸ https://doi.org/10.1007/000-dy5)

Fig. 6.2 Audio excerpt of the reading text "The North Wind and the Sun" for acoustic analyses—Case-1 (▸ https://doi.org/10.1007/000-dxc)

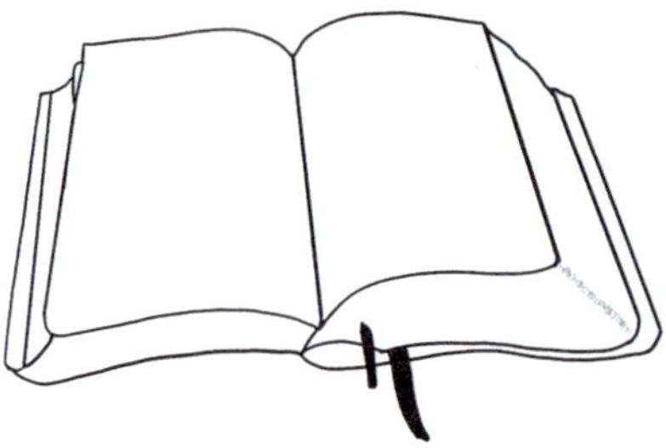

- 6.5 Voice examination protocol-Case-2.xlsm—the already completed voice examination protocol according to Table 3.1 and the correlation matrix according to Table 4.1
- 6.6 Voice quality profile-Case-2.png—voice quality evaluation in the field of acoustics with the software VOXplot
- 6.7 Voice range profiles-Case-2.png—voice function evaluation of SRP and VRP with the software Vox Phonetography
- 6.8 VHI-VFI-VTD forms-Case-2.pdf—the three completed questionnaires in the field of self-evaluation
- 6.9 Voice examination protocol-Case-3.xlsm—the already completed voice examination protocol according to Table 3.1 and the correlation matrix according to Table 4.1
- 6.10 Voice quality profile Case 3.png—voice quality evaluation in the field of acoustics with the software VOXplot

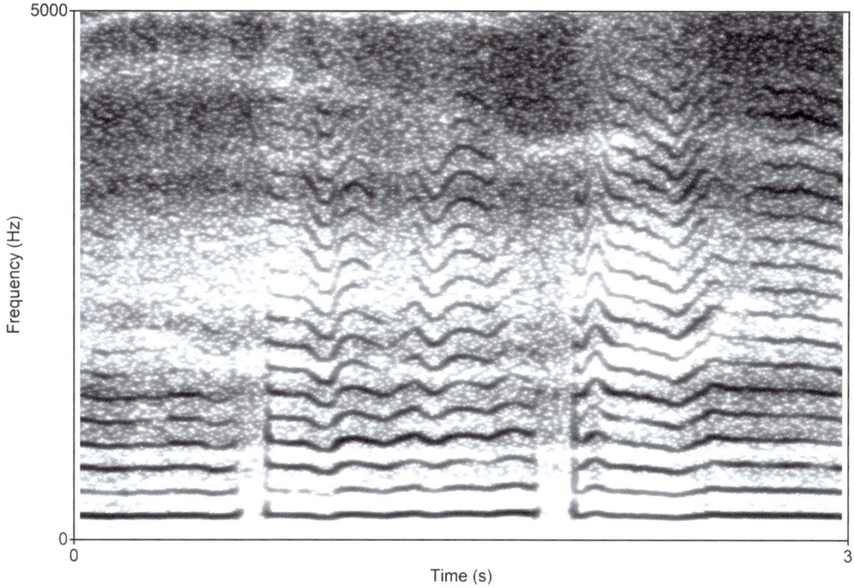

Fig. 6.3 Audio of the 3-second sustained phonation of the vowel /a:/ for acoustic analyses—Case-1 (▸ https://doi.org/10.1007/000-dxd)

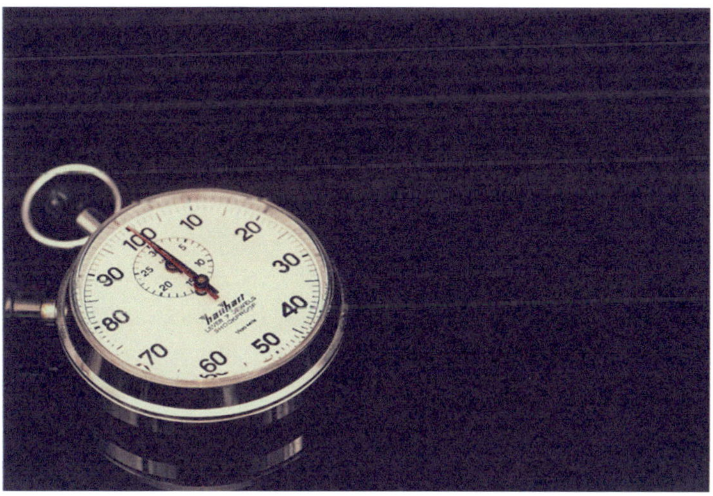

Fig. 6.4 Audio recording for maximum phonation time performance—Case-1 (▸ https://doi.org/10.1007/000-dxe)

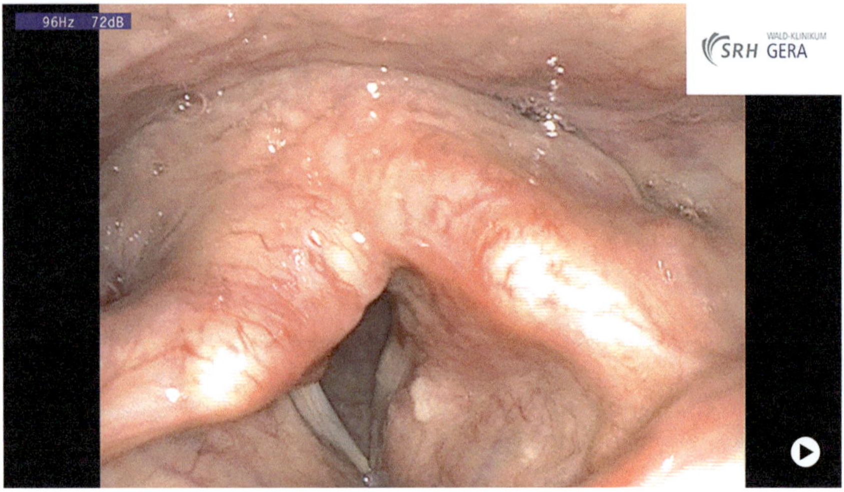

Fig. 6.5 Stroboscopic video recording for visual analysis—Case-2 (▸ https://doi.org/10.1007/000-dxf)

Fig. 6.6 Audio excerpt of the reading text "The North Wind and the Sun" for acoustic analyses—Case-2 (▸ https://doi.org/10.1007/000-dxg)

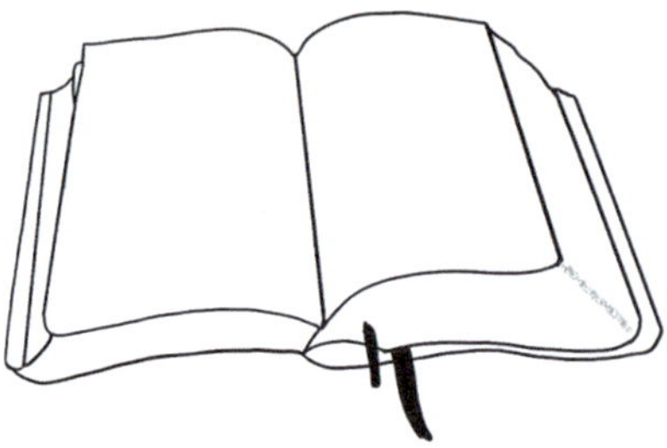

- 6.11 Voice range profiles Case 3.png—voice function evaluation of SRP and VRP with the software Vox Phonetography
- 6.12 Forms VHI-VFI-VTD Case 3.pdf—the three completed questionnaires in the field of self-evaluation
- 6.13 Voice examination protocol Case 4.xlsm—the already completed voice examination protocol according to Table 3.1 and the correlation matrix according to Table 4.1
- 6.14 Voice quality profile Case 4.png—voice quality evaluation in the field of acoustics with the software VOXplot
- 6.15 Voice range profiles Case 4.png—voice function evaluation of SRP and VRP with the software Vox Phonetography
- 6.16 Forms VHI-VFI-VTD Case 4.pdf—the three completed questionnaires in the field of self-evaluation

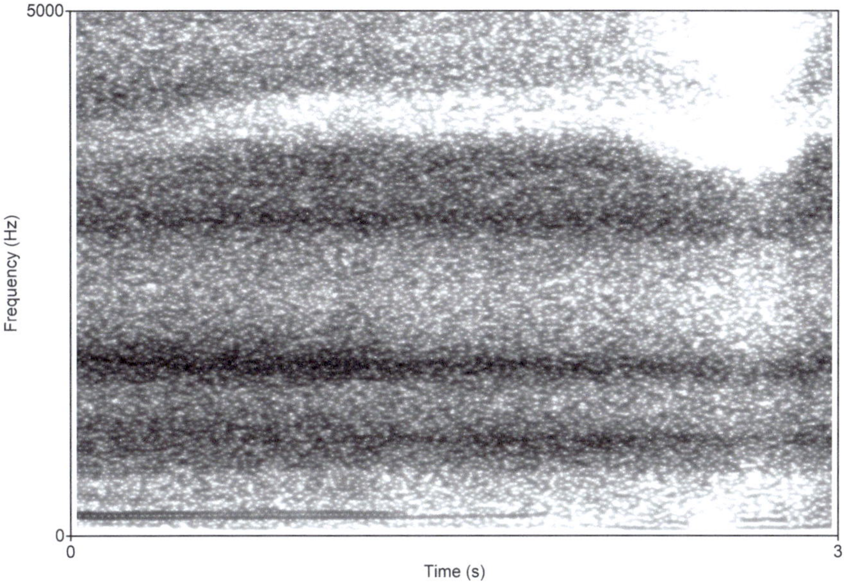

Fig. 6.7 Audio of the 3-second sustained phonation of the vowel /a:/ for acoustic analyses—Case-2 (▸ https://doi.org/10.1007/000-dxh)

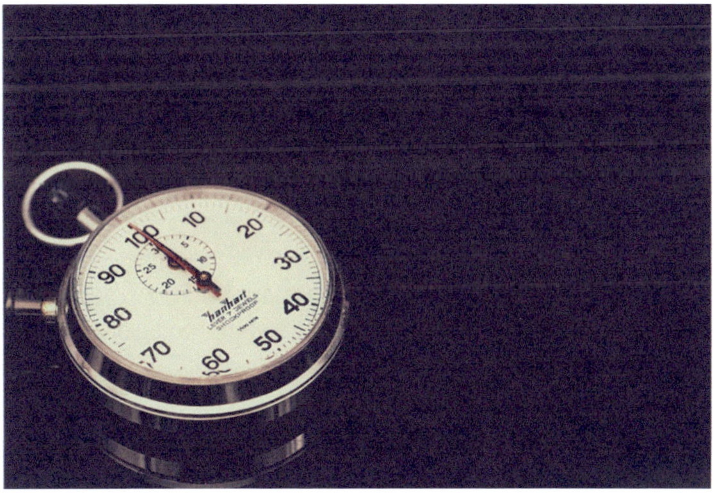

Fig. 6.8 Audio recording for maximum phonation time performance—Case-2 (▸ https://doi.org/10.1007/000-dxj)

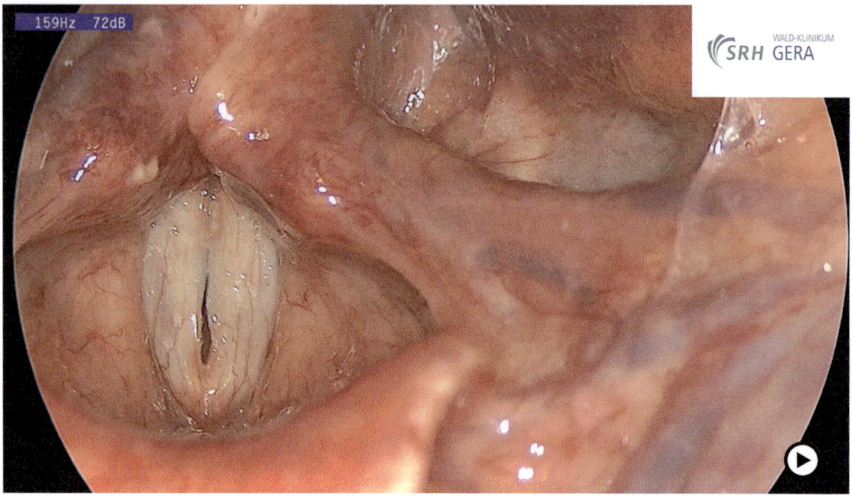

Fig. 6.9 Stroboscopic video recording for visual analysis—Case-3 (▸ https://doi.org/10.1007/000-dxk)

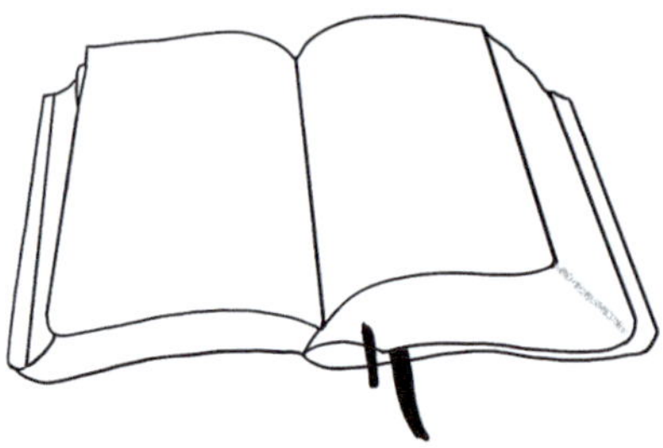

Fig. 6.10 Audio excerpt of the reading text "The North Wind and the Sun" for acoustic analyses—Case-3 (▸ https://doi.org/10.1007/000-dxm)

- 6.17 Voice examination protocol Case 5.xlsm—the already completed voice examination protocol according to Table 3.1 and the correlation matrix according to Table 4.1
- 6.18 Voice quality profile Case 5.png—voice quality evaluation in the field of acoustics with the software VOXplot
- 6.19 Voice range profiles Case 5.png—voice function evaluation of SRP and VRP with the software Vox Phonetography
- 6.20 Forms VHI-VFI-VTD Case 5.pdf—the three completed questionnaires in the field of self-evaluation
- 6.21 Voice examination protocol Case 6.xlsm—the already completed voice examination protocol according to Table 3.1 and the correlation matrix according to Table 4.1
- 6.22 Voice quality profile Case 6.png—voice quality evaluation in the field of acoustics with the software VOXplot

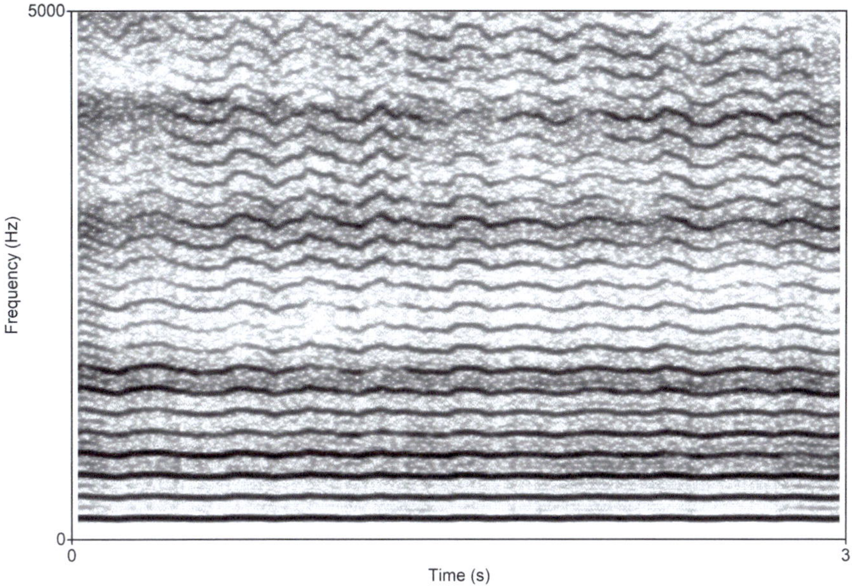

Fig. 6.11 Audio of the 3-second sustained phonation of the vowel /a:/ for the acoustic analyses—Case-3 (▸ https://doi.org/10.1007/000-dxn)

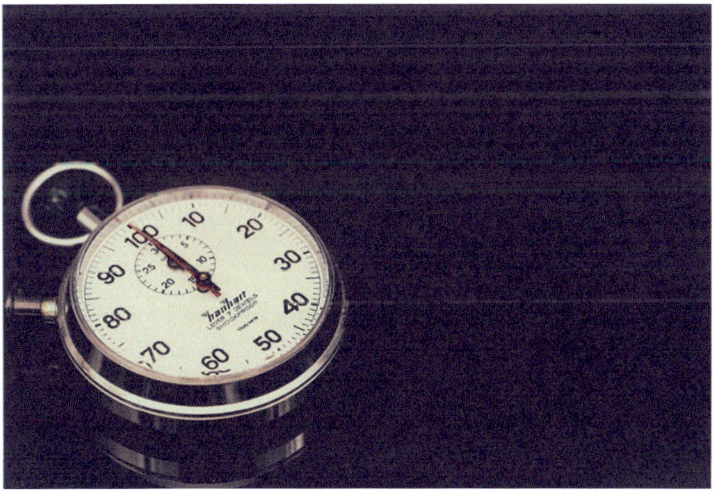

Fig. 6.12 Audio recording for the maximum phonation time performance—Case-3 (▸ https://doi.org/10.1007/000-dxp)

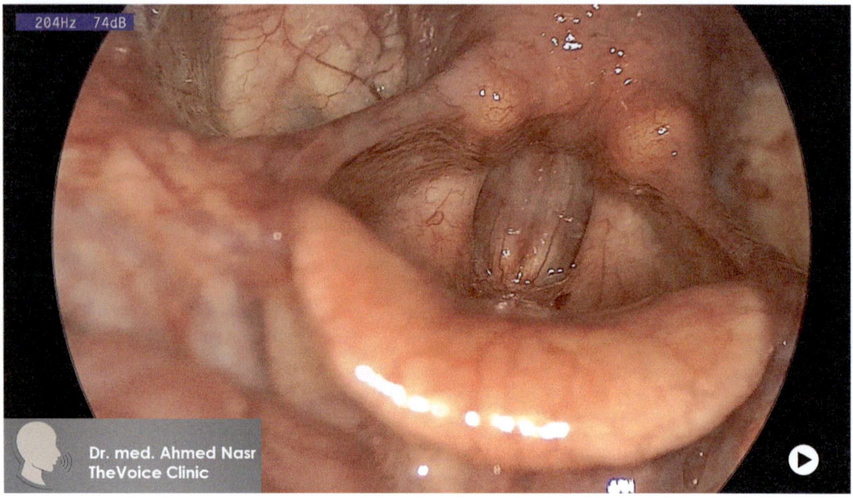

Fig. 6.13 Stroboscopic video recording for visual analysis—Case-4 (▸ https://doi.org/10.1007/000-dxq)

Fig. 6.14 Audio excerpt of the reading text "The North Wind and the Sun" for the acoustic analyses—Case-4 (▸ https://doi.org/10.1007/000-dxr)

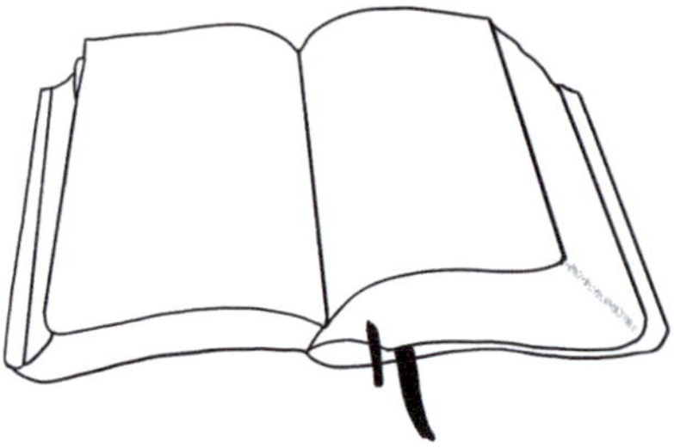

- 6.23 Voice range profiles Case 6.png—voice function evaluation of SRP and VRP with the software Vox Phonetography
- 6.24 Forms VHI-VFI-VTD Case 6.pdf—the three completed questionnaires in the field of self-evaluation
- 6.25 Voice examination protocol Case 7.xlsm—the already completed voice examination protocol according to Table 3.1 and the correlation matrix according to Table 4.1
- 6.26 Voice quality profile Case 7.png—voice quality evaluation in the field of acoustics with the software VOXplot
- 6.27 Voice range profiles Case 7.png—voice function evaluation of SRP and VRP with the software Vox Phonetography
- 6.28 Forms VHI-VFI-VTD Case 7.pdf—the three completed questionnaires in the field of self-evaluation

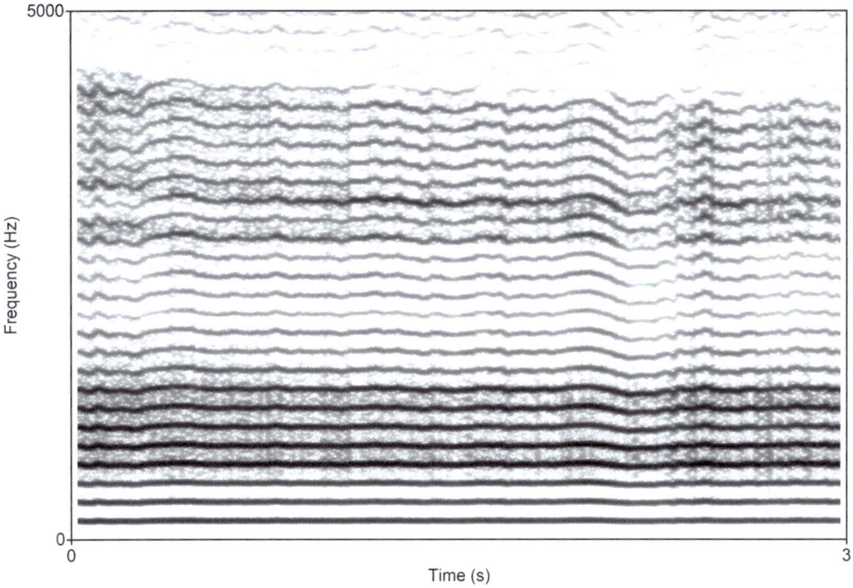

Fig. 6.15 Audio of the 3-second sustained phonation of the vowel /a:/ for the acoustic analyses—Case-4 (▸ https://doi.org/10.1007/000-dxs)

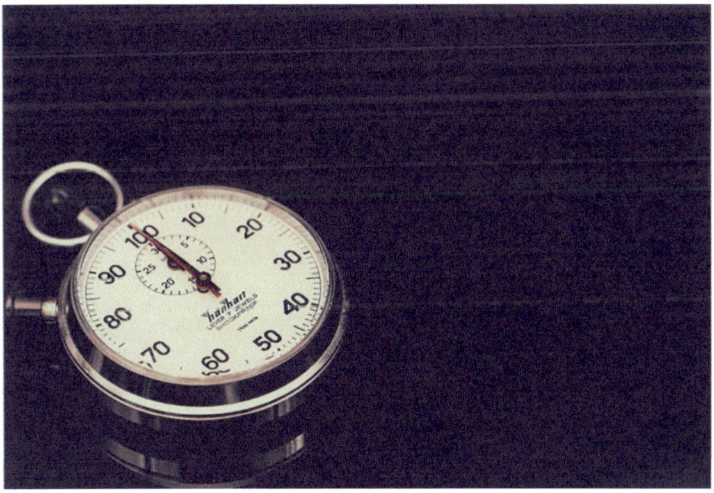

Fig. 6.16 Audio recording for the maximum phonation time performance—Case-4 (▸ https://doi.org/10.1007/000-dxt)

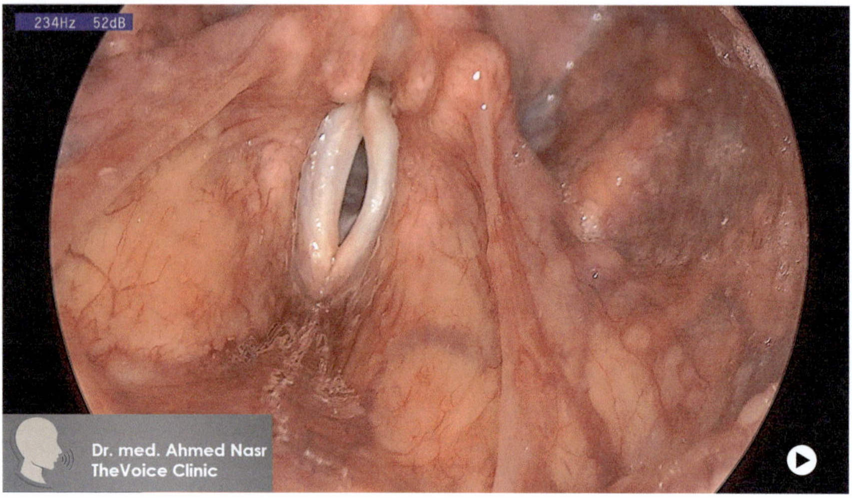

Fig. 6.17 Stroboscopic video recording for visual analysis—Case-5 (▸ https://doi.org/10.1007/000-dxv)

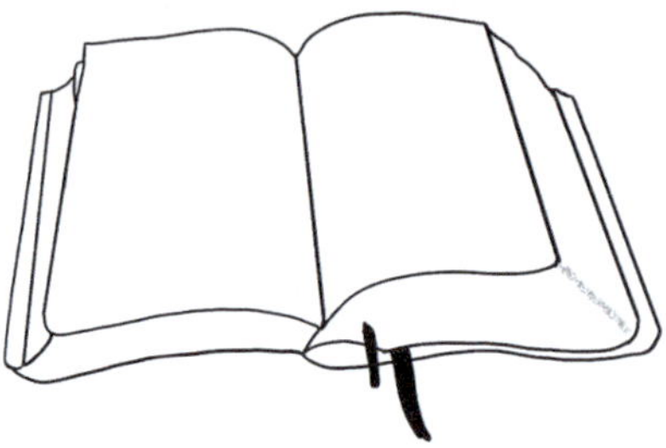

Fig. 6.18 Audio excerpt of the reading text "The North Wind and the Sun" for acoustic analyses—Case-5 (▸ https://doi.org/10.1007/000-dxw)

6.1 Case 1: Chronic Laryngitis with Bilateral Leukoplakia

Brief description: A woman, 63 years old, working as a market vendor with an outdoor stall, has chronic laryngitis and bilateral leukoplakia. Common associated factors in patients with chronic laryngitis are nicotine abuse, gastroesophageal reflux, and inhalative corticosteroid therapy (Reiter and Brosch 2009). The patient in Case 1 has a long history of these three factors, with still frequent nicotine abuse and inhalative corticosteroid therapy due to chronic obstructive pulmonary disease (also associated with nicotine).

The analysis in Fig. 6.29 shows the following evaluation after the voice examination (all measurements can be viewed in detail online for download).

Based on the description of the dysphonia severity degree, as described in Sects. 3.3 and 4.2, this patient has moderate dysphonia severity with the main

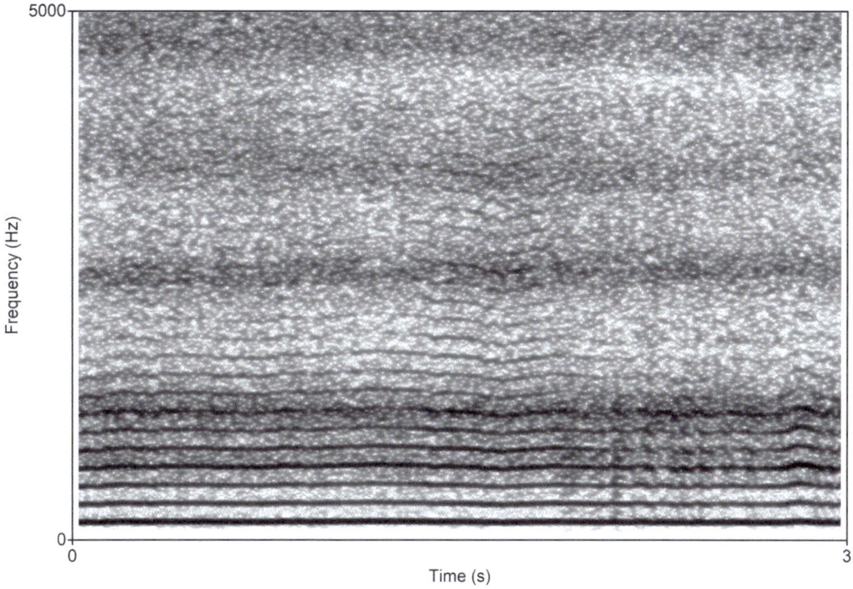

Fig. 6.19 Audio of the 3-second sustained phonation of the vowel /a:/ for acoustic analyses—Case-5 (▸ https://doi.org/10.1007/000-dxx)

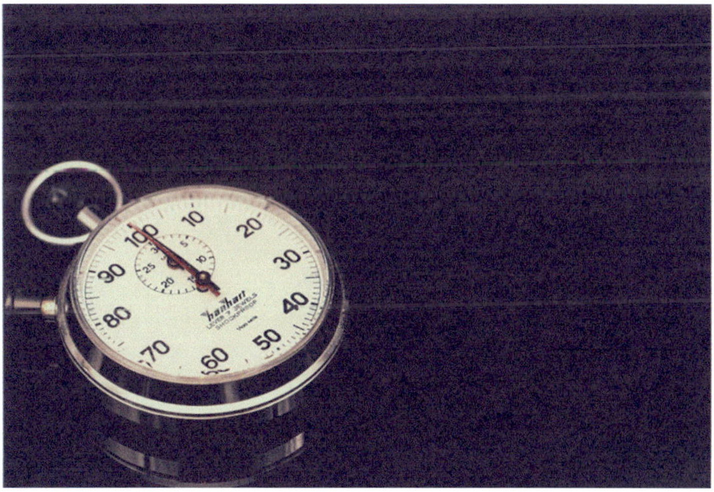

Fig. 6.20 Audio recording of the maximum phonation time performance—Case-5 (▸ https://doi.org/10.1007/000-dxy)

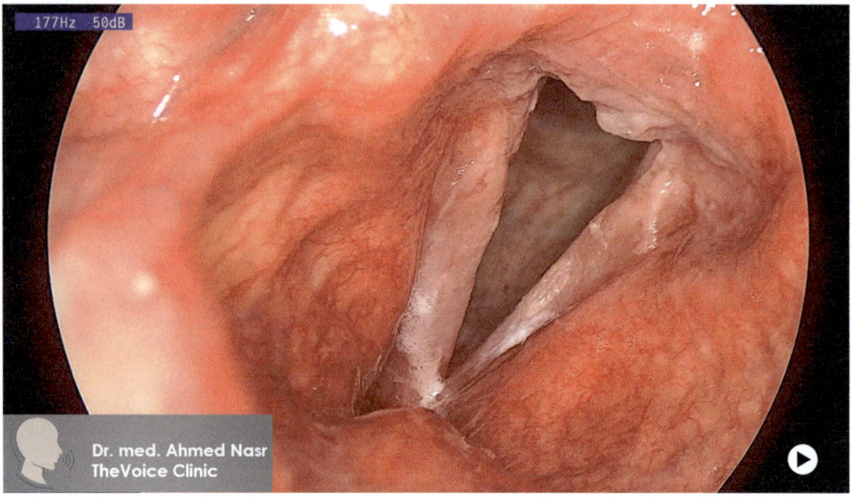

Fig. 6.21 Stroboscopic video recording for visual analysis—Case-6 (▸ https://doi.org/10.1007/000-dxz)

Fig. 6.22 Audio excerpt of the reading text "The North Wind and the Sun" for acoustic analyses—Case-6 (▸ https://doi.org/10.1007/000-dy0)

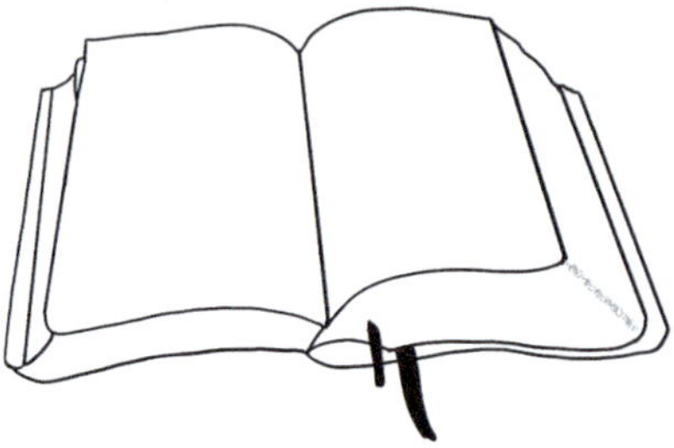

impairment in voice quality (100%) in relation to voice function (58%). Only 19% of all measurements of the voice diagnostic protocol are within the physiological range. An initial suggestion based on the correlation matrix (see Sect. 4.2) shows that the parameters glottal closure, VHI-T, and DSI are key parameters that can be crucial for treatment as primary critical voice parameters. Additionally, the same number of connection points from the correlation matrix as the DSI has the VRP-boundaries, MPT, and VFI cluster 1. Additional information about the patient can be found in the overview of the individual ICF components (see Table 6.1).

Primary goals according to Sect. 3.3

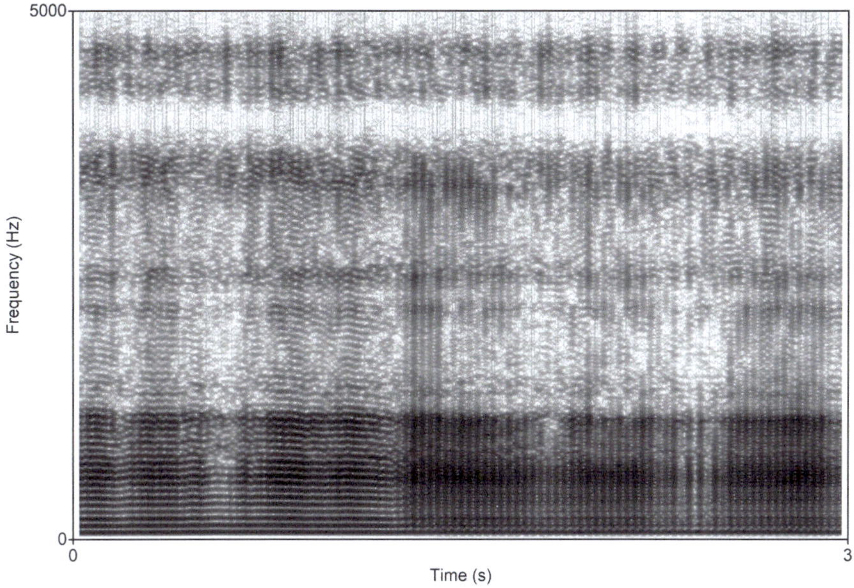

Fig. 6.23 Audio of the 3-second sustained phonation of the vowel /a:/ for acoustic analyses—Case-6 (▸ https://doi.org/10.1007/000-dy1)

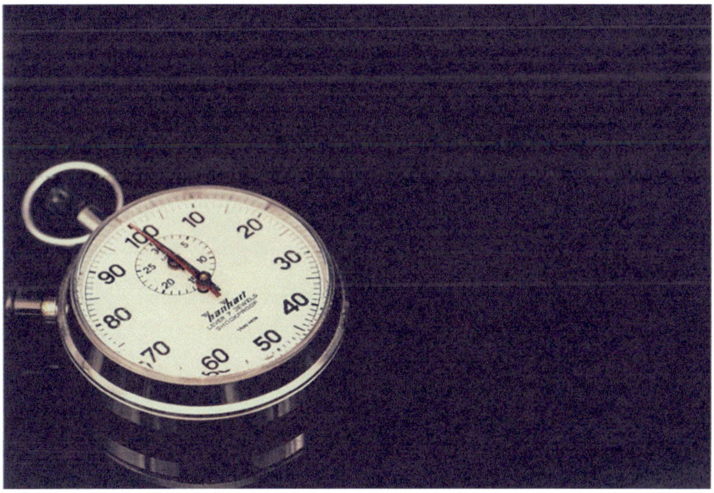

Fig. 6.24 Audio recording of the maximum phonation time performance—Case-6 (▸ https://doi.org/10.1007/000-dy2)

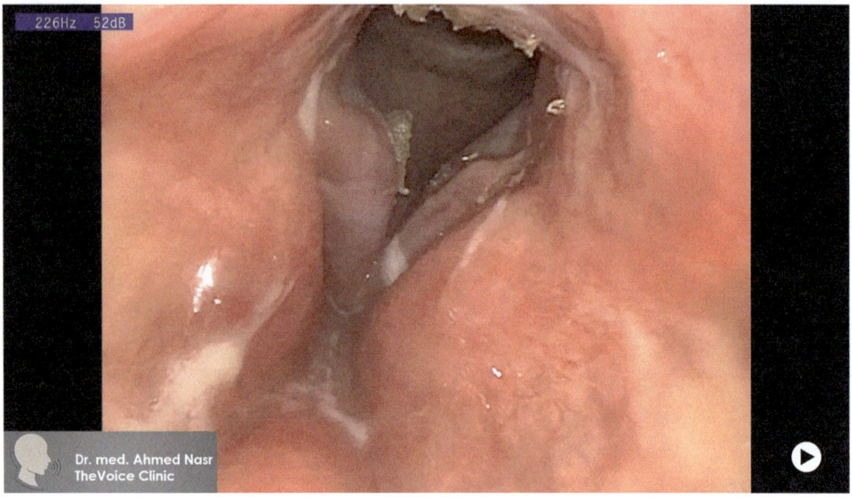

Fig. 6.25 Stroboscopic video recording for visual analysis—Case-7 (▸ https://doi.org/10.1007/000-dy3)

Fig. 6.26 Audio excerpt of the reading text "The North Wind and the Sun" for acoustic analyses—Case-7 (▸ https://doi.org/10.1007/000-dy4)

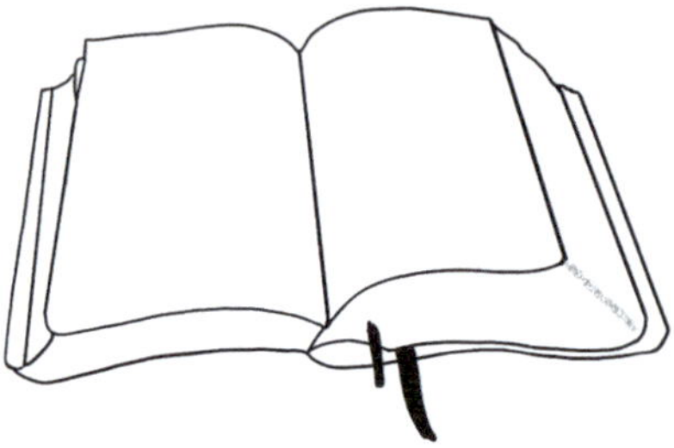

1. Reduction of general voice disorder symptoms:
   - Critical parameters of stroboscopy, VHI, and DSI

2. Improvement of voice quality in case of glottal closure insufficiency:
   - Critical parameters are the glottal closure in stroboscopy, B of GRB, ABI, GNE, CPPS, and maximum phonation time

Although the patient showed abnormalities in various voice parameters (regularity/symmetry as well as supraglottic compensation in stroboscopy, AVQI, VRP parameters, MPT, VFI cluster 1, VTD-T), a laryngeal hypertonus was only slightly noticeable in static/dynamic palpation. This can be explained on the one hand by a varying severity in the different voice parameters and on the other hand, the patient is able to compensate for the voice pathology. Thus, no further primary goals can be clearly formulated for the time being, and the focus remains on the top two primary goals.

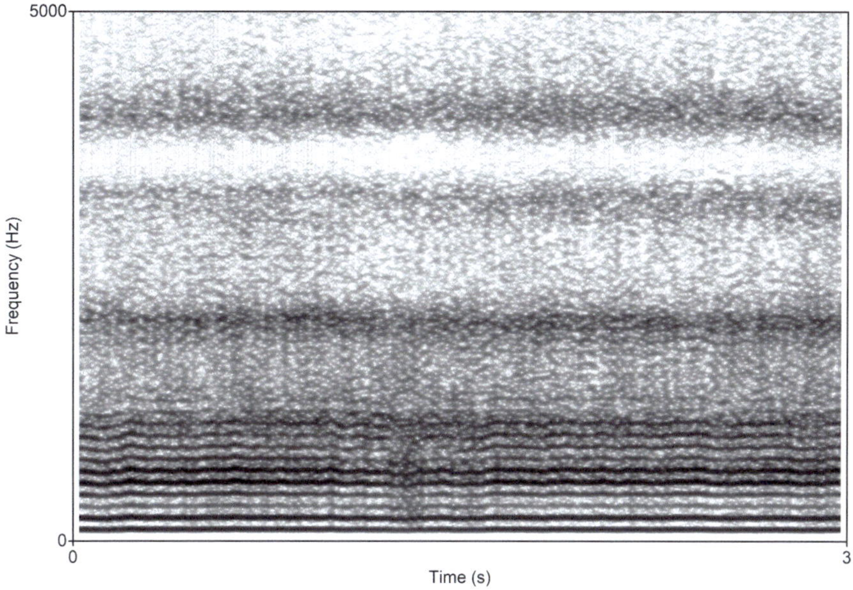

Fig. 6.27 Audio of the 3-second sustained phonation of the vowel /a:/ for acoustic analyses—Case-7 (▸ https://doi.org/10.1007/000-dxb)

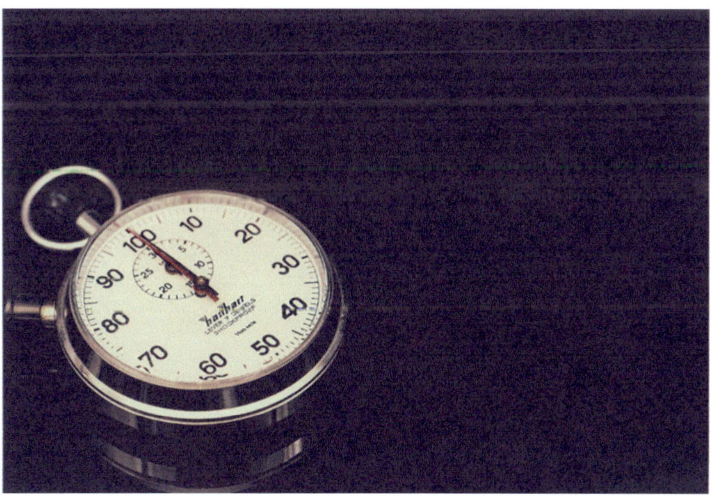

Fig. 6.28 Audio recording of the maximum phonation time performance—Case-7 (▸ https://doi.org/10.1007/000-dy6)

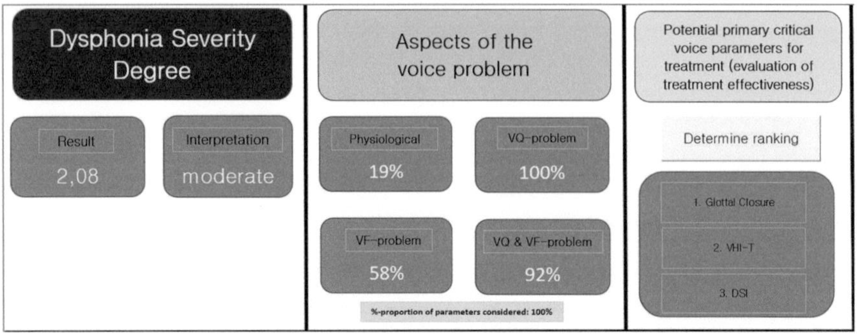

Fig. 6.29 Excerpt from the Excel macro (dashboard) for the multidimensional examination protocol (see Chap. 3) for Case-1

Table 6.1 Overview of individual ICF components with codes and descriptions for the patient

ICF Components	Code	Description
Body Functions	B126	Temperament and Personality Functions
	B152	Emotional Functions
	B310	Voice Function
	B3100	Production of Voice
	B3101	Voice Quality
Body Structures	S3400	Body Structures of the Vocal Folds
Activity and Participation	D330	Speaking
	D350	Conversing
	D845	Acquiring, Keeping, and Terminating Employment
	D850	Remunerative Employment
	D9205	Social Activities
Environmental Factors	E225	Climate
	E2250	Temperature
	E2251	Humidity
	E250	Ambient Noise
	E2500	Intensity of Noise
Personal Factors	Pf1	Sociodemographic Factors/General Personal Data
	Pf4	Mental Personal Factors
	Pf6	Lifestyle
	Pf7	Work-Related Personal Factors

As a top-3 assessment of the primary critical voice parameters according to Sect. 4.2, the following order can be established:

1. *Voice quality, especially the breathiness of the voice*
2. *VRP- boundaries*
3. *VHI-T*

Explanations for the choice of parameters and their ranking:

1. Voice quality (hoarseness) is indicative in this moderate organic dysphonia of the patient due to the majority of aspects of the voice problem. The focus of the voice quality problems is on breathiness (B of GRB, ABI, GNE, and CPPS) due to: a) the most connection points within the correlation matrix through the glottal closure insufficiency, which is significantly correlated with breathiness, b) the perceptual as well as acoustic-objective assessment, breathiness is most pronounced compared to roughness.
2. The VRP- boundaries is one of the most crucial voice function parameters, which stands out from the 58% of voice function problems and has the third most connection points in the correlation matrix. In particular, the pathological semitone range is indicative here, as the patient shows very good intensity range (and thus sufficient voice control) in both the SRP and the VRP.
3. In the VHI-T, the highest value of 120 was indicated and serves as a key parameter in this voice disorder due to the variety of various pathological parameters that can be best summarized by the VHI-T and has the second most connection points in the correlation matrix.

If these top-3 parameters can be significantly improved after the primary treatment, other voice parameters should also be positively influenced by the avalanche effect, thus significantly increasing the number of physiological parameters, which currently stands at 19%.

Voice treatment options

Since a tumor could currently be ruled out by a biopsy (histopathology of the leukoplakia confirmed a fungal infection), the finding should be considered a side effect of inhalative corticosteroid therapy, and a change in the treatment of COPD should be discussed with a pulmonologist. Reflux was ruled out, and a primarily conservative voice therapy was suggested (Reiter and Brosch 2009; Stein and Noordzij 2013). An initial step could be voice hygiene based on various individual characteristics according to the ICF factors of body functions (e.g., B126, B152), environmental factors (e.g., E250), and personal factors (Pf6) with an important focus on nicotine abuse. Furthermore, a physiological and/or eclectic voice therapy (with or without device-assisted aids) is recommended as described in Sects. 5.3.1 and 5.3.2. Specific voice therapy programs that could achieve targeted significant improvements based on the top-3 would be the Vocal Function Exercises, the Comprehensive Voice Rehabilitation Program, and the resonance therapy concepts.

6.2 Case 2: Unilateral Vocal Fold Paresis (Right)

Brief description: A woman, 54 years old, employed as a clerk with regular customer contact (tending to be a professional speaker), exhibits a unilateral vocal fold hypomobility on the right side following a cervical spine surgery (iatrogenic cause).

The analysis in Fig. 6.30 shows the following evaluation after the voice examination (all measurements can be viewed in detail online for download).

After evaluations of the severity of dysphonia (see Sects. 3.3 and 4.2), the patient reaches a severe dysphonia severity. Overall, the voice quality (86%) is more affected than the voice function (75%). However, due to the severity, with high aphonia segments, the parameters that include both aspects are the most noticeable (92%). Only a small proportion of 16% of all measurements of the voice diagnostic protocol is physiological. An initial suggestion based on the correlation matrix (see Sect. 4.2) shows that the parameters glottal closure, MPT, and VHI-T are key parameters that can be crucial for treatment as primary critical voice parameters. MPT and VHI-T have the same number of connection points from the correlation matrix. Subsequently, the parameters with the same number of connection points from the correlation matrix include breathiness, DSI, VRP-boundaries, and VFI cluster 1. Further information about the patient is shown in the overview of the individual ICF components (see Table 6.2).

Primary goals according to Sect. 3.3

1. Reduction of general voice disorder symptoms:
   - Critical parameters of stroboscopy, VHI, and DSI
2. Improvement of voice quality in glottal closure insufficiency:
   - Critical parameters are the glottal closure in stroboscopy, B of GRB, ABI, GNE, CPPS, and max. phonation time
3. Improvement of phonation duration in glottal closure insufficiency:
   - Critical parameters: glottal closure in stroboscopy, max. phonation time, VRP-dynamic, VRP-semitone range; VRP-boundaries

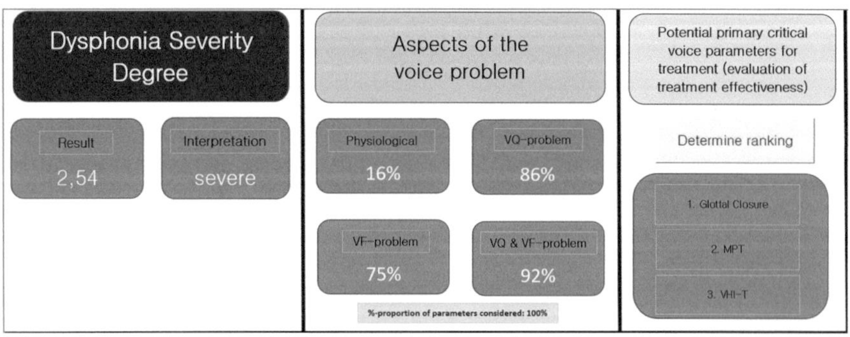

Fig. 6.30 Excerpt from the Excel macro (dashboard) for the multidimensional examination protocol (see Chap. 3) for Case-2

Table 6.2 Overview of individual ICF components with codes and descriptions for the patient

ICF Components	Code	Description
Body Functions	B310	Voice Function
	B3100	Production of Voice
	B3101	Voice Quality
Body Structures	S340	Structures of the Larynx
	S3400	Structures of the Vocal Foldss
Activity and Participation	D330	Speaking
	D350	Conversing
	D845	Acquiring, Keeping, and Terminating Employment
	D850	Remunerative Employment
	D9205	Social Activities
Environmental Factors	E250	Ambient Noise
	E2500	Intensity of Noise
Personal Factors	Pf2	Body Functions and Structures
	Pf3	Personal Factors Related to the Illness
	Pf4	Mental Personal Factors
	Pf7	Work-Related Personal Factors
	Pf8	Other Personal Factors

4. Improvement of speaking loudness (intelligibility).
    - Critical parameters for speaking loudness (intelligibility): SRP-I, VRP-intensity range

As a top-3 assessment of the primary critical voice parameters according to Sect. 4.2, the following order can thus be established:

1. *Glottal closure*
2. *MPT*
3. *VRP-boundaries with particular focus on the intensity range*

Explanations for the choice of parameters and their ranking:

1. The glottal configuration shows a right intermediate vocal fold position in phonation with compensatory overcorrection from the left and occasionally bilateral vibration capability of the paralyzed vocal fold. The glottal closure insufficiency is the leading symptom of this recurrent nerve paresis, explaining the severe breathiness up to aphonia and thus the significantly more severe voice quality issues. The glottal closure insufficiency also has the most connections within the correlation matrix, indicating a strong link with the extremely short phonation time and significantly reduced loudness.

2. Due to the high proportion of aphonia, the maximum phonation time becomes a stronger focus of treatment, as the patient cannot even achieve 4 seconds. Additionally, the MPT, like in Top-1, is another connecting feature to the glottal closure insufficiency.
3. Besides the voice quality aspects, which are particularly associated with the glottal closure insufficiency, the third significant feature of this recurrent nerve paresis is the low intensities in VRP and SRP. To increase the SRP-I, the general possibilities of the intensity range (especially the VRP-I-max) need to be improved, which applies to both the chest voice and the head voice, to expand the voice range contour of the small voice range.

If these top-3 parameters can be significantly improved after primary treatment, other voice parameters should also be positively influenced by the avalanche effect, thereby significantly increasing the number of physiological parameters, which currently stands at 16%.

Voice treatment options
The onset of the recurrent laryngeal nerve paresis is less than 3 months ago, and a complete unilateral vocal fold paralysis on the right is excluded based on the stroboscopic findings, as partial mobility on the right was confirmed, thus defining a vocal fold paresis. In cases of iatrogenic unilateral vocal fold paresis, a recovery rate of up to 89% can be observed if medical intervention via augmentation is considered (Husain et al. 2019). Thus, early symptom relief through augmentation of the paretic vocal fold (see Sect. 5.2.1) can be achieved and is also advisable in this case due to the intermediate position of the paretic vocal fold and the resulting significant glottal closure insufficiency. To be able to use this before awaiting the natural recovery period (6 to 12 months), a resorbable material (temporary) should be used. By increasing the volume of the right vocal fold, the glottal closure insufficiency will be reduced, and the left vocal fold will regain contact with the right vocal fold during phonation.

Currently, the patient only shows higher values of increased muscle tone (4 points) in the static area of palpation, which has not yet extended to the dynamic area (0 points). By considering performing an augmentation promptly, it should also be avoided that the patient exerts more pressure, tension, and effort to increase intelligibility.

A conservative voice therapy should follow the medical treatment to significantly improve the further symptoms, prevent or eliminate inappropriate compensatory behavior in voice production, and restore the voice to its usual strength and robustness as before the onset of vocal fold paresis (Maryn et al. 2020). Here, a physiological voice therapy or a voice therapy with device-assisted aids can be recommended, as described in Sects. 5.3.1 and 5.3.2. Specific voice therapy programs that could achieve significant improvements based on the Top-3 would be the Vocal Function Exercises, resonance therapy concepts, Novafon Local Vibration Voice Therapy, and Water Resistance Therapy.

6.3 Case 3: Functional Dysphonia with Bronchial Asthma

Brief description: A 66-year-old woman, a speech-language pathologist by profession shortly before retirement (professional speaker), has functional dysphonia with bronchial asthma, which is being treated medically (including with inhaled corticosteroid therapy) by the pulmonologist. The incidence of dysphonias as a side effect of inhaled corticosteroid applications ranges between 5% to 58% (Chmielewska and Akst 2015).

The analysis in Fig. 6.31 shows the following evaluation after the voice examination (all measurements can be viewed in detail online for download).

The patient records a slight dysphonia severity according to evaluations of the dysphonia severity degree (see Sects. 3.3 and 4.2). Overall, voice quality (57%) is more affected than voice function (17%). Voice quality parameters and the combination of parameters from voice quality and voice function are comparable in the percentage frequency of the voice problem. Overall, 56% of the voice parameters are physiological. An initial suggestion based on the correlation matrix (see Sect. 4.2) identifies the three key parameters glottal closure, VHI-T, and MPT, which can be primary critical voice parameters for treatment guidance. Further information about the patient is shown in the overview of the individual ICF components (see Table 6.3).

Primary goals according to Sect. 3.3

1. Reduction of general voice disorder symptoms:
   - Primarily critical parameters of the VHI
2. Improvement of *voice quality* and *voice condition,* caused by irregular vocal fold vibration, through passive and active exercises for laryngeal tone regulation:
   - Critical parameters of voice quality: Regularity/symmetry of stroboscopy, R of GRB, AVQI, dynamic evaluation of palpation
   - Critical parameters of voice condition: MPT

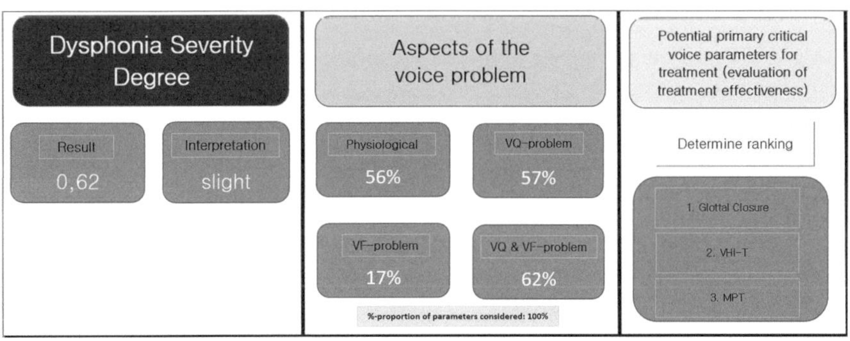

Fig. 6.31 Excerpt from the Excel macro (dashboard) for the multidimensional examination protocol (see Chap. 3) for Case-3

Table 6.3 Overview of the individual ICF components with codes and descriptions for the patient

ICF Components	Code	Description
Body Functions	B152	Emotional Functions
	B3101	Voice Quality
Activity and Participation	D330	Speaking
	D350	Conversing
	D845	Acquiring, Keeping, and Terminating Employment
	D850	Remunerative Employment
	D920	Recreation and Leisure
	D9204	Hobbies
	D9205	Social Activities
Environmental Factors	E2501	Quality of Noise
	E260	Quality of Air
Personal Factors	Pf1	Sociodemographic Factors/General Personal Data
	Pf2	Body Functions and Structures
	Pf3	Personal Factors Related to the Illness
	Pf7	Work-Related Personal Factors

As a top-3 assessment of the primary critical voice parameters according to Sect. 4.2, the following order can be determined:

1. *MPT*
2. *Voice quality (especially the AVQI and/or G of the GRB scale)*
3. *Palpation*

Explanations for the choice of parameters and their ranking:

1. The MPT is a central measure of voice condition and voice function, which in this patient shows one of the highest connection points alongside the VHI-T within the correlation matrix and shows a significant abnormality below 10 s. Since the MPT is also associated with glottal closure insufficiency and this reached the most connection points in the correlation matrix, the consequence of glottal closure insufficiency, such as breathiness, is not clearly classified and is therefore not directly considered as a final choice for the top-3 decision. Additionally, the MPT parameter is the most noticeable single parameter in 17% of voice function problems.
2. Voice quality is a leading symptom in the aspects of this voice problem (57%) of the patient. Perceptually, roughness is present, but acoustically, breathiness reaches increased abnormalities. Thus, in this hoarseness, it cannot be clearly

determined to what extent breathiness and/or roughness is underlying. The general voice quality is guiding here. Overall, this is expressed perceptually by the G of the GRB scale and objectively-acoustically by the AVQI.

3. The palpation values reached the highest values compared to the other pathological results from the voice examination protocol (static: 4 out of 8; dynamic: 5 out of 9). Connection points from the correlation matrix with the increased palpation values can be demonstrated with the VHI-T and roughness.

Voice treatment options

The development of functional dysphonia accompanying bronchial asthma can be triggered by obstructive ventilation disorder, chronic cough stimulus, and exacerbated by inhalative corticosteroid therapies. Conservative voice therapy should help to reduce laryngeal hyperfunction, thereby improving respiratory techniques and vocal hygiene (Hackenberg et al. 2010). On the one hand, voice quality can be improved in combination with the MPT through Vocal Function Exercises. On the other hand, voice anomalies regarding voice quality and palpatory abnormalities can be treated using Manual Circumlaryngeal Therapy. Both methods are equally suitable for the initial phase of treatment.

6.4 Case 4: Functional Dysphonia with Suspected Allergy-Induced Laryngitis

Brief description: A woman, 57 years old, working as a kindergarten teacher (professional speaker), presents with functional dysphonia with additional suspicion of allergy-induced laryngitis, which needs further investigation.

The analysis in Fig. 6.32 shows the following evaluation after the voice examination (all measurements can be viewed in detail online for download).

The patient records a slight dysphonia severity according to evaluations of the dysphonia severity degree (see Sects. 3.3 and 4.2). In particular, mixed parameters

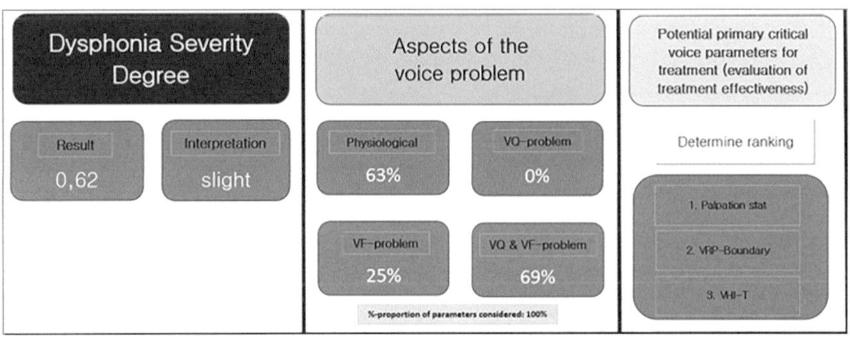

Fig. 6.32 Excerpt from the Excel macro (dashboard) for the multidimensional examination protocol (see Chap. 3) for Case-4

for voice quality and voice function are noticeable (69%). Parameters that relate only to voice quality are not affected (0%) and deviations in voice function are only detectable to 25%. A large portion of the voice parameters (63%) is physiological, thus indicating a favorable baseline after the voice examination. An initial suggestion based on the correlation matrix (see Sect. 4.2) shows three key parameters: static palpation, VRP-boundaries, and VHI-T, which can be potential primary critical voice parameters for the treatment. The same number of connection points as the three previously mentioned key parameters from the correlation matrix has the VFI cluster 1. Subsequently, the MPT follows from the correlation matrix with the second highest number of connection points. Further information about the patient is shown in the overview of the individual ICF components (see Table 6.4).

Primary goals according to Sect. 3.3

1. Reduction of general voice disorder symptoms:
   - Critical parameter of the VHI
2. Improvement of voice condition through passive and active exercises for laryngeal muscle tone regulation:
   - Critical parameters of voice condition: MPT, VFI-cluster 1

As a top-3 assessment of the primary critical voice parameters according to Sect. 4.2, the following order can thus be determined:

1. *VHI-T*
2. *VFI-cluster 1*
3. *MPT*

Table 6.4 Overview of the individual ICF components with codes and descriptions for the patient

ICF Components	Code	Description
Body Functions	B152	Emotional Functions
	B310	Voice Function
	B3100	Producing Voice
Activity and Participation	D330	Speaking
	D845	Acquiring, Keeping, and Terminating Employment
	D850	Remunerative Employment
	D9205	Social Activities
Environmental Factors	E250	Ambient Noise
	E2500	Intensity of Noise
Personal Factors	Pf1	Sociodemographic Factors/General Personal Data
	Pf4	Mental Personal Factors
	Pf7	Work-Related Personal Factors

Explanations for the choice of parameters and their ranking:

1. One of the most severely affected individual parameters in the evaluation of the patient's voice diagnostics is the VHI-T, which also showed the most connection points from the correlation matrix, as well as constituting an important component of the voice problem (69%) from the combination of voice quality and voice function parameters. Due to the low dysphonia severity degree with a majority of a physiological evaluation of all examined voice parameters, the VHI-T is generally an optimal gauge to evaluate the success of the therapy from the patient's perspective.
2. Regarding the patient's profession and the current findings, the symptom of vocal fatigue is a leading symptom in the patient's individual voice disorder, which can best be expressed by the VFI-cluster 1. Confirmed with the same number of connection points as the VHI-T from the correlation matrix, the VFI-cluster 1 thus emerges as another key component.
3. The MPT is a central measure of voice condition and voice function, which in this patient shows the second highest number of connection points within the correlation matrix. Additionally, this parameter is the most noticeable in voice function problems.

Voice treatment options

If the symptoms of dysphonia do not improve after conservative voice therapy and/or reflux treatment (e.g., using proton pump inhibitors), the suspected allergy-related laryngitis as a co-factor of the voice problems should be clarified and, if necessary, primarily treated medically (Roth and Ferguson 2010). Allergic or reflux-related voice problems and laryngeal abnormalities cannot always be clinically distinguished (Roth and Ferguson 2010). Therefore, conservative voice therapy is primarily recommended for this patient. Due to the favorable initial situation with mild dysphonia severity and short maximum phonation time as well as lack of voice robustness due to rapid vocal fatigue, a voice conditioning therapy program is recommended. Vocal Function Exercises would be the first choice, as this voice therapy was the only one in a meta-analysis to significantly increase the MPT, and the concept with a high number of repetitions with corresponding drill in execution is a core element that thus distinguishes the demonstrable success (see Sect. 5.3.2). The principles and exercises of Vocal Function Exercises can also be applied to other semi-occluded Vocal Tract Exercises, such as Water Resistance Therapy. After significant improvement of MPT and VFI-cluster 1, it can be assumed that the VHI-T would also significantly improve due to the avalanche effect, which is used as a general gauge of this functional voice disorder to evaluate the success of the therapy.

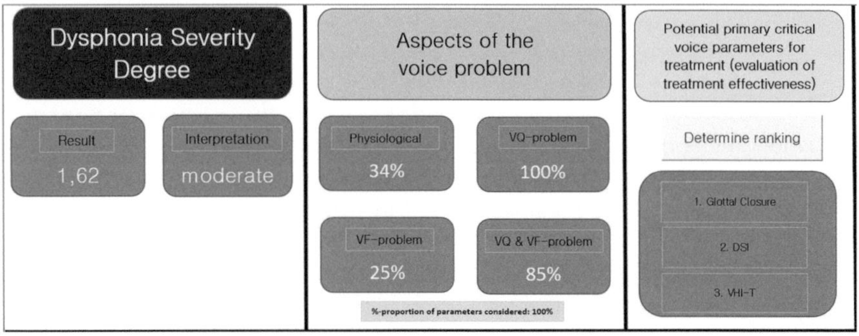

Fig. 6.33 Excerpt from the Excel macro (dashboard) for the multidimensional examination protocol (see Chap. 3) for Case-5

Table 6.5 Overview of the individual ICF components with codes and descriptions for the patient

ICF Components	Code	Description
Body Functions	B3101	Voice Quality
Body Structures	S3400	Body Structures of the Vocal Folds
Activity and Participation	D350	Conversing
	D9205	Social Activities
Environmental Factors	E410–e499	Attitudes
Personal Factors	Pf3	Personal Factors Related to the Illness
	Pf8	Other Personal Factors

6.5 Case 5: Vocalis Atrophy

Brief description: A man, 51 years old, a truck driver by profession, suffers from idiopathic vocalis atrophy.

The analysis in Fig. 6.33 shows the following evaluation after the voice examination (all measurements can be viewed in detail online for download).

According to the dysphonia severity assessment, the patient has moderate dysphonia severity (see Sects. 3.3. and 4.2). In particular, the voice quality is affected (100%), but the voice function only by 25%. The voice parameters are physiological by 34%. As a first suggestion based on the correlation matrix (see Sect. 4.2.), three key parameters emerge: glottal closure, DSI, and VHI-T, which can be guiding as primary critical voice parameters for treatment. Since DSI and VHI-T have the same number of connection points from the correlation matrix, they are followed by AVQI, VRP- boundaries, and VFI-cluster 1 with the same number of connection points. Further information about the patient is shown in the overview of the individual ICF components (see Table 6.5).

Primary goals according to Sect. 3.3

1. Reduction of general voice disorder symptoms:
   - Critical parameters of stroboscopy and VHI
   - Improvement of voice quality in case of glottal closure insufficiency: Critical parameters are the glottal closure in stroboscopy, B of GRB, ABI, GNE, and CPPS
2. Improvement of *voice quality* and *throat discomfort,* caused by irregular vocal fold vibration, through passive and active exercises for laryngeal muscle tone regulation:
   - Critical parameters of voice quality: Regularity/symmetry of stroboscopy, R of GRB, AVQI, dynamic evaluation of palpation
   - Critical parameters of throat paresthesia: VTD-T

As a top-3 assessment of the primary critical voice parameters according to Sect. 4.2, the following order can thus be established:

1. *Glottal closure*
2. *AVQI*
3. *VRP-boundaries*

Explanations for the choice of parameters and their ranking:

1. Glottal closure insufficiency is a significant feature of vocalis atrophy with resulting deviation in voice quality related to breathiness (Omori et al. 1997), which is also confirmed in this patient. This parameter also has the most connection points in the correlation matrix.
2. In addition to the typical features of vocalis atrophy (breathiness), this patient also shows a comparable degree of voice quality deviation due to roughness. The leading parameter for voice quality deviations is the AVQI due to the third-highest number of connection points in the correlation matrix. It remains unclear whether the high regularity and symmetry values from the stroboscopy represent a compensation in phonation. This could occur alongside moderately noticeable laryngeal discomfort and noticeable dynamic palpatory findings, all of which can be associated with deviations in voice quality.
3. A weakly pronounced chest voice is also a common feature in vocalis atrophy (Vilkman et al. 1995), which is also confirmed in the VRP-boundaries (discongruity) and thus best represents the voice function problems of 25%. The VRP-boundaries also has the third-highest number of connections in the correlation matrix and confirms the final choice for the top-3 assessment of the primary critical voice parameters. The circumstance of the discongruity voice range profile contour can also be a consequence of a too high SRP-F0. It is assumed that once the chest voice is expanded in the dynamic range (Q3), the SRP-F0 can also be lowered (consciously, e.g., through symptomatic voice therapy or unconsciously through the previous course of therapy).

If these top-3 parameters can be significantly improved after the primary treatment, other voice parameters should also be positively influenced by the avalanche effect, thus significantly increasing the number of physiological parameters, which currently stand at 34%.

Voice treatment options
The glottal closure insufficiency is of central importance for the voice quality problem in this vocalis atrophy. Since the patient has already received a prescription for conservative voice therapy and the result of this follow-up still shows an obvious persistent dysphonia, a medical intervention such as vocal fold augmentation (see Sect. 5.2.1) is recommended. If conservative voice therapy is continued, it would be sensible to specifically address the voice quality problem and the VRP contour. Regarding the voice quality aspects of this patient, targeted voice therapy programs such as Vocal Function Exercises are recommended, and resonance therapy concepts concerning the VRP-boundaries.

6.6 Case 6: Reinke's Edema

Brief description: A 53-year-old man, a restaurant manager by profession (not a professional speaker), has Reinke's edema with leukoplakia and suspected reflux due to postcricoid mucosal changes. Additionally, there is a long and still frequent nicotine abuse, as the most significant risk factor for the development of Reinke's edema (Dewan et al. 2022; Jones and Song 2023).

The analysis in Fig. 6.34 shows the following evaluation after the voice examination (all measurements can be viewed in detail online for download).

Although some areas in the multidimensional voice examination protocol for this Reinke's edema were assessed as severely disturbed (e.g., DSI and VTD-T) and other areas such as amplitude, mucosal wave, and VHI-T as normal, the patient overall achieves a mild dysphonia severity (see Sects. 3.3 and 4.2). The grading of Reinke's edema is determined, for example, with a grading scale from 1 to 4 (see Sect. 5.1.4). The patient presented here has developed Reinke's edema grade 1 (obstructing <25% of the glottic gap). The most affected aspect for him is voice quality (71%) in relation to voice function, which shows 50% problems. 41% of the voice parameters from the examination protocol are physiological. As a first suggestion based on the correlation matrix (see Sect. 4.2), three key parameters are present such as regularity/symmetry, SC (ventricular voice), and VRP-boundaries, which can be indicative as primary critical voice parameters for treatment. The same number of connection points in the correlation matrix as the aforementioned top-3 parameters is shown by VFI-cluster 1. The subsequent parameters with the second highest number of connection points include roughness, breathiness, AVQI, DSI, palpation dynamics, semitone range from VRP, and MPT. Further information about the patient is shown in the overview of the individual ICF components (see Table 6.6).

Primary goals according to Sect. 3.3

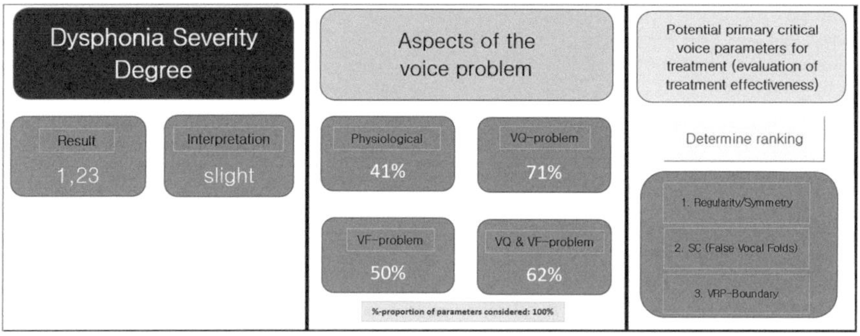

Fig. 6.34 Excerpt from the Excel macro (dashboard) for the multidimensional examination protocol (see Chap. 3) for Case 6

1. Reduction of general voice disorder symptoms:
   - Critical parameters of stroboscopy and DSI
2. Improvement of *voice quality* and *voice condition* and *laryngeal discomfort,* caused by an *irregular vocal fold vibration* and *supralaryngeal constriction,* through passive and active exercises for laryngeal muscle tone regulation:
   - Critical parameters of voice quality: Regularity of stroboscopy, R of GRB, AVQI, dynamic evaluation of palpation
   - Critical parameters of voice condition: VFI-cluster 1
   - Critical parameters of throat paresthesia: VTD-T
3. Improvement of *speaking pitch:*
   - Critical parameters for speaking pitch: SRP-F0, VRP-semitone range

As a top-3 assessment of the primary critical voice parameters according to Sect. 4.2, the following order can thus be determined:

1. *Regularity/Symmetry*
2. *VRP-boundaries, especially the semitone range*
3. *VTD-T*

Explanations for the choice of parameters and their ranking:

1. Pivotal in this organic voice pathology due to Reinke's edema is, among other things, the regularity/symmetry of the vocal fold vibration (Watanabe et al. 2016; Dewan et al. 2022), which also shows high connection points in the correlation matrix for this patient. This irregularity of the vocal fold vibration caused by the morphological changes of the vocal folds in the Reinke space is the cause of the roughness and the lower SRP-F0 (Watanabe et al. 2016; Tavaluc and Tan-Geller 2019), as was also confirmed in this patient.

Table 6.6 Overview of individual ICF components with codes and descriptions for the patient

ICF Components	Code	Description
Body Functions	B126	Temperament and Personality
	B3101	Voice Quality
Body Structures	S3400	Body Structures of the Vocal Folds
Activity and Participation	D330	Speaking
	D350	Conversing
	D845	Acquiring, Keeping, and Terminating Employment
	D9205	Social Activities
Environmental Factors	E250	Ambient Noise
	E2500	Intensity of Noise
	E2501	Quality of Noise
	E260	Air Quality
	E410-e499	Attitudes
Personal Factors	Pf2	Body Functions and Structures
	Pf3	Personal Factors Related to the Illness
	Pf6	Lifestyle
	Pf7	Work-Related Personal Factors

2. Due to the morphological changes of the vocal folds, a significant lowering of the semitone voice range of the VRP contour is clearly recognizable (especially VRP-F0-high noticeable), which also has effects on the significant lowering of the SRP-F0.
3. VTD-T is, alongside the DSI, the most affected single parameter of the voice examination in the patient. Since the high deviation in the DSI is explained by the roughness (PPQ5) and VRP-boundaries restriction and these are already sufficiently represented in Top-1 and Top-2, the focus for this patient is on laryngeal discomfort. Normally, the voice disorder is sufficiently characterized by the VHI (Behlau et al. 2016), but in this individual case, the VHI evaluation corresponds to a normal assessment, but not in the case of laryngeal discomfort, which are perceived as a severe impairment.

Voice treatment options

In the literature, symptomatic treatment is suggested for the treatment of Reinke's edema with a focus on addressing the causes, as in this case of nicotine abuse (Tavaluc and Tan-Geller 2019). Additionally, leukoplakia is visible on the left vocal fold, which needs to be further medically examined (e.g., by biopsy) as well as further clinical investigation of the suspicion of reflux. Medical interventions for Reinke's edema include phonosurgical measures, such as suction and excision of the mucosal excess using "cold" surgery or laser reduction, possibly supported by intralesional steroid injection (Jones and Song 2023). Surgery is recommended when voice therapy measures are exhausted, the VHI is still very noticeable, and/or the lesion leads to dyspnea (Tavaluc and Tan-Geller 2019). Medical interventions can improve certain symptoms of dysphonia but cannot establish normophonia (Tavaluc and Tan-Geller 2019). For the current patient, conservative voice therapy is thus advisable due to the still Grade I edema, normal VHI, and no reported dyspnea.

A beginning should be made with vocal hygiene due to the person-related factors (Pf6) of the ICF components with an important focus on necessary nicotine abstinence.

Furthermore, a physiological and/or symptomatic voice therapy is recommended as described in Sects. 5.3.1 and 5.3.2. Specific voice therapy programs that could achieve significant improvements based on the top-3 would be the stretch-and-flow phonation and resonance therapy concepts.

6.7 Case 7: Mix of Various Organic Voice Pathologies: a) Chronic Laryngitis, b) Reinke's Edema, c) Vocal Fold Polyp with Crusting

Brief description: A man, 65 years old, part-time bus driver (not a professional speaker), exhibits a mix of various organic voice pathologies, such as a) chronic laryngitis, b) Reinke's edema, c) vocal fold polyp with crusting. The patient has a frequent nicotine abuse, which is a significant cause of all three organic voice disorders (Reiter and Brosch 2009; Vasconcelos et al. 2019; Tavaluc and Tan-Geller 2019).

The analysis in Fig. 6.35 shows the following evaluation after the voice examination (all measurements can be viewed in detail online for download).

According to the dysphonia severity assessment, the patient has moderate dysphonia severity (see Sects. 3.3 and 4.2). The essential feature of this mixed voice pathology is the voice quality (100%) with equally high proportions of mixed

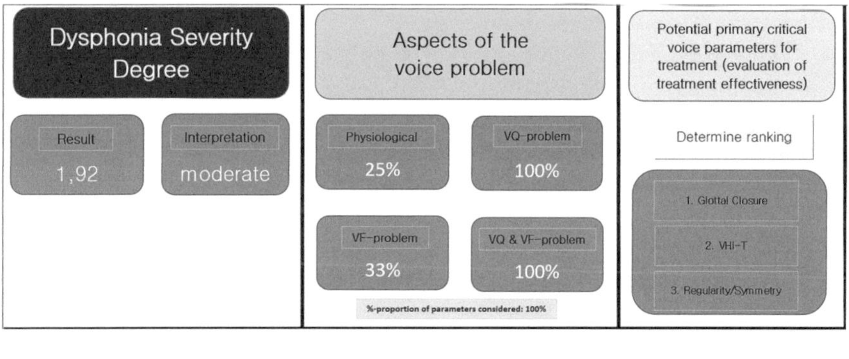

Fig. 6.35 Excerpt from the Excel macro (dashboard) for the multidimensional examination protocol (see Chap. 3) for Case-7

Table 6.7 Overview of the individual ICF components with codes and descriptions for the patient

ICF Components	Code	Description
Body Functions	B3100	Production of Voice
	B3101	Voice Quality
Body Structures	S340	Body Structures of the Larynx
	S3400	Body Structures of the Vocal Folds
Activity and Participation	D350	Conversing
	D920	Recreation and Leisure
	D9205	Social Activities
Environmental Factors	E310-e399	Support and Relationships
	E410-e499	Attitudes
Personal Factors	Pf1	Sociodemographic Factors/General Personal Data
	Pf2	Body Functions and Structures
	Pf4	Mental Personal Factors
	Pf6	Lifestyle
	Pf8	Other Personal Factors

parameters for voice quality and voice function (100%). The voice function is slightly affected (33%). Also, only 25% of the voice parameters are physiological. An initial suggestion based on the correlation matrix (see Sect. 4.2.) highlights the three key parameters: glottal closure, VHI-T, and regularity/symmetry, which can be critical primary voice parameters for treatment. The same number of connection points in the correlation matrix as regularity/symmetry have DSI, VRP-boundaries, and VFI-cluster 1. Further information about the patient is shown in the overview of the individual ICF components (see Table 6.7).

Primary goals according to Sect. 3.3

1. Reduction of general voice disorder signs:
   - Critical parameters of stroboscopy, VHI and/or DSI
2. Improvement of *voice quality* and *voice condition* and *laryngeal discomfort,* caused by an *irregular vocal fold vibration* and supralaryngeal constriction through passive and active exercises for laryngeal muscle tone regulation:
   - Critical parameters of voice quality: Regularity/symmetry of stroboscopy, R of GRB, AVQI, dynamic evaluation of palpation
   - Critical parameters of voice condition: VRP parameters, MPT
   - Critical parameters of paresthesia in the throat: VTD-T
3. Improvement of speaking pitch (intelligibility):
   - Critical parameter for speaking pitch: SRP-F0

As a top-3 assessment of the primary critical voice parameters according to Sect. 4.2, the following order can thus be established:

1. *Regularity/symmetry*
2. *VHI-T*
3. *DSI*

Explanations for the choice of parameters and their ranking:

1. Combinations of these three organic voice pathologies are often characterized by an irregularity/asymmetry of vocal fold vibration (Watanabe et al. 2016; Yamauchi et al. 2016; Dewan et al. 2022), which was also evident in this case. Thus, many connection points in the correlation matrix to this critical parameter are also shown. Since the areas VQ (especially roughness) and VQ & VF are affected 100% in this patient, the regularity/symmetry from the stroboscopic finding proves to be a comprehensive parameter.
2. The VHI-T is, besides the stroboscopic parameter symmetry, the most affected in this patient. Additionally, the VHI-T shows the most connection points in the correlation matrix. Due to the multiple organic occurrence of various voice disorders, the VHI-T proves to be a general gauge for improving the patient's vocal situation.
3. The DSI also extends as a comprehensive measure for detecting voice disorders and is highlighted here due to the versatility of the patient's symptoms and pathologies. The individual parameters of the DSI, which are particularly noticeable, such as the VRP- I-min, MPT, and PPQ5, take a special position here.

Voice treatment options

Due to multiple synchronous organic voice pathologies, a primarily conservative voice therapy, accompanied by treatment of nicotine abuse through indirect voice therapy, should be initiated in this case to limit the number of organic voice pathologies. Further conservative treatment approaches, as in Case-1 for chronic laryngitis and Case-5 for Reinke's edema, are also recommended in this case. Additionally, there is a polypoid new formation of the right vocal fold (posterior), where a crust has formed over it. This should be clarified histologically. The Reinke's edema is significantly larger on the right than on the left, and if conservative voice therapy does not achieve the desired success, medical intervention or phonosurgical measures, such as suction and excision of the mucosal excess using "cold" surgery or laser reduction, possibly supported by intralesional steroid injection, are recommended (Jones and Song 2023). Further vocal and laryngoscopic reevaluation at short intervals is urgently advised to avoid missing a tumor and to check for any further need for medical intervention.

References

Behlau M, Madazio G, Moreti F, Oliveira G, Dos Santos Lde M, Paulinelli BR, Couto Junior Ede B (2016) Efficiency and cutoff values of self-assessment instruments on the impact of a voice problem. J Voice 30(4):506.e9–506.e18. https://doi.org/10.1016/j.jvoice.2015.05.022

Chmielewska M, Akst LM (2015) Dysphonia associated with the use of inhaled corticosteroids. Curr Opin Otolaryngol Head Neck Surg 23(3):255–259. https://doi.org/10.1097/MOO.0000000000000153

Dewan K, Chhetri DK, Hoffman H (2022) Reinke's edema management and voice outcomes. Laryngoscope Investig Otolaryngol. 7(4):1042–1050. https://doi.org/10.1002/lio2.840

Hackenberg S, Hacki T, Hagen R, Kleinsasser NH (2010) [Voice disorders in asthma]. Laryngorhinootologie 89(8):460–464. https://doi.org/10.1055/s-0030-1249694

Husain S, Sadoughi B, Mor N, Sulica L (2019) Time course of recovery of iatrogenic vocal fold paralysis. Laryngoscope 129(5):1159–1163. https://doi.org/10.1002/lary.27572

Jones NN, Song SA (2023) Reinke Edema. In StatPearls. StatPearls Publishing

Maryn Y, Dedry M, Szmalec A, Desuter G (2020) [Behavioural treatment of unilateral vocal fold paralysis of the recurrent laryngeal nerve: Literature overview]. Sprache Stimme Gehör. 44(1):34–43. https://doi.org/10.1055/a-0949-7863

Omori K, Slavit DH, Matos C, Kojima H, Kacker A, Blaugrund SM (1997) Vocal fold atrophy: quantitative glottic measurement and vocal function. Ann Otol Rhinol Laryngol 106(7 Pt 1):544–551. https://doi.org/10.1177/000348949710600702

Reiter R, Brosch S (2009) [Chronic laryngitis--associated factors and voice assessment] . Laryngorhinootologie 88(3):181–185. https://doi.org/10.1055/s-0028-1100390

Roth DF, Ferguson BJ (2010) Vocal allergy: recent advances in understanding the role of allergy in dysphonia. Curr Opin Otolaryngol Head Neck Surg 18(3):176–181. https://doi.org/10.1097/MOO.0b013e32833952af

Tan M, Bryson PC, Pitts C, Woo P, Benninger MS (2017) Clinical grading of Reinke's edema. Laryngoscope 127(10):2310–2313. https://doi.org/10.1002/lary.26647

Tavaluc R, Tan-Geller M (2019) Reinke's Edema. Otolaryngol Clin North Am 52(4):627–635. https://doi.org/10.1016/j.otc.2019.03.006

Stein DJ, Noordzij JP (2013) Incidence of chronic laryngitis. Ann Otol Rhinol Laryngol 122(12):771–774. https://doi.org/10.1177/000348941312201207

Vasconcelos D, Gomes AOC, Araújo CMT (2019) Vocal fold polyps: Literature review. Int Arch Otorhinolaryngol. 23(1):116–124. https://doi.org/10.1055/s-0038-1675391

Vilkman E, Alku P, Laukkanen AM (1995) Vocal-fold collision mass as a differentiator between registers in the low-pitch range. J Voice 9(1):66–73. https://doi.org/10.1016/s0892-1997(05)80224-3

Yamauchi A, Yokonishi H, Imagawa H, Sakakibara K, Nito T, Tayama N, Yamasoba T (2016) Quantification of vocal fold vibration in various laryngeal disorders using high-speed digital imaging. J Voice 30(2):205–214. https://doi.org/10.1016/j.jvoice.2015.04.016

Watanabe T, Kaneko K, Sakaguchi K, Takahashi H (2016) Vocal-fold vibration of patients with Reinke's edema observed using high-speed digital imaging. Auris Nasus Larynx 43(6):654–657. https://doi.org/10.1016/j.anl.2016.02.007

Glossary

Ablation Removal of tissue by heating, for example by a laser

Absolute voice rest total prohibition of speaking, including whispering and quiet speaking

Abusus Missuse, excessive use

Acoustics The study of sound, is used here as a field of investigation in voice diagnostics to objectively measure the voice in its function or quality

Aerodigestive tract refers to a complex of organs that collectively extend to the tissues and organs of the upper respiratory tract and the upper part of the digestive tract

Aerodynamics The study of flow processes in gases, especially in the air, is used here as a field of investigation in conjunction with voice production in voice diagnostics

Allergy increased susceptibility to substances or external influences that lead to pathological reactions in the body

Analgesia Insensitivity to pain

Anchor voices Reference voices that serve as a benchmark for assessment in order to make a decision for a new evaluation

Angiomatous Term from pathology, describes the change of the tissue

Aphonia Loss of voice

Articulation Sequence and extent of speech movement, pronunciation

Arytenoid adduction surgical procedure for arytenoid cartilage repositioning

Asthenia Weakness/lack of strength when speaking

Asthma Clinical picture characterized by alternating narrowings of the airways, leading to attacks of shortness of breath, tightness, and coughing

B. Barsties v. Latoszek et al., *Diagnostic and Treatment in Voice Therapy*,
https://doi.org/10.1007/978-3-662-70162-1

Atrophy Shrinking, reduction of volume/mass/extent of the tissue

Auditory-perceptual based on sensory impressions that concern hearing

Augmentation surgical procedure for the enlargement of anatomical structures

Avalanche Effect through targeted Evidence-Based Practice actions and Scientific Clinical Reasoning, a minimal impact of the three most important affected individual voice parameters (Top-3) of the patients should be executed to trigger an exponential effect on other affected parameters from the voice examination

Benign refers to the type of a tumor/swelling that is not a carcinoma/cancer

Benign neoplasms benign organic pathologies

Bevacizumab a humanized monoclonal antibody that is directed against the vascular endothelial growth factor and thereby inhibits the supply of tumors with new blood vessels

Bilateral both sides

Biologic therapy to replace, supplement, or block the body's own messengers and proteins, so that pathological processes are halted, and healing processes in the body are initiated or supported

Biopsy Tissue sample extraction from a conspicuously altered body area

Breathiness Extent of air loss through the glottis (wild air/turbulences in the higher frequency sound range)

Botulinum Toxin Toxin from Clostridium botulinum (BOTOX™)

Calcification Calcification or deposition of calcium in an organ or tissue

Calibration the comparison and adjustment of a measured value with the correct value under specified conditions, referring here to volume measurement (e.g., decibel meter vs. voice range profile measurement systems)

Carcinoma malignant (malignant) tumor (swelling)

Cidofovir a nucleotide analogue that is used as an antiviral agent for the treatment of infections caused by DNA viruses

Chest voice Full vibration of the vocal foldss; a series of (lower) tones of the same timbre, whose resonance can be clearly felt in the sternum

Chronic Obstructive Pulmonary Diseases (COPD) chronic obstructive pulmonary disease due to narrowing of the airways

Clipping refers to the process of overdriving when the level of an incoming audio signal is too high, which can no longer be processed and as a result, excess signal components are "clipped"

Commissure Connection

Comorbidity simultaneous occurrence of different diseases

Compression Applying pressure to a tissue

Computed Tomography (CT) special 3D X-ray examination with cross-sectional images of the body

Contraction a shortening of the length of muscles with an increase in muscle tension

Correlation statistical term for the mutual relationship of at least two characteristics

Corticosteroids (Corticoids) a general term for hormones that are produced in the adrenal cortex, as well as partially artificially manufactured as medications such as glucocorticoids (e.g., cortisone)

Cricothyroid muscle Laryngeal muscle that is needed during contraction to achieve and control a higher pitch with the voice

Cricothyroid space Space between the thyroid cartilage (Cartilago thyroidea) and the cricoid cartilage (Cartilago cricoidea)

Cyst benign organic voice disorder, which is a cavity filled with fluid and lined with epithelium; has a transparent or yellowish appearance and can, depending on size and extent, hinder the complete closure of the vocal cords

dB Decibel (unit of measurement for sound pressure/intensity)

Dehiscence pathological separation of two adjacent tissue structures

Dexamethasone a synthetic glucocorticoid that has anti-inflammatory and immunosuppressive effects

Diagnosis Determination/identification of the nature of a disease through medical examination(s)

Dignity a classification of tumors, in which one distinguishes between benign and malignant tumors

Diplophonia Registration of two simultaneous frequencies (high and low) in the vocal sound during phonation; this phenomenon of voice quality is attributed to roughness

Direct voice therapy/exercise/technique Therapy/exercise/technique that aims to change the voice directly

Disease Illness

Distant metastases the cancer cells have settled in other, more distant organs than the malignant primary tumor

Dorsal belonging to the back side

Dystonia Movement disorders that have their cause in the brain and are accompanied by involuntary, long-lasting muscle contractions

EBM-Level Evidence-Based Medicine Level or evidence-based medicine for the description and categorization of the quality of clinical studies from Level 1 (literature reviews) to Level 5 (expert opinions)

EBP Evidence-Based Practice encompasses the aim to meet, on the one hand, the wishes and expectations of the patient and, on the other hand, the area of expertise of the treating therapist through the latest scientific findings in therapy

Eclectic Voice Therapy a voice therapy that combines different techniques from various concepts and forms of therapy

Edema Fluid accumulation in the upper layer of the lamina propria of the vocal folds (e.g., Reinke's space)

Electroglottography non-invasive measurement method for analyzing vocal fold movement, for which two skin electrodes are symmetrically placed over the two thyroid cartilage wings and the impedance of the vibrating vocal folds is measured between the electrodes during phonation

ELS European Laryngological Society

EMG Electromyography, invasive measurement method that measures the activity of muscle potentials/muscle activities

Endolarynx Interior of the larynx

Endoscope an optical instrument to look inside the body

Epithelial tissue belonging to the epithelium

Epithelium top cell layer of the skin and mucous membrane tissue

Euton Tonus of optimal tension

Excision the removal of tissue or a portion of tissue in surgery

F0 Fundamental frequency of the vocal folds

Falsetto register Range of the head voice

Fibrose benign proliferation or increase of connective tissue, resulting in tissue hardening (often as a reaction or repair process following an iatrogenic cause)

Focal pertaining to or originating from a focus or disease site

Frequency Number of oscillations in a unit of time

Frequentist the term "frequentist" describes in statistics the interpretation of the probability of an event as the relative frequency that occurs in a large number of identical, repeated, independent random experiments

Functional Dysphonia Voice disorder that shows no signs of organic changes/ pathology of the vocal folds, but different changes in voice function and/or voice quality can be measured

Glissando continuous sliding change of pitch

Globus sensation "Lump in the throat" or "frog in the throat" sensation/ discomfort

Glottal closure Vocal fold closure

Glottal Fry creaking, but here very low frequency (approx. 50 Hz) of the vocal fold vibration: pulse register

Glottal insufficiency incomplete vocal fold closure during phonation

Glottis Glottal gap between the two vocal foldss in the larynx

Handicap Term from WHO terminology, which refers to the (social or economic) disadvantage of a person due to an impairment or disability

Hemangiomatous the presence of numerous hemangiomas (blood vessel tumors) simultaneously

Hematoma Vascular injury with bleeding into the tissue ("bruise" or "contusion")

Heterogeneity statistical term for describing random variations ("scatter" between studies)

Histology medical subfield that deals with the fine tissue, microscopic aspect of pathological changes in the body

Hoarseness (Grade) Overall severity or degree of voice abnormality (general) at the glottal level

Hyaluronidase an enzyme that dissolves hyaluronic acid

Hyperkeratosis Cornification/thickening of the epithelium; at this level, the cells are heavily loaded with keratin, a protein that gives them a dry and very hard character

Hyperkinesia describes the pathologically increased mobility or motor activity of the skeletal muscles

Hypertension/Hypertonus/hypertonic Muscle hypertension/-tonus with the two main forms spasticity (cramp) and rigidity (stiffness); describes the tension state of the muscle, which is pathologically increased

Hypervascularization Signs of the increased metabolic demand of a tissue, which occur, among other things, in the context of repair processes (wound healing), in chronic inflammations, and in the growth zone of malignant tumors

Hz Hertz (repetition of a pattern per second)

Iatrogenic Diseases that were caused or worsened by medical actions

ICC Intra Class Correlation Coefficient is a statistical measurement method to test reliability; the ICC ranges from 0.00 (i.e., completely lacking reliability) to 1.00 (i.e., perfect reliability); a general guideline indicates ICC values above 0.75 as good reliability and ICC values below 0.75 as poor to moderate reliability

ICF (formerly ICDIH, International Classification of Functioning, Disability and Health) International Classification of Functioning, Disability and Health, which describes a classification framework with a standardized set of terms for describing human functioning and the problems that occur in the process

Indirect Voice Therapy voice therapy method that focuses significantly on the development of favorable conditions for phonation, e.g., through vocal hygiene

Infiltration describes the penetration of solid or liquid substance (infiltrate) into biological tissue; the spread of tumor cells or pathogens into tissue is also referred to as infiltration

Inhalative refers to the inhalation of gaseous substances or aerosols

Intensity Measure of the sound pressure level (e.g., of a voice), measured in dB

Intensity Degree of force or strength, in the case of the voice: the loudness, which is measured in dB

Interarytenoid region between the arytenoid cartilages on the inner side of the posterior wall of the larynx

Interferon-Alpha Drug that consists of natural interferon alpha, which is obtained from the leukocyte fraction of human blood after induction with the Sendai virus

Intra- or Inter-rater Reliability Degree of pre-post agreement related to the same individual (Intra) or to a group (Inter)

Intubation Insertion of a tube (endotracheal tube) into the airways to ensure breathing

Invasive (e.g., for diagnostic purposes) a procedure that penetrates the body

kPa Kilopascal (pressure unit)

KTP Laser Potassium titanyl phosphate laser

Lamina propria a layer of the vocal folds between the epithelium and the vocalis muscle

Laryngeal concerning the larynx

Laryngeal mirror Mirror with a special angle that allows the observation of the vocal cords through the mouth

Laryngitis Inflammation of the vocal cords and/or the larynx

Laryngopharynx Section of the laryngeal pharynx

Laryngoscopy instrumental examination procedure for the visual assessment of the vocal cords and the larynx

Larynx anatomical structure that defines the upper, expanded part of the trachea, in which the cartilage rings have developed in a special way, and thus performs certain functions (primarily = protective function of the lower airways, e.g., when swallowing; secondarily = by closing the glottis, the prerequisite for, e.g., the Valsalva maneuver, coughing, and voice production is enabled), so that this part is considered an independent organ (larynx)

Laser Acronym for light amplification by stimulated emission of radiation (German: Lichtverstärkung durch stimulierte Emission von Strahlung)

Latency Period between an event and the occurrence of a visible reaction to it

Lesion a tissue damage that is caused by an injury or disease

Leukoplakie white-colored plaques on the vocal folds, which are to be considered as a premalignant lesion (precursor of a malignant tumor)

Lipom benign fatty tumor

Magnetic Resonance Imaging (MRI) Magnetic resonance imaging is a measurement method that is free of X-ray radiation and visually represents the interior of the body (e.g., muscles and tendons, brain tissue, as well as the abdominal and pelvic area and the vessels)

Maligne malignant (carcinoma/cancer)

Manual Therapy/Approach Therapy/approach with the hand that applies pressure and/or displacement (on the larynx)

Medial towards the middle

Meta-analysis statistical method that combines the results of several studies on the same question and calculates a more meaningful result from it

Metastases spatially separated, similar secondary tumors from the primary tumor, which arise through the dissemination of viable tumor cells

Modal register Range of the chest voice

Morphology The study of form, shape, and structure; in medicine, the term refers to the description of the external shape of living organisms or their components

Motility Ability for active movement

Mucosal wave wave-like movement of the mucous membrane of the vocal fold during phonation, initiated by, among other things, the Bernoulli effect (flowing liquids and gases exert less pressure on their surroundings than stationary ones; the higher the speed, the lower the pressure)

Mutation falsetto Voice disorder during the period of puberty (mutation falsetto voice) with the main symptom of an excessively high speaking pitch in the falsetto register

Myoelastic the muscle activity regulates the position of the vocal folds in such a way that the elastic properties of the vocal folds provide the appropriate basic state for the oscillation process of phonation

Nasalizing a resonance technique to make the speech sound resonate more through the nose

Nervus laryngeus superior Nerve branch of the vagus nerve, which is responsible for the motor innervation of the cricothyroid muscle, the sensory innervation of the cricothyroid joint, and the anterior subglottic region

Network meta-analysis statistical method that is structured similarly to a meta-analysis, but it allows the estimation of effect sizes for all comparisons of interventions that are connected within a network

Nicotine abuse Smoking, nicotine dependence

Normophonia healthy voice production, clear voice, no voice disorder

Noxen various substances or events (e.g., chemical or biological) that cause harm to a biological organism

Odynophonia Pain when speaking

Oncology medical specialty that deals with benign and malignant types of tumors as well as cancer diseases

Ordinal scale these parameters have an assigned rank order (here exclusively from 0 to 3, i.e., from normal to severe)

Organic voice disorder Voice disorder that is based on an organic change, such as benign swellings

Oropharynx anatomical region of the mouth part of the pharynx

Oscillogram graphical representation of the temporal course of a deflection (here: the vocal energy)

Pacemaker Laryngeal pacemakers are implants that, for example, stimulate the nerves of the abductor muscle of the vocal cords, allowing patients to breathe freely if this muscle should be paralyzed

Palpation Assessment of muscle tension by palpation (diagnostics)

Paraglottic beside the vocal cords

Paralysis/Paresis complete/partial paralysis

Parkinson's disease a chronically progressive, neurodegenerative disease that, among other things, leads to stiff muscles (rigor), slowed movements (bradykinesia), and uncontrollable trembling (tremor), which can also alter speech and voice

Pathological Deviation from the norm, diseased

Perception/perceptive based on sensory impressions

pH-metry is an invasive measuring device for determining and displaying the pH value (a measure of the acidic or basic character of an aqueous solution, in this case, saliva secretion)

Phonation Voice production

Phonosurgery medical surgery using various techniques on and around the vocal folds

Phonotrauma Inflammatory reaction of the vocal fold mucosa due to biomechanical stress and changes during high vocal effort

Physiological physiology is the study of the life phenomena of living beings, which is described here as the norm in function and/or quality of vocal performance

Pitch perceived height of the voice; frequency in vibrations per second (Hz) as an acoustic correlate

Pitch instability Pitch jumps or breaks

Pneumotachographs medical device used for performing spirometry and thus checking lung function as well as determining dynamic respiratory volumes

Posterior Backside

Post mortem after death

Prevalence medical statistic of a metric, for example, for the frequency of diseases

Presbyphonia Voice changes due to aging

Primary focus of treatment refers to the initial phase, the beginning/start of an intervention (medical or voice therapy) in terms of the manner of treatment and choice of methods

Primary treatment see "primary focus of treatment" (synonym)

Professional speaker Group of people who rely heavily on their voice for their profession and for whom voice problems significantly impair the performance of their job

Prophylactic preventive against a disease

Prosody Form of emphasis or expressive features in speech

Pulmonary concerning the lungs

Quantifiability describable/expressible through quantity, number, or value measure

Quefrency an anagram of "frequency"; calculated from signal processing, where the signal is first transferred to the frequency domain of the Fourier transform, then the magnitude spectrum is logarithmically compressed and transformed back into the "quefrency" domain

Reclination generally refers to the backward tilting in medicine

Reconstruction surgical restoration of tissue form and function after trauma or tumor operations

Recurrent laryngeal nerve paralysis Paralysis of the recurrent laryngeal nerve (provides motor innervation to the intrinsic muscles of the larynx except for the cricothyroid muscle)

Recurrence rate Relapse rate, which describes the frequency of the reoccurrence of a disease after temporarily successful therapy

Reflux Backflow of stomach contents/acid to the mouth

Reinnervation the restoration of nerve supply (innervation) after denervation (interruption of nerve pathways)

Relative voice rest Voice conservation with partial use of the voice or voice rehabilitation through voice therapy measures, e.g., after a medical procedure on the vocal folds

Reliability Reliability of a measurement method

Register Series of pitches with the same timbre (tone color, determined by the overtones)

Register boundaries Separation of registers such as modal or falsetto register

Rehabilitation Restoration through various interventions to eliminate, alleviate, or mitigate the physical, psychological, and social consequences of a disability or an activity limitation

Reinke's space filled space with loose connective tissue, disordered elastin fibers embedded in a gelatinous ground substance, located beneath the epithelial layer of the vocal fold

Resection surgical removal of specific tissue parts of an organ or also of a tumor

Resonator oscillating system such as, for example, the trachea or vocal tract

Resorbable dissolved/liquid substances are absorbed by the body

Respiration concerning breathing

Rhinolaryngoscope invasive flexible endoscopes that are guided through the nose to the larynx and can visually assess these structures

Rhinosinusitides Inflammations of the paranasal sinuses as well as the mucous membrane of the nose

Roughness irregular fluctuations of speed and/or amplitude of the vocal fold vibration resulting in a rough voice quality

SD Spasmodic Dysphonia

Sensitivity Percentage of correct positive results of an examination/test procedure in the presence of the disease/disorder, i.e., if 90 out of 100 patients are detected using the procedure, the procedure has a sensitivity of 90 %

Shunt valve Voice prosthesis

Sinusitis Inflammation of the paranasal sinuses

Sinus morgagni Space that is located between the vocal cords and the vestibular folds

Sleep apnea Condition in which breathing repeatedly stops for short periods during sleep, caused by relaxed muscles of the upper airways

Source-Filter Model according to Fant (1960), the conceptual model that the vocal tract (resonator) functions as a linear acoustic filter and the vocal folds are considered as the raw sound production (source) and thus the speech sound production is composed of these two sub-mechanisms

Sonography Ultrasound examination

Spasm Cramp, contraction of the muscles, caused by sudden and very forceful movements

Specificity Percentage of negative results of an examination/test procedure, e.g., "no findings", to correctly identify patients without the disease. A test with 100% specificity therefore correctly identifies all patients without the disease.

Spectrogram/Spectrography three-dimensional graphical representation of a spectrum, which shows the time course at different frequencies and its amplitude (intensity); for voice assessments, a narrow-band spectrogram is recommended in the settings

Spirometer a medical device for determining lung volumes

Squamous epithelial cells (keratinocytes) important structural cells of the epidermis (the outer layer of the skin); squamous cell carcinoma is a cancer of these cells

Stenosis congenital or acquired narrowing in hollow organs (e.g., trachea) that hinders the normal passage of the contents (in this case, air)

Steroids ring-shaped molecules that belong to the fats and play an important role in human metabolism

Stoma artificial body opening

Strain pressed vocal sound

Stroboscopy instrumental medical examination to accurately assess the vocal fold movement

Subglottic pressure Air pressure below the vocal folds

Supraglottic compensation Narrowing above the vocal cords due to hypertonic muscle contraction (e.g., through the activation of the ventricular folds), which affects the voice quality and/or causes discomfort

Symmetry describes the uniformity of the vocal fold vibration

Symptom Signs or manifestations of illness

T4-Laryngeal carcinoma the letter *T* refers to the primary tumor (primary tumor) and the numbers 1 to 4 represent an increasing ordinal size and spread of the tumor: T1 denotes a small tumor, while, for example, T2 stands for a larger one in the ranking.

Tactile-perceptive based on sensory impressions that concern touching/feeling

Test–Retest Procedure this procedure examines whether repeated measurements under unchanged conditions achieve the same measurement results

Testosterone male sex hormone

Thorax Chest

Thyroid space Space between the hyoid bone and the thyroid cartilage

Thyroplasty surgical procedure on the laryngeal skeleton to achieve, for example, a vocal fold medialization (Type I)

Tonus State of tension of a body structure, particularly the state of tension of the muscles (muscle tone)

Trachea Windpipe

Tracheobronchial belonging to the trachea and the bronchi

Tracheobronchitiden simultaneous inflammation of the mucous membranes in the trachea and the air-conducting parts of the lungs (bronchi)

Trans* encompasses in medicine all terms related to gender identity disorders such as, for example, transidentity or transsexualism, which thus does justice to most affected individuals and their individual perceptions, as a (complete) alignment of their body or determination of a gender is not necessarily sought

Transglottal through the glottis

Transnasal endoscopy in this visual measurement method, a flexible endoscope is inserted into the patient's nose

Transoral Endoscopy in this visual measurement method, a rigid endoscope is inserted through the patient's mouth

Trauma any type of wound or injury that has been caused by an external force on living tissue

Tremor pathological unconscious movement (here at the voice level) with a modulation of 4 to 6 Hz

Tumor Swelling

Unilateral one-sided

Validity Quality criterion for measurement methods for the substantive agreement of an empirical measurement

Ventricular Concerning false vocal folds

Ventricular folds Structure above the vocal folds that typically should not play a role in physiological voice production

Ventricular Phonation Voice production with the ventricular folds/false vocal folds

Videokymography Real-time video playback in two-dimensionality of the vibration of the vocal folds, which allows a detailed analysis of the vocal fold closure at different levels

Vital capacity the maximum volume of air that a person can exhale at once after maximum inhalation

Vocalis deep layer of the vocal folds, which consists of muscle tissue

Vocalis atrophy Muscle atrophy of the Musculus vocalis (vocal foldd muscle)

Vocal folds pairwise arranged structure with myoelastic properties in the larynx, which can vibrate and produce sounds

Vocal tract Airway between the glottis and the mouth or nose

Voice function specific measurement parameters of voice examination, which belong to the category of vocal performance, namely pitch, volume, and endurance

Voice Range Profile an acoustic measuring instrument that graphically measures the frequency-dependent sound level registration of a voice with respect to the speaking voice range profile (SRP) or the general vocal performance of pitch and volume (VRP)

Voice therapy usually voice therapeutic interventions based on a conservative form of therapy

Voice quality specific measurement parameters of voice examination that assess the quality of the voice sound at the glottal level (excluded are measurement methods that are monodimensional, i.e., those that have a direct objective equivalent in subjective assessment, such as pitch, which is acoustically measured in Hz)

VRP Voice Range Profile

Whistle register High-pitched register that follows the falsetto and is "incorrectly" assessed as vocal energy in voice range profiles, because the overtone energy is louder than the vocal energy and thus pitches beyond 2000 Hz can be reached

WHO World Health Organization

MIX
Papier aus verantwortungsvollen Quellen
Paper from responsible sources
FSC® C105338

If you have any concerns about our products,
you can contact us on
ProductSafety@springernature.com

In case Publisher is established outside the EU,
the EU authorized representative is:
Springer Nature Customer Service Center GmbH
Europaplatz 3, 69115 Heidelberg, Germany

Printed by Libri Plureos GmbH
in Hamburg, Germany